Current Topics in Neuroendocrinology Volume 9

Editors

Detlev Ganten, Heidelberg · Donald Pfaff, New York

Current Topics in Neuroendocrinology

Vol. 1: Sleep. Clinical and Experimental Aspects
1982. 47 figures. VII, 129 pages. DM 95,–. ISBN 3-540-11125-5
Neurobiology of REM Sleep. A Possible Role for Dopamine · Endocrine and Peptide Functions in the Sleep-Waking Cycle · Sleep Regulation: Circadian Rhythm and Homeostasis · Haemodynamic Changes During Sleep in Man

Vol. 2: Adrenal Actions on Brain
1982. 25 figures. V, 153 pages. DM 95,–. ISBN 3-540-11126-3
Glucocorticoids and Hippocampus: Receptors in Search of a Function · Glucocorticoids and the Developing Nervous System · Feedback Actions of Adrenal Steroid Hormones · Electrophysiologic and Clinical Aspects of Glucocorticoids on Certain Neural Systems · Adrenal Steroids and Behavioral Adaptation: Relationship to Brain Corticoid Receptors

Vol. 3: Central Cardiovascular Control. Basic and Clinical Aspects
1983. 71 figures. V, 192 pages. DM 106,–. ISBN 3-540-11350-9
Functional and Anatomic Aspects of Central Nervous Cardiovascular Regulation · Autonomic Nervous System and Blood Pressure Control in Normotensive and Hypertensive Conditions · Reflex Control of Circulation in Normotensive and Hypertensive Humans · Corticotropin-Releasing Factor: Central Nervous System Effects on the Sympathetic Nervous System and Cardiovascular Regulation · Neuropeptides and Central Blood Pressure Regulation · Centrally Acting Drugs as a Tool to Study Central Mechanisms of Blood Pressure Control · The Blood-Brain Barrier and its Role in the Control of Circulating Hormone Effects on the Brain

Vol. 4: Neurobiology of Vasopressin
1985. 53 figures. V, 203 pages. DM 98,–. ISBN 3-540-11351-7
Biosynthesis of Vasopressin · Electrophysiological Studies of the Magnocellular Neurons · Volume Regulation of Antidiuretic Hormone Secretion · Vasopressin, Cardiovascular Regulation and Hypertension · Neuroanatomical Pathways Related to Vasopressin

Vol. 5: Actions of Progesterone on the Brain
1985. 61 figures. V, 216 pages. DM 98,–. ISBN 3-540-13433-6
Antiprogestins · Progesterone Receptors in Brain and Hypophysis · Effects of Estrogen and Progesterone as Revealed by Neurophysiological Methods · Progesterone Receptors in CNS Correlated with Reproductive Behavior · Estradiol-Progesterone Interactions in the Reproductive Behavior of Female Rats · Behavioral Effects on Humans of Progesterone-Related Compounds During Development and in the Adult

Vol. 6: Neurobiology of Oxytocin
1986. 38 figures. V, 175 pages. DM 98,–. ISBN 3-540-15341-1
Biosynthesis of Oxytocin in the Brain and Peripheral Organs · Regulation of Oxytocin Release · Proteolytic Conversion of Oxytocin, Vasopressin, and Related Peptides in the Brain · Oxytocin and Behavior · Oxytocin as an Ovarian Hormone · Oxytocin and the Milk-Ejection Reflex

Vol. 7: Morphology of Hypothalamus and its Connections
1986. 94 figures. VI, 314 pages. DM 148,–. ISBN 3-540-16919-9
The Pituitary Portal System · Functional Ultrastructure of Gonadotropes: a Review · Ultrastructure of Anterior Pituitary Cells · Catecholamine-Peptide Interactions in the Hypothalamus · Neuroendocrine Projections to the Median Eminence · Afferents onto Neuroendocrine Cells · Interconnectedness of Steroid Hormone-Binding Neurons: Existence and Implications · Ultrastructure of Regulatory Neuroendocrine Neurons and Functionally Related Structures · Synaptogenesis and Neuronal Plasticity to Gonadal Steroids: Implications for the Development of Sexual Dimorphism in the Neuroendocrine Brain

Vol. 8: Neuroendocrinology of Mood
1988. 80 figures. VI, 335 pages. DM 175,–. ISBN 3-540-17892-9
Principles for the Hormone Regulation of Wiring Transmission and Volume Transmission in the Central Nervous System · Clinical Studies with Corticotropin Releasing Hormone: Implications for Hypothalamic-Pituitary-Adrenal Dysfunction in Depression and Related Disorders · Biological Rhythms and Mood Disorders · Recurrent Affective Disorders: Lessons from Limbic Kindling · The Mechanisms of Action of Antipsychotics and Antidepressant Drugs · Catecholamines and Mood: Neuroendocrine Aspects · Serotonin and Mood: Neuroendocrine Aspects · Cholinergic Mechanisms in Mood: Neuroendocrine Aspects · The Psychobiology of Neurotensin · Cholecystokinin and Mood · Opioid Peptides and Mood: Neuroendocrine Aspects · The Neuroendocrinology of Anorexia Nervosa · Effects of Peripheral Thyroid Hormones on the Central Nervous System: Relevance to Disorders of Mood

D. Ganten and D. Pfaff (Eds.)

Stimulus-Secretion Coupling in Neuroendocrine Systems

Coeditor: B. Pickering

Contributors
I.M. Cooke, H. Duve, D.K. Hartline, G.I. Hatton
W.J. Malaisse, R.W. Newcomb, L.J. Parry
D.A. Poulain, F. Strumwasser, E.L. Stuenkel
A.J.S. Summerlee, D.T. Theodosis, A. Thorpe

With 69 Figures

Springer-Verlag Berlin Heidelberg New York
London Paris Tokyo

Editors

Dr. DETLEV GANTEN, M.D., Ph.D.
Pharmakologisches Institut
Universität Heidelberg
Im Neuenheimer Feld 366
6900 Heidelberg/FRG

Dr. DONALD PFAFF, Ph.D.
Rockefeller University
York Avenue, and 66th Street
New York, NY 10021/USA

Coeditor

Dr. BRIAN PICKERING, Ph.D.
Department of Anatomy
Medical School
Bristol BS8 1TD
England, U.K.

The picture on the cover has been taken from Nieuwenhuys R., Voogd J., van Huijzen Chr.: The Human Central Nervous System. 2nd Edition. Springer-Verlag Berlin Heidelberg New York 1981

ISBN 3-540-19043-0 Springer-Verlag Berlin Heidelberg New York
ISBN 0-387-19043-0 Springer-Verlag New York Berlin Heidelberg

Library of Congress Cataloging in Publication Data. Stimulus-secretion coupling in neuroendocrine systems/D. Ganten and D. Pfaff (eds.), coeditor, B. Pickering; contributors, I. M. Cooke ... [et al.]. p. cm. – (Current topics in neuroendocrinology; v. 9) Includes bibliographies and index. ISBN 0-387-19043-0 (U.S.) 1. Neuroendocrinology. 2. Secretion. 3. Paraneurons. I. Ganten, D. (Detlev), 1941–. II. Pfaff, Donald W., 1939–. III. Pickering, Brian T. IV. Cooke. I. M. (Ian M.) V. Series. QP356.4.S75 1988 591.1'88 – dc 19 88-15923

Typesetting, printing and binding: Brühlsche Universitätsdruckerei, Giessen
2121/3130-543210 – Printed on acid-free paper

Table of Contents

Cellular Reorganization in Neuroendocrine Secretion *

G. I. HATTON

Contents

1 Introduction

Cellular reorganization accompanying changes in the physiological state of organisms is an emerging concept based upon rather recent discoveries. Old notions of central nervous systems as being structurally static after development are giving way to conceptualizations involving reorganization of the participating elements as function demands. All aspects of nervous systems should perhaps be thought of as at least having the potential for change and reorganization. Recent developments suggest that any arrangement of elements extant at a given time, or under one set of conditions, should be warily viewed as only one organization among many possible. The inseparability of structure and function has never been more undeniable. Research involving neuroendocrine systems has provided some of the more exciting and provocative ideas of the depth and extent of the reorganization that the nervous system may undergo in response to physiological challenges. It will be the aim of this chapter to present the evidence for function-related cellular reorganization in a neurosecretory system for which the phenome-

* Support from NIH research grants NS 09140 and NS 16942 is gratefully acknowledged
Neuroscience Program Michigan State University East Lansing, Mi 48824, USA

Current Topics in Neuroendocrinology, Vol. 9

non is well documented. In addition, the mechanisms involved in the cellular reorganization, to the extent that they are known or can at least be speculated on, will be discussed. Finally, evidence for function-related cellular reorganization in neurosecretory systems for which evidence is just beginning to appear will be reviewed.

Cellular reorganization is a broad term under which may be subsumed a variety of changes in virtually any aspect of neurosecretion. In the context of this volume, dealing with stimulus-secretion coupling, it is appropriate to focus on those events that appear to be directly related to neuroendocrine secretion resulting from physiological stimulation. For the sake of comprehensiveness, we will discuss reorganizations that occur within neurosecretory cells and changes in the relationships of these cells (or of portions of them) to one another, along with reorganization involving the neurosecretory neurons and other structures (e.g., glia, blood vessels, basal lamina) that are integral parts of neurosecretory systems.

2 A Model Neurosecretory System

It seems fair to say that the magnocellular neuropeptidergic system of the hypothalamus has achieved the status of a model system. That is, we know a good deal about the stimulus conditions that activate the neurons of this system; we can record its electrophysiological responses to stimuli and relate them to both biosynthetic and secretory events; we can measure its peptide output; many of the physiological actions of its main secretions on peripheral tissues are well characterized; and the basic organization of the cellular elements comprising this system has permitted studies of events occurring at different levels, from the hypothalamus to the posterior pituitary. All of these factors have helped us to gain more understanding of how at least one mammalian neurosecretory system works. Time and further effort will reveal the extent to which we can apply what has been and will be learned about this model system to other systems in the brain.

2.1 General Features of the Hypothalamo-Neurohypophysial System

In Fig. 1 are shown the brain region in which the hypothalamo-neurohypophysial system (HNS) is located and the general relationships among the major components of the HNS. Many of the magnocellular neurons of this system are condensed into two cell masses, the paraventricular (PVN) and the supraoptic (SON) nuclei. The remaining HNS magnocellular neurons are found in so-called accessory groups and along blood vessels throughout this region of the hypothalamus (Fisher et al. 1979). Some of these latter features, along with the main nuclei, are shown in Fig. 2. While the PVN and SON have been most thoroughly studied, it seems that the magnocellular neurons in the accessory groups have similar characteristics. This peculiar arrangement of what appear to be altogether similar cells remains something of a mystery. Most if not all magnocellular neurons of these accessory groups join with those of the SON and PVN to send at least one axonal

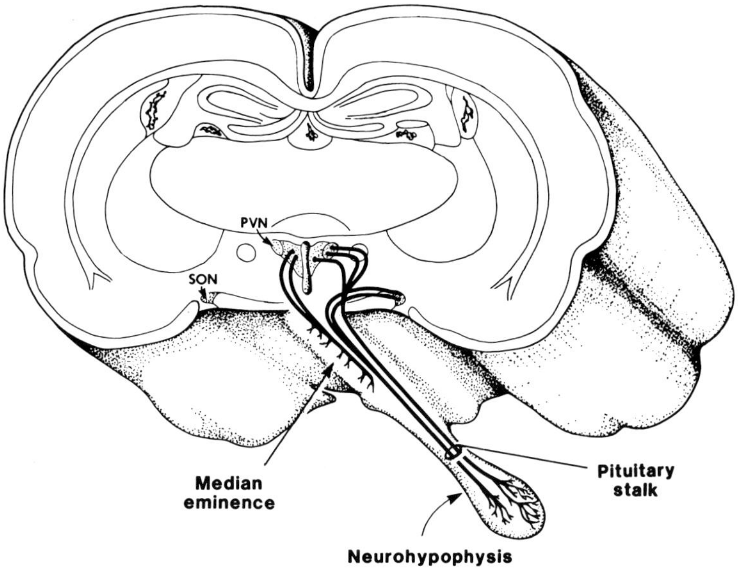

Fig. 1. Semidiagrammatic representation of the rat hypothalamo-neurohypophysial system. Projections of the supraoptic (*SON*) and paraventricular (*PVN*) nuclei to the neurohypophysis are shown. Also shown are PVN projections to the external zone of the median eminence. Not shown are the many intra- and extrahypothalamic projections of the magnocellular neurons

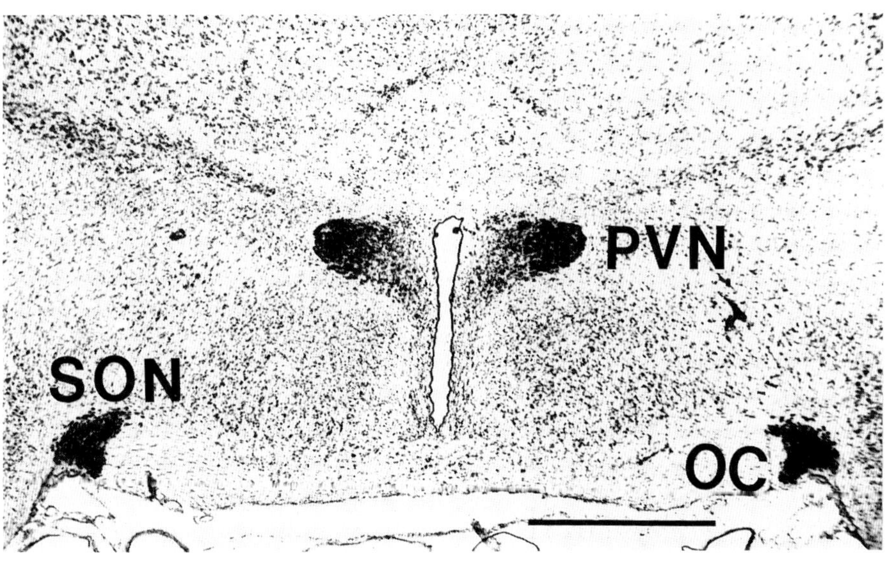

Fig. 2. Photomicrograph of a Nissl-stained, coronal section through the optic chiasm (*OC*) at the level of the supraoptic (*SON*) and paraventricular (*PVN*) nuclei. *Scale bar* 1 mm

projection to the neurohypophysis. There the secretory axons terminate near the basal lamina that separates the neural compartment from the perivascular spaces surrounding fenestrated capillaries. Depolarization of these terminals, occurring under physiologically appropriate conditions, results in release of peptides which then enter the blood. Most of what is released from these sites within the neurohypophysis is thought to enter the general circulation. It seems likely, however, that neurohypophysial peptides, oxytocin (OXT), vasopressin (VP) and perhaps dynorphin (DYN), may also enter the hypophysial portal blood, influencing the adenohypophysis, and/or affect targets in the neurohypophysis itself. In addition to the neurosecretory terminals in the posterior pituitary, there are terminals containing a variety of potential transmitters and/or modulators (e.g., noradrenaline, GABA, dopamine and enkephalins). There is some controversy over whether opioid peptides are colocalized with VP or OXT (Martin et al. 1983; Nordmann et al. 1986; van Leeuwen et al. 1983; Watson et al. 1982), but there is currently no disagreement on their existence in the neurohypophysis.

2.2 Anatomical Considerations

No attempt will be made here to give a detailed account of HNS anatomy. Nor will we stray much from the rat, since most of what is known about cellular reorganization of the HNS comes from that species. Rather, what follows is a selective description of the anatomical elements, and their juxtapositions, that play important roles in the reorganization of this system in response to naturally occurring stimulus conditions.

The magnocellular neurons (15–30 μm in diameter) of the PVN and SON are tightly packed, as can be seen in Fig. 2 and tend to be grouped within each nucleus according to hormone type, although there is a considerable amount of intermixing (Hou-Yu et al. 1986 b). In the main portions of the rat SON, the more ventral and caudal neurons tend to be those containing VP, while the OXT-containing neurons are found in the more rostral and dorsal parts of the nucleus. In the PVN, the lateral portions are occupied by VP cells, and OXT cells are found more anteromedially and in the extreme caudal portion. With their principal axes at about 45 ° to the brain's ventral surface (Armstrong et al. 1982; Hatton and Walters 1973), SON neurons project their primary dendrites, in a more or less parallel fashion, into the ventral glial lamina and toward the pial surface (Armstrong et al. 1982; Perlmutter et al. 1984 b). This glial laminar zone contains much glial membrane and astrocytic cell bodies that have been shown immunocytochemically to send long processes among the tightly packed SON dendrites and somata (Salm and Hatton 1980). Under basal conditions these glial processes interpose themselves between otherwise adjacent dendritic and somatic membrane of SON neurons (see. Fig. 3 A and Hatton and Tweedle 1982; Perlmutter et al. 1984 b; Theodosis et al. 1981; Tweedle and Hatton 1976, 1977, 1984 a).

Similar neuron-glia relationships have been observed in the PVN (Gregory et al. 1980). PVN neurons have dendritic trees that generally project toward the third ventricle (Armstrong et al. 1980; van den Pol 1982). Their axons cascade from the nucleus in the general direction of the SON. Some give rise to collaterals

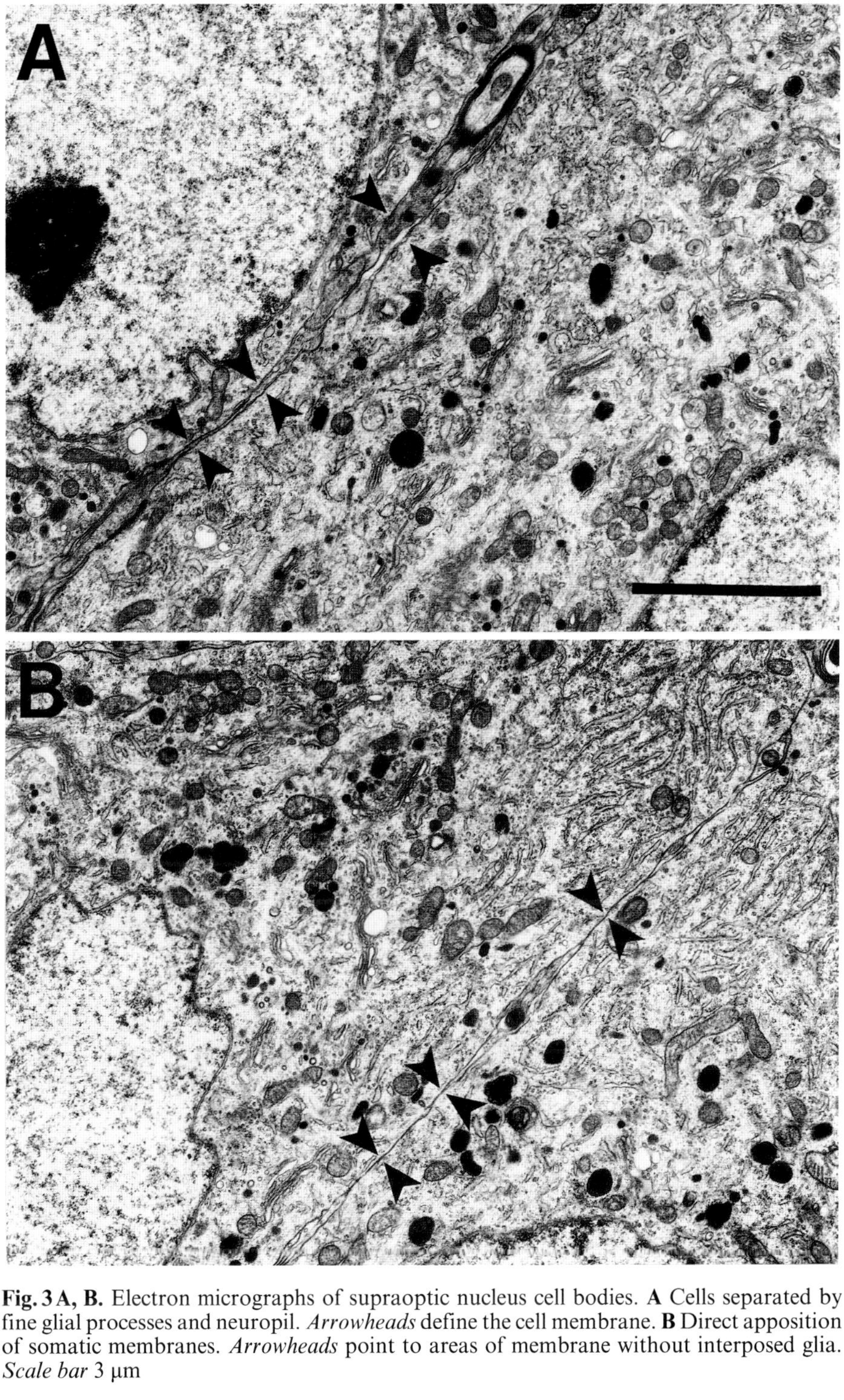

Fig. 3 A, B. Electron micrographs of supraoptic nucleus cell bodies. **A** Cells separated by fine glial processes and neuropil. *Arrowheads* define the cell membrane. **B** Direct apposition of somatic membranes. *Arrowheads* point to areas of membrane without interposed glia. *Scale bar* 3 µm

in the perifornical area (Hatton et al. 1985). Magnocellular PVN projections go to the external zone of the median eminence (Pittman et al. 1981; Vandesande et al. 1977), the neurohypophysis along with SON axons, the dorsal motor vagal complex, the nucleus of the solitary tract (Conrad and Pfaff 1976; Swanson and Kuypers 1980), and the spinal cord (Armstrong et al. 1980; Swanson 1977). SON axonal projections exit the nucleus dorsomedially, some giving rise to collaterals close to the nucleus (Mason et al. 1984). The parent axons then turn caudally as they enter the internal layer of the median eminence and, along with PVN fibers, continue on to the neurohypophysis.

The neurohypophysial neurosecretory terminals also have rather intimate relationships with the resident glia (called pituicytes) which have been shown to contain the astrocytic marker, glial fibrillary acidic protein (Salm et al. 1982; Suess and Pliška 1981). Under the same basal conditions in which astrocyte processes are interposed between the dendrites and somata of the magnocellular neurons, the pituicytes have been shown to completely surround and/or engulf many of the axons and terminals in the posterior pituitary (Dreifuss et al. 1975; Tweedle and Hatton 1980a, 1980b, 1982, 1987). Also under these conditions, pituicytes tend to occupy a relatively large portion of the basal lamina, thus interposing themselves between it and the neurosecretory terminals. Recently, scanning electron micrographs of torn tissue preparations have clearly revealed axon terminals within pituicytes, confirming our previous findings (Hatton et al. 1984, Fig. 2).

Afferents to the magnocellular nuclei have recently been described, but much work remains. For example, there is evidence for subfornical organ and nucleus medianus inputs to the SON and PVN (Lind et al. 1982; Miselis et al. 1979; Renaud et al. 1983; Sgro et al. 1984); the medial preoptic area appears also to provide afferents (Carithers et al. 1981; Carithers and Johnson 1984; Sladek and Johnson 1983; Swanson 1976; Tribollet et al. 1985); and there is reason to believe that there is an olfactory bulb input to at least the supraoptic portion of this system (Dougherty et al. 1986; Heimer 1978; Hollowell et al. 1986; Scalia and Winans 1975). There is a cholinergic input to the SON from neurons just outside of the nucleus (Hatton et al. 1983; Mason et al. 1983; Meyer and Brownstein 1980); angiotensinergic inputs appear to be operative in excitation of this system (Sladek and Joynt 1979); catecholaminergic inputs have now been shown by a number of workers using different methods (Alonso and Assenmacher 1984; Day and Renaud 1984; Sladek and McNeill 1980; Swanson et al. 1981; Tweedle and Hatton 1984b); and excitation by histamine has been reported (Armstrong and Sladek 1985).

2.3 Physiology

Adequate evidence exists supporting the notion that neurosecretion is coupled, albeit in complex ways, to the electrical activity of the hormone-containing cell (for reviews see Finlayson and Osborne 1975; Mason and Bern 1977; Poulain and Wakerley 1982). In the rat HNS, studies of dehydration, hemorrhage and suckling (the three most commonly used stimulus complexes) have relatively consistently suggested that increases in hormone release are accompanied by specific alterations in the patterns of neuronal firing observed at the level of the cell bodies in the hypothalamus. Further, these alterations are different for OXT-containing and VP-containing cells, even when, as with dehydration, both cell types are activated by the same set of stimulus conditions (Brimble and Dyball 1977; Wakerley et al. 1978). In the unstimulated state, cells of the SON, for instance, that have been antidromically identified as having terminals in the neurohypophysis, generally exhibit slow (0.5–1 Hz), unpatterned activity. On osmotic stimulation, two activated states have been seen to emerge and predominate. One major cell type simply fires faster and continuously at >4 Hz. These so-called fast-continuous firing neurons have been shown, in lactating, nursing mother rats, to burst (60–80 Hz) about 15 s prior to each milk ejection. Such observations led to the conclusions that (a) these are oxytocinergic neurons and (b) they must be roughly synchronized in order to provide enough hormone release to produce the observed intramammary pressure rise. In a recent series of elegant experiments, direct evidence establishing relative synchrony among oxytocinergic neurons has been obtained (Belin et al. 1984; Belin and Moos 1986). The mechanisms of such synchrony remain unknown. Dogma and general paucity of data would have us believe it is due solely to chemical synaptic input, but non-chemical synaptic and perhaps non-synaptic events are also apt to be involved. OXT-containing neurons respond to hypertonic stimulation with an increase in their fast-continuous firing rates, with no change in firing pattern.

The activity of the other major magnocellular neuron type shows no consistent relationship to the milk ejection reflex in actively suckling mothers. When stimulated osmotically, such as following intraperitoneally administered hypertonic NaCl injections, these neurons generally become "phasic." This activity is characterized by variable periods of silence (10–40 s) punctuated by equally variable (and roughly equal in their range of durations) bursts of action potentials. Magnocellular neurons showing this pattern when activated have long been thought to be vasopressinergic. Recent direct evidence from imunocytochemical analyses of intracellularly marked phasic cells have confirmed this hypothesis (Cobbett et al. 1986; Yamashita et al. 1983). VP neurons are generally not thought to be synchronized, although there is some evidence for synchrony (Thomson 1984). All the evidence points to their at least having thresholds of excitability that are coordinated, so that under conditions of increased VP demand most VP-containing SON or PVN neurons are found to be in an activated state. This may be accomplished partly by a direct membrane-depolarizing effect of elevated osmotic pressure of the extracellular fluid (Mason 1980). Mechanisms responsible for coordination of excitability, or synchrony of VP or OXT neurons, have not yet been identified with certainty. In Sect. 4 of this chapter, candidate mechanisms for these phenomena will be proposed.

Both the fast-continuous and phasic patterns of firing have been observed under in vitro conditions in 400- to 500-μm-thick brain slices (Hatton 1982; Hatton et al. 1978; Mason 1983) and in cultured explants (Armstrong and Sladek 1982; Gähwiler and Dreifuss 1980). Indeed, phasic activity in PVN neurons has been shown to persist in the absence of chemical synaptic transmission (Hatton 1982), perhaps supporting earlier notions of pacemaker cells (Gähwiler and Dreifuss 1980). Membrane currents intrinsic to these neurons appear to be largely responsible for the plateau potentials upon which the phasic bursts are superimposed (Andrew and Dudek 1984) and for the generation and termination of the bursts.

Dehydration and lactation are, of course, conditions that are associated with these activated firing patterns in OXT and VP neurons. Such conditions also produce increases in protein synthetic activity of these neurons, specifically, though not exclusively, the biosynthesis of prohormone molecules for OXT, VP and DYN (Gainer et al. 1977; Sherman et al. 1986 a).

3 Reorganization Within Neurosecretory Neurons

3.1 Numbers of Cellular Organelles

Dogma once held that "neurons with more than one nucleolus per nucleus are extremely rare in the normal brain" (Konigsmark 1970). This turns out not to be the case for neuroendocrine cells of the hypothalamus when observed under conditions of physiologically induced increase in hormone demand. When stimulated to release more hormone from their terminals during dehydration, the PVN, SON and accessory groups show an increase in the number of neurons having more than one nucleolus per nucleus (Hatton 1976; Hatton and Walters 1973; Hoblitzell et al. 1976). Of some interest here may also be that rodents that are close genetic relatives, but live in habitats differing with respect to water availability, also differ markedly in both the number of SON neurons with multiple nucleoli and the maximum numbers of nucleoli per cell. Desert species, fed their natural diets, commonly have four or five, whereas species adapted to more mesic habitats tend to have one or, when stimulated by dehydration, at most two nucleoli per nucleus (Hatton et al. 1972).

Since nucleoli are organelles involved in the production of ribosomal RNA, it is hardly odd that stimulation of protein synthesis induces some nucleolar response. When stimulated thus, some of the neurons are observed to have one nucleolus which is simply enlarged, while other, neighboring and similar neurons have produced additional nucleoli. This is curious. Given that they are made at nucleolar organizer regions on chromosomes, de novo production of nucleoli would seem to require altered genetic expression. This, therefore, represents a profound reorganization in those cells. What is special about the cells responding to stimulation with neucleolar proliferation remains unknown, as does whether the newly produced and original nucleoli are functionally identical to one another. That this cellular reorganization was more than a special circumstance of imposed dehydration is evidenced by its occurrence as a circadian fluctuation. The SONs (but not the PVNs) of rats were found to contain significantly more cells with multiple nucleoli at the beginning than at the end of the rats' 12-h active period (Armstrong and Hatton 1978). This strongly suggests that this type of reorganization is a normal, recurrent daily phenomenon.

3.2 Altered Organelle Function

Peptidergic neurons synthesize a variety of products, but there are two important groups of these that are packaged for transport down their axons in membrane-bound vesicles. One group, the neurosecretory vesicles, contain the neuropeptide product to be released, along with the necessary enzymes to complete its processing. The other group is lysosomes, generally large vesicles containing lytic enzymes and vested with membrane-recycling and mopping-up operations. Under basal conditions the responsibility for providing membranes for these two vesicle types is assumed by two different regions of the Golgi apparatus (for a review see Castel et al. 1984). Lysosomes are packaged on the GERL (Golgi-associated endoplasmic reticulum giving rise to lysosomes). Histochemical studies by Broadwell and Oliver (1981) have shown that, upon appropriate stimulation (e.g., dehydration), SON neurons reorganize the arrangement that exists under basal conditions. When called upon to maximize hormone synthesis and release, the GERL virtually ceases to package lysosomes and switches over to packaging neurosecretory vesicles. When basal conditions are re-established, (i.e., upon rehydration) the GERL returns to its regular duties. It seems likely that these changes in observed lysosome/hormone-containing vesicles are due to a more fundamental change at the level of mRNA. Message relating to preprohormone production appears to be increased with stimulation (Sherman et al. 1986 b). A corresponding decrease in expression of lysosome-related message would be expected to present the GERL with little choice but to package the available product.

3.3 Altered Message

It has been known for many years that adrenal steroids exerted negative feedback control over corticotrophin-releasing hormone (CRH). Accordingly, adrenalectomy removes this feedback and increased release of CRH and adrenocorticotrophic hormone (ACTH) occur. One of the more exciting findings in recent years has been the discovery that, following adrenalectomy, CRH-containing neurons in the PVN begin to exhibit VP-like immunoreactivity (Sawchenko et al. 1984). This phenomenon has not gone unchallenged (Piekut and Joseph 1985), but one possible implication is that a new message has been turned on in these cells, perhaps via gene depression in the absence of steroid feedback. That this may be more than just an oddity of adrenalectomized animals (Wolfson et al. 1985) is suggested by recent work showing that this message switchover may be expressed at certain restricted times of the diurnal cycle (Baldino et al., personal communication). A recent study has shown that chronic behavioral stress can affect the expression of peptide in certain PVN neurons. Conditioned emotional responses to pairings of white noise and inescapable foot shock for 72 h in rats resulted in an increase in the numbers of PVN neurons showing immunoreactivity to both CRH and OXT antisera (Hou-Yu et al. 1986 a). This finding supports earlier studies implicating OXT, in addition to VP, as a cofactor with CRH in stress (Gibbs 1984). In a larger sense these findings appear to be revealing a most remarkable capacity of individual cells to respond to altered hormone demands by the manufacture and presumed release of totally different products as conditions dictate. The functional significance of these changes in peptide production are far from clear at this early time. Perhaps the addition of VP or OXT to the CRH release only at certain times could serve as cofactors or upregulated receptor agonists and, thus, enhance ACTH output. Needless to say, other possibilities abound.

4 Intercellular Reorganization

Much of the reorganization that is known to take place in response to increased hormone demand involves changes in the relationships between and among cells. Both the neurons and their associated astroglia appear to play important roles in the neurosecretory system's responses. Several different types of intercellular reorganization accompanying increasing secretory activity have been investigated to date. Some of these involve relationships of neurons to other neurons, the formation of intercellular junctions allowing electrotonic interactions or the formation of new specialized chemical synapses. Other types involve selective interrelations between neurons or parts of neurons (e.g., their dendrites, somata or axon terminals) and the glia in the vicinity. These latter types often also change the relationship of neural elements to structures such as blood vessels or basal laminae. Evidence gathered so far indicates that the observed reorganization may have important effects on neuronal metabolism, electrical activity and, of course, hormone release.

4.1 Direct Somatic Appositions and Dendritic Bundles

Normally, the cell bodies of the SON and PVN are separated by fine glial processes (see Fig. 3 A). When hormone demand is increased via dehydration, at parturition or during lactation, these processes appear to retract, allowing the neurons to make direct soma-somatic appositions (Hatton and Tweedle 1982; Theodosis et al. 1981; Tweedle and Hatton 1976, 1977). An example of this activated state is shown in Fig. 3 B. In similar fashion, glia also remove themselves from between adjacent dendrites, resulting in dendritic membrane apposition and allowing the formation of dendritic bundles (see Fig. 4). Since SON neurons have relatively few (two to four) dendrites and bundles containing as many as twelve dendrites have been observed (Perlmutter et al. 1984 b), such bundling must involve different neurons. Therefore, large amounts of somatic and dendritic membrane surface from different neurons come into direct apposition without intervening glial processes. The resulting narrow intercellular distances along these appositions have been estimated to be 7–9 nm, or about the width of a plasma membrane (Hatton et al. 1984; Tweedle and Hatton 1976, 1977).

What are the functional implications of these cellular reorganizations that occur under conditions of increased hormone synthesis and release? One established role of astrocytic glia is the uptake and spatial buffering of extracellular potassium, $[K^+]_0$, that rises during neuronal firing (for reviews see Orkand 1977; Walz and Hertz 1983). The relative absence of these K^+ wicks between significant portions of adjacent SON somata and dendrites could result in significant increases in $[K^+]_0$. Due to the minute size of the intercellular cleft, the actual changes in $[K^+]_0$ cannot be measured using currently available ion-selective microelectrodes, whose tiny tips are orders of magnitude larger than would be needed for accurate measurement of ion concentrations. A reasonable estimate, however, would be that actively firing neurons would cause a several millimolar rise in $[K^+]_0$ in a 7- to 9-nm intermembrane space. Correspondingly, the membrane along these appositions would be depolarized by this raised $[K^+]_0$ by several millivolts. Therefore, these partially depolarized neurons would show increased excitability (i.e., be closer to firing threshold). This mode of partially depolarizing large numbers

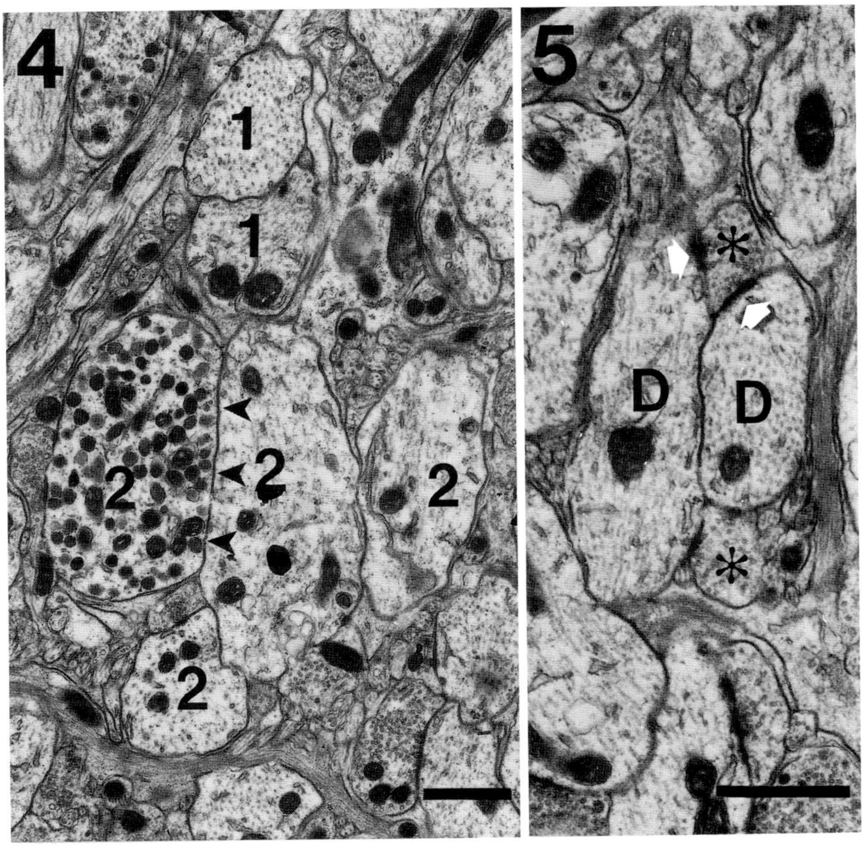

Fig. 4. Electron micrograph of dendritic bundles (dendrites in direct apposition without intervening glial processes). A bundle of two (*1*) and a bundle of four (*2*) dendrites in the supraoptic dendritic zone are shown. *Arrowheads* point to direct apposition between two dendrites, one of which contains neurosecretory vesicles. *Scale bar* 1 μm

Fig. 5. Electron micrograph of supraoptic cell dendrites (*D*) in apposition and being contacted by two double synapses (∗). *Arrowheads* point to the postsynaptic densities of the upper double synapse. *Scale bar* 1 μm

of SON cells may be one mechanism for coordinating the excitabilities (without actual synchronization) of both VP and OXT neurons during dehydration.

Another consequence of elevated $[K^+]_0$ after glial retraction in the activated SON would be increased protein synthesis. Lipton and Heimbach (1977, 1978) have shown that significant increases in protein synthetic activity (predominantly in neurons) occur in brain slices with elevations equal to or greater than 1.6 m*M* $[K^+]_0$. Such a consequence of elevated $[K^+]_0$ would be very useful to peptidergic neurons being called upon to manufacture and release increased amounts of their secretory products.

In addition to removal of $[K^+]_0$ from the extracellular space, thereby contributing to repolarization of neurons after each action potential, astrocytes may actually directly exert inhibitory influences on nearby neurons. There is reason to believe, for instance, that astrocytes may be able to exude such inhibitory amino acids as taurine, in which many glia are rich (see Hösli et al. 1986 for review), into the perineuronal space (Shain and Martin 1984). Of special interest here is the finding that the SON is particularly rich in taurine (Palkovits et al. 1986). Other molecules associated with astrocytes, such as the S-100 protein, may also cause inhibition upon incorporation into neurons (Hydén et al. 1987). Therefore, glial retraction from between and among neurons would remove these potential sources of inhibition at times of physiologically increased hormone demand.

A fourth possible functional sequela of large amounts of somatic and dendritic membrane in direct apposition might be the formation of electrical fields developing around groups of neurons. This has been shown in hippocampus, where the large pyramidal cell bodies and their parallel dendrites support synchronizing field potentials (Taylor and Dudek 1982, 1984a, 1984b). In the activated, reorganized SON, the morphological preconditions are ripe for the development of field effects which might be generated by appropriate inputs, but this has yet to be demonstrated experimentally.

4.2 Double Synapses

One presynaptic terminal simultaneously contacting two postsynaptic elements (somata and/or dendrites) has been called a "double synapse" (see Fig. 5). First described in the SON by Lafarga et al. (1975), it was proposed that such synapses might have something to do with synchronizing the firing of the neurons they contact. The abundance of double synapses in the lactating rat, compared to their paucity in virgin females, was discovered by Theodosis et al. (1981) and confirmed by Hatton and Tweedle (1982). Subsequently, it was also shown that the double synapses observed in lactating animals disappear within a month after the mother has weaned the pups (Theodosis and Poulain 1984). Lest it be thought that the double synapses on SON cell bodies are a phenomenon peculiar to the complex state of lactation, it should be noted that such synapses can be induced to form in males. Chronic dehydration produced by substitution of 2% NaCl solution for normal drinking water for 8–10 days results in double synapse formation. This is also reversible in about 14 days by allowing the dehydrated animals to again drink tap water (Tweedle and Hatton 1984a). So, the formation of double syn-

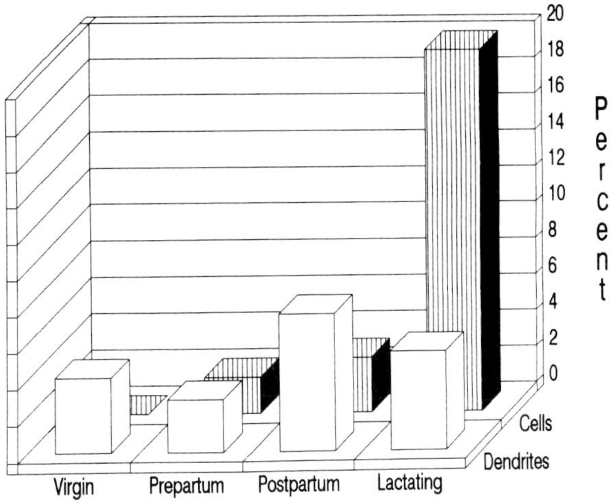

Fig. 6. Percentage of supraoptic cell bodies and dendrites contacted by double synapses (one terminal simultaneously contacting two postsynaptic elements) in female rats in four different reproductive states. Since only those double synapses occurring in one ultrathin section are counted, the percentages shown probably underestimate the true values. *Prepartum*, day 21 of gestation; *postpartum*, 4–24 h after parturition; *lactating*, 14 days of lactation with six or more pups

apses in the somatic region of the SON appears to be dependent upon the chronic nature of the stimulus situation rather than upon its special characteristics.

Double synapses also can be found in the dendritic zone of the SON (Perlmutter et al. 1984b, 1985). Several features of these synapses and their modulation by conditions activating SON neurons differ from the somatic region, however. First, axodendritic double synapses are not as rare as are axosomatic ones under basal conditions. About 2% of SON dendrites are normally contacted by double synapses, whereas this number is virtually zero in the somatic region (see Fig. 6). Second, the axodendritic double synapses are most numerous immediately after parturition and appear to be on the decline during lactation, while axosomatic double synapses are only abundant during lactation. Third, noradrenaline is probably the neurotransmitter in axodendritic double synapses and not in axosomatic ones (Tweedle and Hatton 1984b). There is suggestive evidence that some of the latter may contain dopamine (Buijs et al. 1984), OXT (Theodosis 1985) and/or GABA (Theodosis et al. 1986), but all of these findings on transmitters are still in need of confirmation. Finally, the stimulus conditions that induce the formation of double synapses at the two regions differ. Unlike the situation at the somatic region, chronic dehydration is not accompanied by an increase in the frequency of axodendritic double synapses in the SON (Perlmutter et al. 1985). The reasons for this last difference are not altogether clear, but doubtless the synapses at the two regions of the cell have different influences on their postsynaptic neurons.

At one level of understanding, the functional significance of double synapses is quite straightforward: they coordinate in time and intensity the message delivered to two postsynaptic elements. This could, as originally suggested by Lafarga et al. (1975) and further entertained by Theodosis et al. (1981), be at least part of the synchronizing influence on SON cell firing. In particular, the synchrony among OXT cells during the milk ejection reflex might be facilitated by activation of the axosomatic double synapses, presuming that they are excitatory, that are a prominent feature only during lactation.

Even the GABAergic double synapses described by Theodosis et al. (1986) would be expected to participate in the synchrony of OXT neurons, since there is a powerful and prolonged inhibition (on the order of seconds; see, e.g., Belin and Moos 1986) following the synchronized burst of action potentials that precedes the milk ejection reflex. It is more difficult to define the exact role of the axodendritic double synapses whose course of formation and disappearance is somewhat earlier in time. In order to begin to make valid predictions concerning the function of these synapses, one would need to know not only the transmitter (and possible coreleased peptide) in the presynaptic terminal, but the type of receptor(s) on the postsynaptic elements. Nevertheless, the degree of cellular reorganization displayed by this system is well illustrated by the appearance and disappearance of double synapses, associated with particular portions of the neuron, in relation to specific physiological events.

There may be a distinct, causal relationship between glial retraction and reinsertion, on one hand, and double synapse formation and disappearance, respectively, on the other. Evidence for this comes from the observation that the number of terminal boutons apparently remains the same, while the number of synapses increases in the SON (Perlmutter et al. 1984b, 1985). One way this could occur is for boutons making conventional single synaptic contacts to form a second contact when glial retraction allows the bouton membrane to come into apposition with another potential postsynaptic element.

4.3 Electrical Coupling

That some SON and PVN magnocellular neurons were electrically coupled to one another was suggested by Andrew et al. (1981). Intracellular injections of the fluorescent dye, lucifer yellow CH (LY; Stewart 1978), into individual neurosecretory cells of the SON and PVN in brain slices frequently resulted in more than one stained neuron (see Fig. 7). Since LY is a molecule small enough to pass through gap junctions, Andrew and coworkers also sought to demonstrate the presence of these intercellular junctions. Using freeze-fracture methods, they were successful in showing that some magnocellular cell bodies displayed the classical gap junctional morphology. Subsequent work has shown that much of the coupling is through distal dendrites and therefore their relative numbers would not be revealed in freeze-fracture preparations of primarily somatic regions. Nonetheless, these were exciting findings, because the transfer of dye from one neuron to another through gap junctions, although indirect evidence, strongly implies electrical coupling between and/or among these cells. Furthermore, electrotonic current spread among coupled neurons could be an important mechanism in setting the excitability levels of secretory cells. Also, electrical coupling

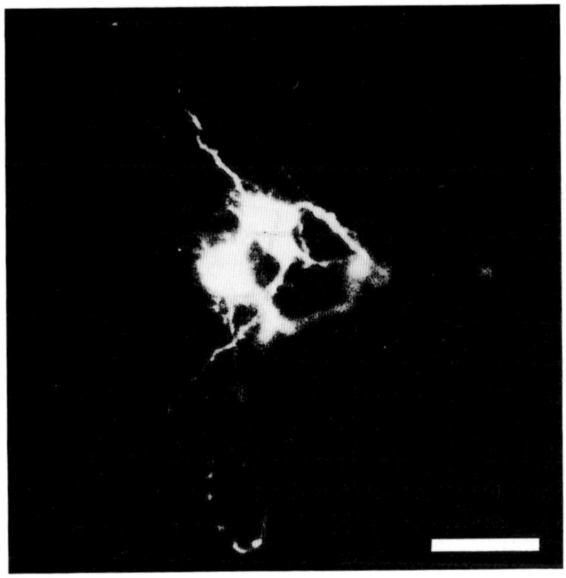

Fig. 7. Fluorescence micrograph of dye-coupling neurons in the paraventricular nucleus. One neuron was intracellularly recorded and injected with lucifer yellow in a hypothalamic slice preparation. Cells were photographed in a cleared, 500-μm-thick tissue slice; thus not all of the neural processes are in focus in one plane. Immunocytochemical identification revealed these cells to be vasopressinergic. *Scale bar* 50 μm

could contribute profoundly to the synchronous firing of OXT neurons during milk ejection. It has now been possible to measure directly the electrical coupling between SON neurons (Hatton and Yang 1986). Since the functional significance of gap junctions and dye coupling depend upon their faithfully representing electrical coupling, we sought to obtain convincing evidence for electrotonic interactions between neurosecretory neurons. Two SON neurons were simultaneously impaled using pairs of microelectrodes, in which one of each pair was filled with 5% LY in 0.25 *M* lithium acetate and the other with 3 *M* potassium acetate. Then, the electrical responses of the two neurons were observed. In many cases, cells showed no evidence of coupling; however, many positive instances were also observed. Taken as evidence for electrical coupling were: fast membrane depolarizations (coupling potentials) in one cell that were synchronized with spontaneously occurring action potentials in the other cell; synchronous changes in the two membrane potentials with current injection; and ability to evoke action potentials in both neurons with current injection in one. In each case where there was evidence for electrical coupling, dye coupling resulted from LY injection via one of the electrodes. All cells were dendrodendritically coupled. That the two electrodes were not in the same neuron was evident since membrane responses between coupled cells were never symmetrical, and interelectrode distances were always too great to allow both electrodes to impale one cell. Capacitative coupling between the electrodes was ruled out by the following observations: cells in the same tissue penetration as the coupled cell showed no responses to membrane voltage changes in the primary cell; no responses were seen when the second electrode was placed extracellularly or in the medium; and similar coupling potentials were also seen when one cell was recorded without a second electrode present. Finally, immunocytochemical identification of the dye-filled cells always confirmed that they were pairs of SON magnocellular neurons (i.e., they contained either VP or OXT). These data indicate that electrical coupling exists among neurosecretory cells in the mammalian brain and that it is reflected in dye coupling.

Intercellular coupling is another of the characteristics of the HNS that shows a marked degree of cellular reorganization when demand for synthesis and release of hormone is increased. For example, if electrical coupling were to participate in the synchrony of bursts shown in the firing of OXT cells during lactation, then one would have to predict that there should be much more coupling of these cells in lactating than in virgin female rats. This prediction is supported in the data of Hatton et al. (1987) in that coupling among OXT cells in the SON of lactating rats was found to be 233% that of virgins. Another example comes from male rats whose circulating plasma VP is significantly reduced by castration and restored to normal levels by testosterone replacement therapy (Crofton et al. 1985). Cobbett et al. (1987) found that the incidence of dye coupling among predominantly VP-containing neurons of the PVN was reduced to one-third of its control value by castration. Also, testosterone replacement completely abolished the effect of castration on coupling. Therefore, the apparent positive relationship between dye coupling and hormone secretion, illustrated in these two examples, supports the hypothesis of a functional role for electrical coupling in the coordination of excitability and in the synchronous activity of SON and PVN neurons. At the same time, these examples also argue against the interpretation of coupling as a spurious or random event, as has been suggested for neocortical coupling by Gutnick et al. (1985). These workers found that dye coupling among neurons in neocortical slices was dependent upon the plane of the slice. Incidence of dye coupling was enhanced in planes that damaged dendrites. Coupling was still only seen to occur among similar cell types, suggesting that selectivity of coupling was not lost. Not determined in that study were other possible effects varying the plane of section, such as altering the excitation/inhibition relationships within the slice which may have contributed to the results. In any case, dye coupling in the SON does not appear to be affected by dendritic damage. Hypothalamic slices cut in a horizontal plane so that no dendrites are injured have as many or more coupled cells as those with dendritic damage (Yang and Hatton 1987).

With regard to synchrony, it should be pointed out that coupling is likely to have the effect of amplifying chemical synaptic input generated by the suckling stimuli. That is, synaptic activation of a given cell would result in activation of all cells to which it was coupled (perhaps seven or more based on experimental evidence). Since OXT cells in lactating rats show predominantly dendrodendritic coupling (Hatton et al. 1987; Hatton and Yang 1986), the somata of coupled cells are at some distance from one another and would rarely be recorded by one extracellular electrode. Therefore, the absence of absolute synchrony among adjacent neurons (Belin and Moos 1986) is not evidence against coupling as one mechanism involved in synchrony.

It is important to note that at least two types of cellular reorganization are likely to be involved in the modulation of electrical coupling. First, neurons cannot form gap junctions if they are separated by astrocytic processes. So, the glial retraction from between adjacent cell bodies and from around at least some portions of the dendrites is a precondition for intercellular junctioning in this system.

Second, the neurons that are in contact must insert gap junction proteins into their membranes and "match up" with those in the membrane of an adjacent neuron. In the case of all OXT and VP neurons studied to date, this match-up has been between and among cells containing the same hormone (Cobbett et al. 1985; Hatton et al. 1987). Not yet known are the mechanisms for this intercellular recognition.

4.4 Pituicyte-Neurosecretory Terminal Interactions

Just as the astrocytes of the SON and its subjacent ventral glial lamina change their relationships with the cell bodies and dendrites of the magnocellular neurons under stimulated conditions, so the pituicytes of the neurohypophysis alter their relationships with the peptidergic terminals. As mentioned in Sect. 2.2 of this chapter, under basal conditions pituicytes tend to surround and/or engulf neurosecretory axons and terminals and to occupy relatively large areas of the basal lamina. It was Wittkowski and Brinkmann (1974) who first presented evidence that, when the HNS was stimulated (by depriving the animal of water), there was an increase in the amount of basal lamina occupied by neural as opposed to pituicyte processes. Stimulation of this sort has also been shown to induce the pituicytes to release the neurosecretory axons and terminals that they surround or engulf, and rehydration reverses this process (Kawamoto and Kawashima 1984; Tweedle and Hatton 1980a). The events occurring around the time of parturition also induce pituicytes to release neurosecretory endings and retreat from the basal lamina (see Fig. 8 and Table 1; Tweedle and Hatton 1982, 1987). Appropriately, parturition is a time when approximately 60% of the VP and OXT in the neurohypophysis is released (Fuchs and Saito 1971). This reorganization of neurohypophysial elements appears to remain throughout the stimulated conditions of lactation (Tweedle and Hatton 1982). By 10 days after weaning the pups, a partial reversion to the control state occurs, in that pituicytes are

Table 1. Changes in pituicyte – neurosecretory terminal relationships under various conditions, differing in hormone demand (means ± SE)

Treatment groups (n)	% Neural contact at the basal lamina	No. enclosed axons per pituicyte
Virgin (4)	70.9 ± 3.6	1.4 ± 0.4
Prepartum (4)	64.4 ± 3.1	1.5 ± 0.4
Postpartum (5)	76.2 ± 2.0 [2]	0.5 ± 0.1 [1, 2]
Lactating (4)	83.9 ± 1.5 [1]	$0.4 \pm 0,1$ [1, 2]
Postweaning (4)	79.0 ± 1.2 [1]	$1.1 \pm 0,2$ [3, 4]

Data from Tweedle and Hatton (1987)
[1] $p < 0.02$ vs control
[2] $p < 0.02$ vs prepartum
[3] $p < 0.02$ vs postpartum
[4] $p < 0.02$ vs lactating

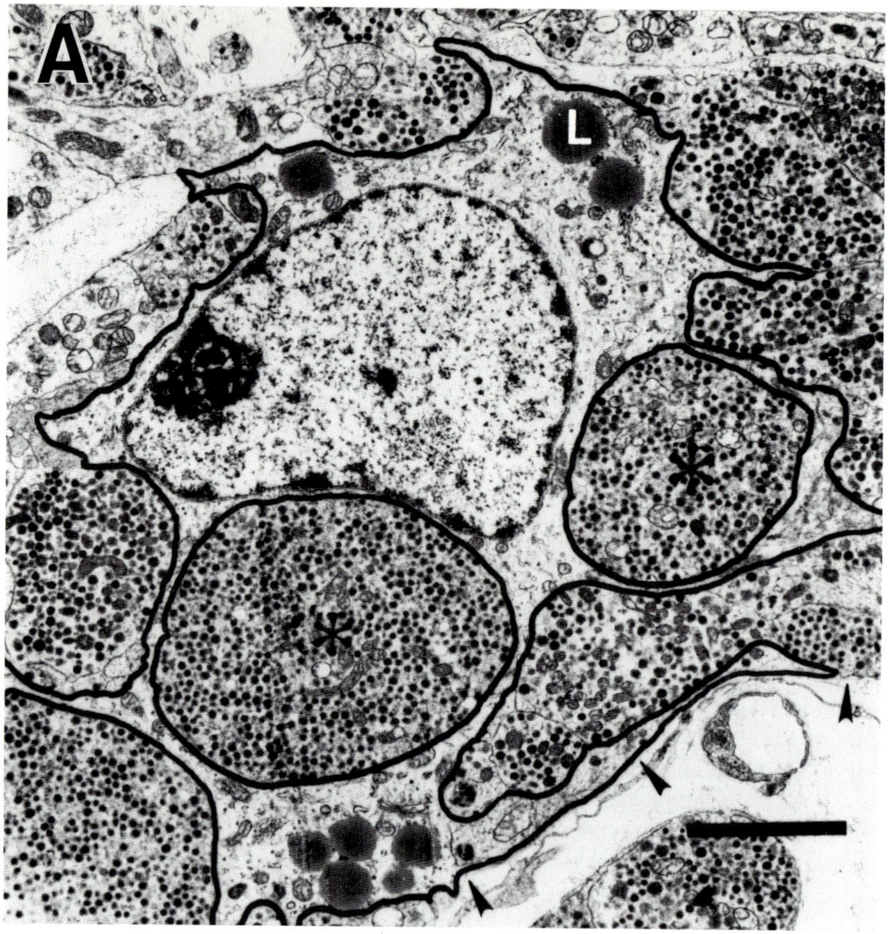

Fig. 8 A, B. Electron micrographs of neurohypophysial pituicytes – identifiable by the presence of lipid inclusions, *L* – and their associated neurosecretory endings. **A** Pituicyte from a prepartum rat engulfing neurosecretory processes (*) which are filled with dense-cored vesicles. *Arrowheads* indicate pituicyte process occupying the basal lamina. **B** Pituicyte from postpartum animal which contains no axonal processes. Neurosecretory terminals (*arrowheads*) abutting the basal lamina are devoid of dense-cored vesicles, having secreted their contents into the perivascular spaces. Pituicyte membranes in both parts of the figure have been darkened for clarification. *Scale bar* 3 µm

again engulfing neurosecretory endings but do not yet occupy their normal extent of basal lamina (see Table 1; Tweedle and Hatton 1987).

There are numerous similarities in both the pituicyte and neural terminal responses to the two types of chronic stimulation represented by lactation and dehydration via saline drinking. One curious difference, however, is worthy of note. During lactation (10–14 days after onset) there is a significant increase in the number of secretory sites (terminals) along the basal lamina, but without any change from controls in the length of each contact. By contrast, after 10 days of

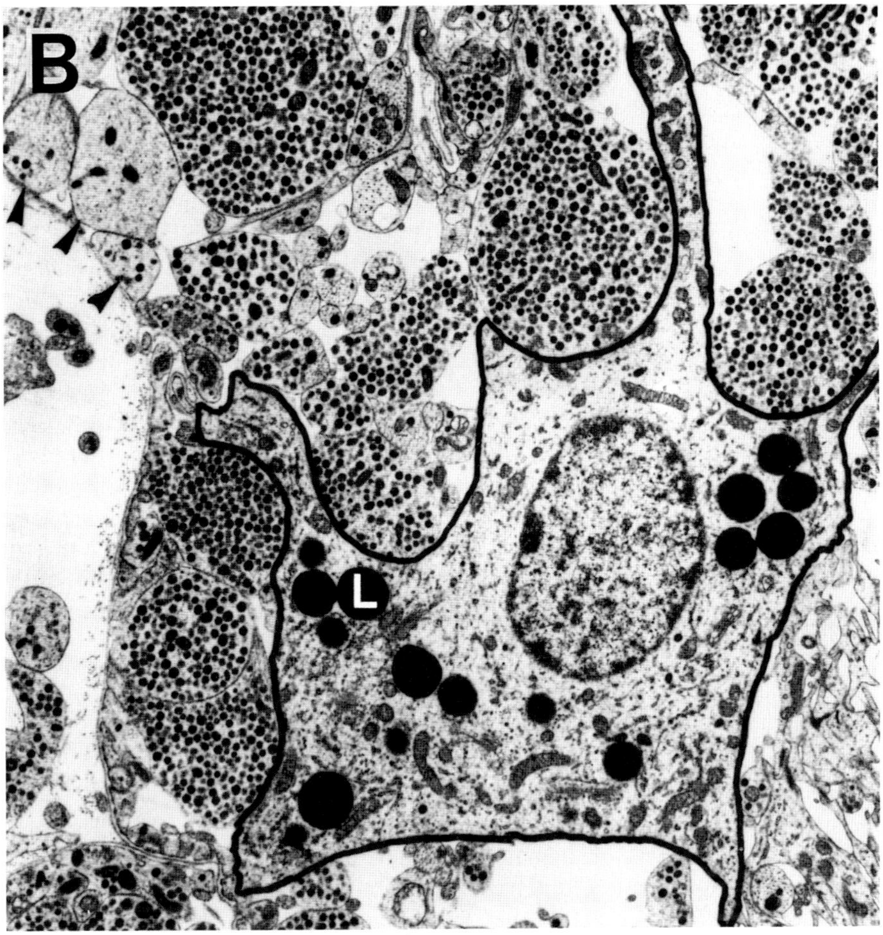

Fig. 8 B

saline treatment the sizes of the neurovascular contacts have increased and the number of them has decreased (Tweedle and Hatton 1987). It is possible that these differences are due to a predominance of neurovascular contact by OXT terminals during lactation and by VP terminals during dehydration. Immunocytochemical studies in which the contents of the terminals are identified are needed to shed light on this possibility.

The mechanisms operative in these reorganizations of neural and pituicyte elements have begun to be investigated. It has been shown, for example, that pituicytes are capable of releasing engulfed axons and receding from the basal lamina in the isolated, osmotically stimulated neurohypophyses maintained in vitro (Perlmutter et al. 1984a). Increasing the osmolality of the in vitro bathing medium within the physiological range (290–340 mOsm/kg) resulted in fewer engulfed secretory axons and more neurovascular contact with the basal lamina. Such osmotic stimulation does not, however, result in increased VP or OXT release. Therefore, it is possible that the pituicytes are themselves osmotically reactive and may respond to the direct action of increased blood osmotic pressure in vivo. Cultured adult rat pituicytes can be induced to undergo shape changes (from flattened to stellate) which are reminiscent of the control and stimulated shapes, respectively, seen in vivo (R.J. Bicknell et al. 1987 unpublished). Agents that will induce this stellation include dibutyryl cAMP or adrenergic agonists that produce receptor-mediated activation of adenylate cyclase. Since noradrenaline is released in the neurohypophysis under various stimulated conditions (Holzbauer et al. 1980), the physiological relevance of these in vitro results becomes apparent. It is interesting to recall, in light of these recent findings, that Ruoff et al. (1976) found that the phosphodiesterase inhibitor, theophylline, markedly increased cAMP accumulation in the neural lobes of saline-dehydrated or lactating rats, but not in control animals. Such increases in cyclic nucleotide were not found in the SON or PVN regions of any of the rats. Possibly these changes were the biochemical reflections of the retracted pituicyte morphology.

The functional significance of pituicyte engulfment of secretory axons and interposition of glial processes between the basal lamina and the neural elements under normal conditions is apparently that these arrangements inhibit hormone release. Facilitation of release, of course, would be an obvious consequence of the pituicyte and neural reorganizations produced by stimulation. It is not known with certainty just how the pituicytes might accomplish the inhibition of hormone release, but any one or a combination of several possible mechanisms may be involved. Action potentials could be kept from propagating into the terminals, thus dissallowing secretion, by the engulfing pituicytes altering the extracellular ionic environment (e.g., via increased calcium). Pituicytes also contain and may release the inhibitory transmitter GABA (Minchin and Nordmann 1975), which they apparently take up when it is released from GABAergic terminals. Another possibility is that engulfment of the neural elements by a pituicyte restricts the extracellular dissipation of released peptide which may then bind autoreceptors on the neurosecretory terminal membrane. This negative feedback would then inhibit further release. Recent evidence suggests that there are VP binding sites on the axons and terminals in the neural lobe (Bunn et al. 1986). This evidence surely gives plausibility to such a negative feedback mechanism operating in pituicyte modulation of secretion.

5 Summary

As a model for the study of neuroendocrine function, the magnocellular hypothalamo-neurohypophysial system has in very recent times revealed many of its secrets relating to the control of its secretions. It has become clear that both the structure and the function of this system are dynamic and capable of remarkable, fully reversible alterations as physiological conditions demand. Cellular reorganization with physiological stimulation occurs at the level of the individual neuron, as well as the level of interactions between and among neurons, neuronal/glial and neuronal perivascular relationships.

Individual neurons in this system respond to increased hormone demand by: (a) either producing additional nucleoli or enlarging the existing one, (b) a change in the function of the GERL from lysosomal to hormonal packaging and/or (c) altering genetic expression of peptides produced. Intercellular reorganization includes a number of changes in the relationships among the structural elements of the system. Fundamental to all of these changes appears to be the mobility of the associated astrocytes. With stimulation, these glia appear to retract from between adjacent neural elements and profoundly affect the system's functional and structural characteristics. Direct soma-somatic and dendrodendritic appositions are permitted by glial retraction, and these may have powerful influences upon electrical events. Also, the formation of new double synapses with prolonged physiological activation may be directly due to glial retraction from between a terminal bouton and a potential postsynaptic cell body or dendrite. Such double synapses are thought to coordinate or synchronize messages from one presynaptic to two postsynaptic elements under appropriate conditions (e.g., lactation). Gap junction formation, which appears to occur at physiologically relevant times, would also be permitted or facilitated by astrocyte retraction. Electrotonic interactions among neurons resulting from the formation of these intercellular junctions may participate in coordinating levels of excitability and in the synchrony of firing shown in this system.

Pituicytes, the astrocytes with the neurosecretory terminals of this system, seem to play an important role in the control of its secretory output. These glia may disallow action potential invasion of the terminals and/or facilitate negative feedback by engulfing the neurosecretory endings. By interposing their processes between the terminals and the basal lamina, they disallow secretion into the perivascular spaces around the capillaries under basal conditions. However, the pituicytes answer the call for hormone secretion by releasing the endings and moving away from the basal lamina. Thus, it seems that there is relatively complete coordination of the various elements of this system and that this coordination is directed at efficient stimulus-secretion coupling.

Acknowledgments. Thanks are due B. K. Modney and M. L. Weiss for helpful comments on an earlier draft of the manuscript. I also thank K. M. Grant, I. L. Taubitz and J. Harper for technical and typing assistance.

References

Alonso G, Assenmacher I (1984) Ultrastructural analysis of the noradrenergic innervation of rat supraoptic nucleus. Neurosci Lett 49:45–50

Andrew RD, Dudek FE (1984) Analysis of intracellularly recorded phasic bursting by mammalian neuroendocrine cells. J Neurophysiol 51:552–566

Andrew RD, MacVicar BA, Dudek FE, Hatton GI (1981) Dye transfer through gap junctions between neuroendocrine cells of rat hypothalamus. Science 211:1187–1189

Armstrong WE, Hatton GI (1978) Morphological changes in the rat supraoptic and paraventricular nuclei during the diurnal cycle. Brain Res 157:407–413

Armstrong WE, Sladek CD (1982) Spontaneous phasic-firing in supraoptic neurons recorded from hypothalamo-neurohypophysial explants in vitro. Neuroendocrinology 34:405–409

Armstrong WE, Sladek CD (1985) Evidence for excitatory actions of histamine on supraoptic neurons in vitro: mediation by an H1-type receptor. Neuroscience 16:307–322
Armstrong WE, Warach S, Hatton GI, McNeill TH (1980) Subnuclei in the rat hypothalamic paraventricular nucleus: a cytoarchitectural, horseradish peroxidase and immunocytochemical analysis. Neuroscience 5:1931–1958
Armstrong WE, Schöler J, McNeill TH (1982) Immunocytochemical, Golgi and electron microscopic characterization of putative dendrites in the ventral glial lamina of the rat supraoptic nucleus. Neuroscience 7:679–694
Belin V, Moos F (1986) Paired recording from supraoptic and paraventricular oxytocin cells in suckled rats: recruitment and synchronization. J Physiol 377:369–390
Belin V, Moos F, Richard P (1984) Synchronization of oxytocin cells in the hypothalamic paraventricular and supraoptic nuclei in suckled rats – direct proof with paired extracellular recordings. Exp Brain Res 57:201–203
Brimble MJ, Dyball REJ (1977) Characterization of the responses of oxytocin- and vasopressin-secreting neurones in the supraoptic nucleus to osmotic stimulation. J Physiol 271:253–271
Broadwell RD, Oliver C (1981) Golgi apparatus, GERL, and secretory granule formation within neurons of the hypothalamo-neurohypophysial system of control and hyperosmotically stressed mice. J Cell Biol 90:474–484
Buijs RM, Geffard M, Pool CW, Hoorneman EMD (1984) The dopaminergic innervation of the supraoptic and paraventricular nucleus. A light and electron microscopical study. Brain Res 323:65–72
Bunn SJ, Hanley MR, Wilkin GP (1986) Autoradiographic localization of peripheral benzodiazepine, dihydroalprenolol and arginine vasopressin binding sites in the pituitaries of control, stalk transected and Brattleboro rats. Neuroendocrinology 44:76–83
Carithers J, Johnson AK (1984) Long term effects on the supraoptic nuclei and neural lobe produced by ablation of the tissue surrounding the preoptic recess. Brain Res 305:123–140
Carithers J, Dellmann HD, Bealer SL, Brody MJ, Johnson AK (1981) Ultrastructural effects of anteroventral third ventricle lesions on supraoptic nuclei and neural lobes of rats. Brain Res 220:13–29
Castel M, Gainer H, Dellmann HD (1984) Neuronal secretory systems. Int Rev Cytol 88:303–459
Cobbett P, Smithson KG, Hatton GI (1985) Dye-coupled magnocellular peptidergic neurons of the rat paraventricular nucleus show homotypic immunoreactivity. Neuroscience 16:885–895
Cobbett P, Smithson KG, Hatton GI (1986) Immunoreactivity to vasopressin- but not oxytocin-associated neurophysin antiserum in phasic neurons of rat hypothalamic paraventricular nucleus. Brain Res 362:7–16
Cobbett P, Yang QZ, Hatton GI (1987) Incidence of dye coupling among magnocellular paraventricular nucleus neurons in male rats is testosterone dependent. Brain Res Bull 18:365–370
Conrad LCA, Pfaff DW (1976) Efferents from medial basal forebrain and hypothalamus in the rat. II. An autoradiographic study of the anterior hypothalamus. J Comp Neurol 169:221–262
Crofton JT, Baer PG, Share L, Brooks DP (1985) Vasopressin release in male and female rats: effects of gonadectomy and treatment with gonadal steroid hormones. Endocrinology 117:1195–1200
Day TA, Renaud LP (1984) Electrophysiological evidence that noradrenergic afferents selectively facilitate the activity of supraoptic vasopressin neurons. Brain Res 303:233–240
Dougherty PJ, Yang QZ, Hatton GI (1986) Synaptically mediated responses recorded intracellularly in rat supraoptic nucleus induced by lateral olfactory tract stimulation. Soc Neurosci Abst 12:1256
Dreifuss JJ, Sandri C, Akert K, Moor H (1975) Ultra-structural evidence for sinusoid spaces and coupling between pituicytes in the rat. Cell Tissue Res 161:33–45

Finlayson LH, Osborne MP (1975) Secretory activity of neurons and related electrical activity. Adv Comp Physiol Biochem 6:165–258

Fisher AWF, Price PG, Burford GD, Lederis K (1979) A 3-dimensional reconstruction of the hypothalamo- neurohypophysial system of the rat. The neurons projecting to the neuro/intermediate lobe and those containing vasopressin and somatostatin. Cell Tissue Res 204:343–354

Fuchs A-R, Saito S (1971) Pituitary oxytocin and vasopressin content of pregnant rats before, during and after parturition. Endocrinology 88:574–578

Gähwiler BH, Dreifuss JJ (1980) Transition from random to phasic firing induced in neurons cultured from the hypothalamic supraoptic area. Brain Res 193:415–425

Gainer HY, Loh PY, Sarne Y (1977) Biosynthesis of neuronal peptides. In: Gainer H (ed) Peptides in neurobiology. Plenum, New York, pp 183–219

Gibbs DM (1984) Dissociation of oxytocin, vasopressin and corticotropin secretion during different types of stress. Life Sci 35:487–491

Gregory WA, Tweedle CD, Hatton GI (1980) Ultra-structure of neurons in the paraventricular nucleus of normal, dehydrated and rehydrated rats. Brain Res Bull 5:301–306

Gutnick MJ, Lobel-Yaakov R, Rimon G (1985) Incidence of neuronal dye-coupling in neocortical slices depends on the plane of section. Neuroscience 15:659–666

Hatton GI (1976) Nucleus circularis: is it an osmoreceptor in the brain? Brain Res Bull 1:123–132

Hatton GI (1982) Phasic bursting activity of rat paraventricular neurones in the absence of synaptic transmission. J Physiol 327:273–284

Hatton GI, Tweedle CD (1982) Magnocellular neuropeptidergic neurons in hypothalamus: increases in membrane apposition and number of specialized synapses from pregnancy to lactation. Brain Res Bull 8:197–204

Hatton GI, Walters JK (1973) Induced multiple nucleoli, nucleolar margination, and cell size changes in supraoptic neurons during dehydration and rehydration in the rat. Brain Res 59:137–154

Hatton GI, Yang QZ (1986) Direct evidence for electrical coupling among rat supraoptic nucleus neurons. Soc Neurosci Abst 12:1257

Hatton GI, Johnson JI, Malatesta CZ (1972) Supraoptic nuclei of rodents adapted for mesic and xeric environments: numbers of cells, multiple nucleoli and their distributions. J Comp Neurol 145:43–60

Hatton GI, Armstrong WE, Gregory WA (1978) Spontaneous and osmotically stimulated activity in slices of rat hypothalamus. Brain Res Bull 3:497–508

Hatton GI, Ho YW, Mason WT (1983) Synaptic activation of phasic bursting in rat supraoptic nucleus neurones recorded in hypothalamic slices. J Physiol 345:297–317

Hatton GI, Perlmutter LS, Salm AK, Tweedle CD (1984) Dynamic neuronal-glial interactions in hypothalamus and pituitary: implications for control of hormone synthesis and release. Peptides 5(Suppl 1):121–138

Hatton GI, Cobbett P, Salm AK (1985) Extranuclear axon collaterals of paraventricular neurons in the rat hypothalamus: intracellular staining, immunocytochemistry and electrophysiology. Brain Res Bull 14:123–132

Hatton GI, Yang QZ, Cobbett P (1987) Dye coupling among immunocytochemically identified neurons in the supraoptic nucleus of lactating rats. Neuroscience 21:923–930

Heimer L (1978) The olfactory cortex and the ventral striatum. Limbic mechanisms. In: Livingston KE, Hornykiewicz O (eds) The continuing evolution of the limbic system concept. Plenum, New York, pp 95–187

Hoblitzell ER, Hatton GI, Armstrong WE (1976) Paraventricular nucleus: changes in the medial and lateral cell groups during dehydration and rehydration in the rat. Brain Res Bull 1:329–332

Hollowell DE, Smithson KG, Hatton GI (1986) Anatomical evidence for olfactory input to the supraoptic nucleus of the rat: an anterograde study employing the lectin *Phaseolus vulgaris* leucoagglutinin (PHA-L). Soc Neurosci Abst 12:1256

Holzbauer M, Sharman DF, Godden U, Mann SP, Stephens DB (1980) Effect of water and salt intake on pituitary catecholamines in the rat and domestic pig. Neuroscience 5:1959–1968

Hösli E, Schousboe A, Hösli L (1986) Amino acid uptake. In: Fedoroff S, Vernadakis A (eds) Astrocytes: biochemistry, physiology and pharmacology of astrocytes, vol 2. Academic, New York, pp 133–153

Hou-Yu A, Kelly DD, Silvermann A-J (1986a) Effects of chronic behavioral stress on corticotropin-releasing hormone and its co-expression with oxytocin in the rat paraventricular nucleus. Soc Neurosci Abst 12:783

Hou-Yu A, Lamme AT, Zimmerman EA, Silverman A-J (1986b) Comparative distribution of vasopressin and oxytocin neurons in the rat brain using a double-label procedure. Neuroendocrinology 44:235–246

Hydén H, Cupello A, Palm A (1987) Increase in chloride ion permeability across the nerve cell membrane after the endogenous antigen S-100 incorporation. Brain Res 404:405–407

Kawamoto K, Kawashima S (1984) Ultrastructural changes and proliferation of pituicytes in mouse posterior pituitary during water deprivation and rehydration. Acta Anat 119:136–141

Konigsmark BW (1970) Methods for counting neurons. In: Nauta WJH, Ebbesson SOE (eds) Contemporary research methods in neuroanatomy. Springer, Berlin Heidelberg New York, pp 315–340

Lafarga M, Palacios G, Perez R (1975) Morphological aspects of the functional synchronization of supraoptic nucleus neurons. Experientia 31: 348–349

Lind RW, von Hoesen GW, Johnson AK (1982) An HRP study of the connections of the subfornical organ of the rat. J Comp Neurol 210:265–277

Lipton P, Heimbach CJ (1977) The effect of extracellular K^+ concentration on protein synthesis in guinea-pig hippocampal slices. J Neurochem 28:1347–1354

Lipton P, Heimbach CJ (1978) Mechanism of extracellular potassium stimulation of protein synthesis in the in vitro hippocampus. J Neurochem 31:1299–1307

Martin R, Geis R, Holl R, Schafer M, Voigt KH (1983) Co-existence of unrelated peptides in oxytocin and vasopressin terminals of rat neurohypophyses: immunoreactive methionine5- enkephalin-, leucine5-enkephalin- and cholecystokinin-like substances. Neuroscience 8:213–227

Mason WT (1980) Supraoptic neurones of rat hypothalamus are osmosensitive. Nature 287:154–157

Mason WT (1983) Electrical properties of neurones recorded from the rat supraoptic nucleus in vitro. Proc Soc Lond [Biol] 217:141–161

Mason CA, Bern HA (1977) Cellular biology of the neurosecretory neuron. In: Kandel ER (ed) Handbook of physiology, vol 1. Waverly, Baltimore, pp 651–689

Mason WT, Ho YW, Eckenstein F, Hatton GI (1983) Mapping of cholinergic neurons associated with rat supraoptic nucleus: combined immunocytochemical and histochemical identification. Brain Res Bull 11:617–626

Mason WT, Ho YW, Hatton GI (1984) Axon collaterals of supraoptic neurones: anatomical and electrophysiological evidence for their existence in the lateral hypothalamus. Neuroscience 11:169–182

Meyer DK, Brownstein MJ (1980) Effect of surgical deafferentation of the supraoptic nucleus on its choline acetyltransferase content. Brain Res 193:566–569

Minchin MCW, Nordmann JJ (1975) The release of 3H gamma-aminobutyric acid and neurophysin from the isolated rat posterior pituitary. Brain Res 90:75–84

Miselis RR, Shapiro RF, Hand PJ (1979) Subfornical organ efferents to neural systems for control of body water. Science 205:1022–1025

Nordmann JJ, Cazalis M, Dayantithi G, Castanas E, Giraud P, Legros J-J, Louis F (1986) Are opioid peptides co-localized with vasopressin or oxytocin in the neural lobe of the rat? Cell Tissue Res 246:177–182

Orkand RG (1977) Glial cells. In: Kandel ER (ed) Handbook of physiology, vol 1. Waverly, Baltimore, pp 855–875

Palkvotis M, Elekes I, Lang T, Patthy A (1986) Taurine levels in discrete brain nuclei of rats. J Neurochem 47:1333–1335

Perlmutter LS, Hatton GI, Tweedle CD (1984a) Plasticity in the neurohypophysis in vitro: effects of osmotic changes on pituicytes. Neuroscience 12:503–511

Perlmutter LS, Tweedle CD, Hatton GI (1984 b) Neuronal glial plasticity in the supraoptic dendritic zone: dendritic bundling and double synapse formation at parturition. Neuroscience 13:769–779
Perlmutter LS, Tweedle CD, Hatton GI (1985) Neuronal/glial plasticity in the supraoptic dendritic zone in response to acute and chronic dehydration. Brain Res 361:225–232
Piekut DT, Joseph SA (1985) Relationship of CRF-immunostained cells and magnocellular neurons in the paraventricular nucleus of rat hypothalamus. Peptides 6:873–882
Pittman QJ, Blume HW, Renaud LP (1981) Connections of the hypothalamic paraventricular nucleus with the neurohypophysis, median eminence, amygdala, lateral septum and midbrain periaqueductal gray: an electro-physiological study in the rat. Brain Res 215:15–28
Poulain DA, Wakerley JB (1982) Electrophysiology of hypothalamic magnocellular neurones secreting oxytocin and vasopressin. Neuroscience 7:773–808
Renaud LP, Rogers J, Sgro S (1983) Terminal degeneration in supraoptic nucleus following subfornical organ lesions: ultrastructural observations in the rat. Brain Res 275:365–368
Ruoff HJ, Mathison R, Lederis K (1976) Cyclic 3′5′-adenosine monophosphate in the hypothalamo-neurohypophysial system of normal, NaCl-treated and lactating rats. Neuroendocrinology 22:18–29
Salm AK, Hatton GI (1980) An immunocytochemical study of astrocytes associated with the rat supraoptic nucleus. Soc Neurosci Abst 6:547
Salm AK, Hatton GI, Nilaver G (1982) Immunoreactive glial fibrillary acidic protein in pituicytes of the rat neurohypophysis. Brain Res 236:471–476
Sawchenko PE, Swanson LW, Vale WW (1984) Co-expression of corticotropin-releasing factor and vasopressin immunoreactivity in parvocellular neurosecretory neurons of the adrenalectomized rat. Proc Natl Acad Sci USA 81:1883–1887
Scalia F, Winans SS (1975) The differential projections of the olfactory bulb and accessory olfactory bulb in mammals. J Comp Neurology 161:35–56
Sgro S, Ferguson AV, Renaud LP (1984) Subfornical organ-supraoptic nucleus connections: an electrophysiologic study in the rat. Brain Res 303:7–13
Shain WG, Martin DL (1984) Activation of beta-adrenergic receptors stimulates taurine release from glial cells. Cell Mol Neurobiol 4:191–196
Sherman TG, Civelli O, Douglass J, Herbert E, Watson SJ (1986 a) Coordinate expression of hypothalamic pro- dynorphin and pro-vasopressin mRNAs with osmotic stimulation. Neuroendocrinology 44:222–228
Sherman TG, McKelvy JF, Watson SJ (1986 b) Vasopressin mRNA regulation in individual hypothalamic nuclei: a northern and in situ hybridization analysis. J Neurosci 6:1685–1694
Sladek CD, Johnson AK (1983) Effect of anteroventral third ventricle lesions on vasopressin release by organ-cultured hypothalamo-neurohypophyseal explants. Neuroendocrinology 37:78–84
Sladek CD, Joynt RJ (1979) Angiotensin stimulation of vasopressin release from the rat hypothalamo-neurohypophyseal system in organ culture. Endocrinology 104:148–153
Sladek JR Jr, McNeill TH (1980) Simultaneous monoamine histofluorescence and neuropeptide immunocytochemistry. IV. Verification of catecholamine-neurophysin interactions through single-section analysis. Cell Tissue Res 210:181–189
Stewart WW (1978) Functional connections between cells as revealed by dye-coupling with a highly fluorescent naphthalimide tracer. Cell 14:741–759
Suess U, Pliška V (1981) Identification of the pituicytes as astroglial cells by indirect immunofluorescence-staining for the glial fibrillary acidic protein. Brain Res 221:27–33
Swanson LW (1976) An autoradiographic study of the efferent connections of the preoptic region in the rat. J Comp Neurol 167:227–256
Swanson LW (1977) Immunohistochemical evidence for a neurophysin-containing autonomic pathway arising in the paraventricular nucleus of the hypothalamus. Brain Res 128:356–363
Swanson LW, Kuypers HGJM (1980) A direct projection from the ventromedial nucleus and retrochiasmatic area of the hypothalamus to the medulla and spinal cord of the rat. Neurosci Lett 17:307–312

Swanson LW, Sawchenko PE, Berod A, Hartman BK, Helle KB, Vanorden DE (1981) An immunohistochemical study of the organization of catecholaminergic cells and terminal fields in the paraventricular and supraoptic nuclei of the hypothalamus. J Compar Neurol 196:271–285

Taylor CP, Dudek FE (1982) Synchronous neural after-discharges in rat hippocampal slices without active chemical synapses. Science 218:810–812

Taylor CP, Dudek FE (1984a) Excitation of hippocampal pyramidal cells by an electrical field effect. J Neurophysiol 52:126–142

Taylor CP, Dudek FE (1984b) Synchronization without active chemical synapses during hippocampal after-discharges. J Neurophysiol 52:143–155

Theodosis DT (1985) Oxytocin-immunoreactive terminals synapse on oxytocin neurones in the supraoptic nucleus. Nature 313:682–684

Theodosis DT, Poulain DA (1984) Evidence for structural plasticity in the supraoptic nucleus of the rat hypothalamus in relation to gestation and lactation. Neuroscience 11:183–193

Theodosis DT, Poulain DA, Vincent J-D (1981) Possible morphological bases for synchronisation of neuronal firing in the rat supraoptic nucleus during lactation. Neuroscience 6:919–929

Theodosis DT, Paul L, Tappaz ML (1986) Immunocytochemical analysis of the GABAergic innervation of oxytocin- and vasopressin-secreting neurons in the rat supraoptic nucleus. Neuroscience 19:207–222

Thomson AM (1984) Correlations between the firing of supraoptic neurones in slices of rat brain. Exp Brain Res 54:217–224

Tribollet E, Armstrong WE, Dubois-Dauphin M, Dreifuss JJ (1985) Extra-hypothalamic afferent imputs to the supraoptic nucleus area of the rat as determined by retrograde and anterograde tracing techniques. Neuroscience 15:135–148

Tweedle CD, Hatton GI (1976) Ultrastructural comparisons of neurons of supraoptic and circularis nuclei in normal and dehydrated rats. Brain Res Bull 1:103–122

Tweedle CD, Hatton GI (1977) Ultrastructural changes in rat hypothalamic neurosecretory cells and their associated glial during minimal dehydration and rehydration. Cell Tissue Res 181:59–72

Tweedle CD, Hatton GI (1980a) Evidence for dynamic interactions between pituicytes and neurosecretory axons in the rat. Neuroscience 5:661–667

Tweedle CD, Hatton GI (1980b) Glial cell enclosure of neurosecretory endings in the neurohypophysis of the rat. Brain Res 192:555–559

Tweedle CD, Hatton GI (1982) Magnocellular neuropeptidergic terminals in neurohypophysis: rapid glial release of enclosed axons during parturition. Brain Res Bull 8:205–209

Tweedle CD, Hatton GI (1984a) Synapse formation and disappearance in adult rat supraoptic nucleus during different hydration states. Brain Res 309:373–376

Tweedle CD, Hatton GI (1984b) Ultrastructure of catecholaminergic synapses in the rat supraoptic nucleus during different hydration states. Soc Neurosci Abstracts 10:209

Tweedle CD, Hatton GI (1987) Morphological adaptability at neurosecretory axonal endings on the neurovascular contact zone of the rat neurohypophysis. Neuroscience 20:241–246

van den Pol AN (1982) The magnocellular and parvocellular paraventricular nucleus of rat: intrinsic organization. J Comp Neurol 206:317–345

Vandesande F, Dierickx K, DeMey J (1977) The origin of the vasopressinergic and oxytocinergic fibres of the external region of the median eminence of the rat hypophysis. Cell Tissue Res 130:443–452

van Leeuwen FW, Pool CW, Sluiter AA (1983) Enkephalin immunoreactivity in synaptoid elements on glial cells in the rat neural lobe. Neuroscience 8:229–241

Wakerley JB, Poulain DA, Brown D (1978) Comparison of firing patterns in oxytocin- and vasopressin-releasing neurones during progressive dehydration. Brain Res 148:425–440

Walz W, Hertz L (1983) Functional interactions between neurons and astrocytes. II. Potassium homeostasis at the cellular level. Prog Neurobiol 20:133–183

Watson SJ, Akil H, Fischli W, Goldstein A, Zimmerman E, Nilaver G, van Wimersma Greidanus TB (1982) Dynorphin and vasopressin: common localization in magnocellular neurons. Science 216:85–87

Wittkowski W, Brinkmann H (1974) Changes of extent of neurovascular contacts and number of neuro-glial synaptoid contacts in the pituitary posterior lobe of dehydrated rats. Anat Embryol 146:157–165

Wolfson B, Manning RW, Davis LG, Arentzen Jr R, Baldino F (1985) Co-localization of corticotropin releasing factor and vasopressin mRNA in neurones after adrenalectomy. Nature 315:59–61

Yamashita H, Inenaga K, Kawata M, Sano Y (1983) Phasically firing neurons in the supraoptic nucleus of the rat hypothalamus: immunocytochemical and electrophysiological studies. Neurosci Lett 37:87–92

Yang QZ, Hatton GI (1987) Dye coupling among rat supraoptic nucleus neurons without dendritic damage: differential incidence in nursing mother and virgin rats. Brain Res Bull 19:559–565

Stimulus-Secretion Coupling in the Oxytocin System *

A. J. S. SUMMERLEE and L. J. PARRY

Contents

1 Introduction

One of the fundamental processes in the functioning of magnocellular neurones is the mechanism of stimulus-secretion coupling, that is the translation of electrical activity of the neurones into the release of precise quantities of neurosecretory product, and we shall be addressing this concept in the oxytocin system in the present chapter. However, we shall broaden the definition to describe the types and modes of stimulation that are responsible for the secretion of oxytocin and its appearance in the blood. It is necessary to start the chapter with a brief review

* Work presented in this chapter was financed by the Medical Research Council
Biomedical Sciences, Ontario Veterinary College, University of Guelph, Guelph NIG ZWI Ontario Canada

of the biochemistry, anatomy and physiology of the oxytocin system and to explain how it is possible to take recordings from identified oxytocin neurones in the hypothalamus.

2 Biosynthesis of Oxytocin

2.1 Biosynthesis

In 1964, Sachs and Takabatake suggested that vasopressin and its associated carrier protein, neurophysin, were produced as parts of a common precursor molecule. Subsequently, it was proposed that oxytocin and its neurophysin were made by a similar mechanism (Pickering and Jones 1971) and this now appears to be a common feature for the method of production of a variety of hypothalamic neuropeptides (see reviews: Brownstein 1983; Richter 1983). In 1982, Land and colleagues (Land et al. 1982) determined the nucleotide sequence of cloned cDNA encoding bovine vasopressin and its neurophysin and this was followed by the determination of the sequence for oxytocin (Fig. 1) and its neurophysin (Ivell and Richter 1984; Ruppert et al. 1984). The oxytocin precursor comprises an initial signal sequence, the hormone itself and the carrier protein (neurophysin I). Unlike the vasopressin precursor, it does not contain a glycoprotein attached to the C-terminus (see reviews: Richter 1983; Pickering 1978; Pickering et al. 1983). Prooxyphysin begins its life associated with the rough endoplasmic reticulum. There the mRNA template is translated. The first 19 amino acid residues contain a hydrophobic middle section, which is typical of precursor signal sequences (Perlman and Halvorson 1983). This putative signal ends in two basic amino acids followed by the nonapeptide sequence of oxytocin, and by glycine, the standard donor of the amino group for C-terminal amidation (Bradbury et al. 1983;

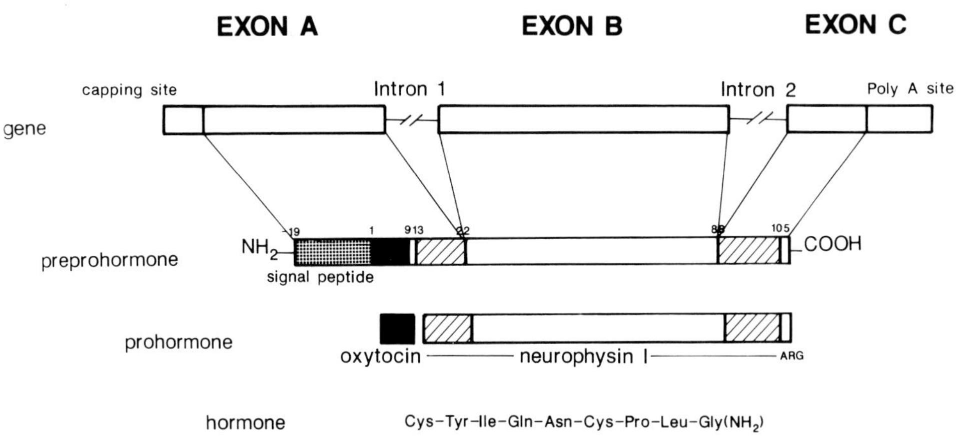

Fig. 1. The structural organization of the oxytocin gene, precursors and the hormone itself. (Redrawn from Richter and Schmale 1984)

Richter 1983). The remainder of the precursor contains neurophysin I and there are no homologous sequences in this part of the molecule when compared with other hypothalamic precursors (Gubler et al. 1983; Furutani et al. 1983; Shen et al. 1982; Seeburg and Adelman 1984), with one major exception: the precursor for neurophysin II, which is associated with vasopressin (Ruppert et al. 1984). Recent analysis of the oxytocin gene encoding the neurohypophysial hormone indicates that it is typical of higher eukaryotic split genes, with functional domains of the protein structure encoded by different exons (Schmale et al. 1983; Ruppert et al. 1984). The gene contains three exons and two introns with exon A including the hormone and exon B, the highly conserved central part of the neurophysin (Fig. 1). Due to similarities in the reading frame and considerable homology between the neurophysin regions of the two precursors for oxytocin and vasopressin (Ruppert et al. 1984), it is likely that the production of the hormones is a consequence of gene duplication (Lincoln and Russell 1986), yet the genes are not expressed together in the same neurone, i.e. neurones produce either vasopressin or oxytocin (and the related neurophysin), but never both. This lack of coexistence was demonstrated by immunocytochemical methods (Dierickx 1980) and has recently been confirmed by in situ hybridization studies using the appropriate cDNA probes (Coghlan et al. 1984). It is conceivable that a cell could switch from producing oxytocin to vasopressin, but this has not been demonstrated.

2.2 Packaging and Processing

After translation of the mRNA template, the precursor is packaged into granules (150–200 nm in diameter) and transported to the neural lobe where it is stored awating release. Sachs and Takabatake (Sachs and Takabatake 1964; Takabatake and Sachs 1964) showed that there was a lag of about 1– 1.5 h between the administration of a radioactively labelled tracer to the synthetic parts of the magnocellular neurones and the appearance of label in the lobe. This means that the precursor is assembled, packaged, processed and transported (a distance of 3 mm) to the terminals in this time. Even allowing virtually no time for the synthesis and processing, the minimum transport velocity would be 2–3 mm/h, which is very rapid axonal transport indeed (Jones and Pickering 1970). It was this rapid transport time that led to the early conclusion that the hormone might be processed whilst in transit (Vogt 1953). More recent work by Gainer (Gainer et al. 1977 a, b; Gainer and Brownstein 1978) has provided convincing evidence for the conversion of the precursor in transit. The signal peptide is removed by cleavage of the Ala-Cys in the rough endoplasmic reticulum soon after assembly, and certainly before packaging (Steiner et al. 1980). The remaining processing occurs within the granule:

1. Separation of the oxytocin peptide from the N-terminus of the neurophysin I, which involves cleavage of a Lys-Arg sequence (Steiner et al. 1980) followed by the action of a carboxy peptidase
2. Cleavage of the Arg-Ala bond between the C-terminus of the neurophysin and the N-terminus

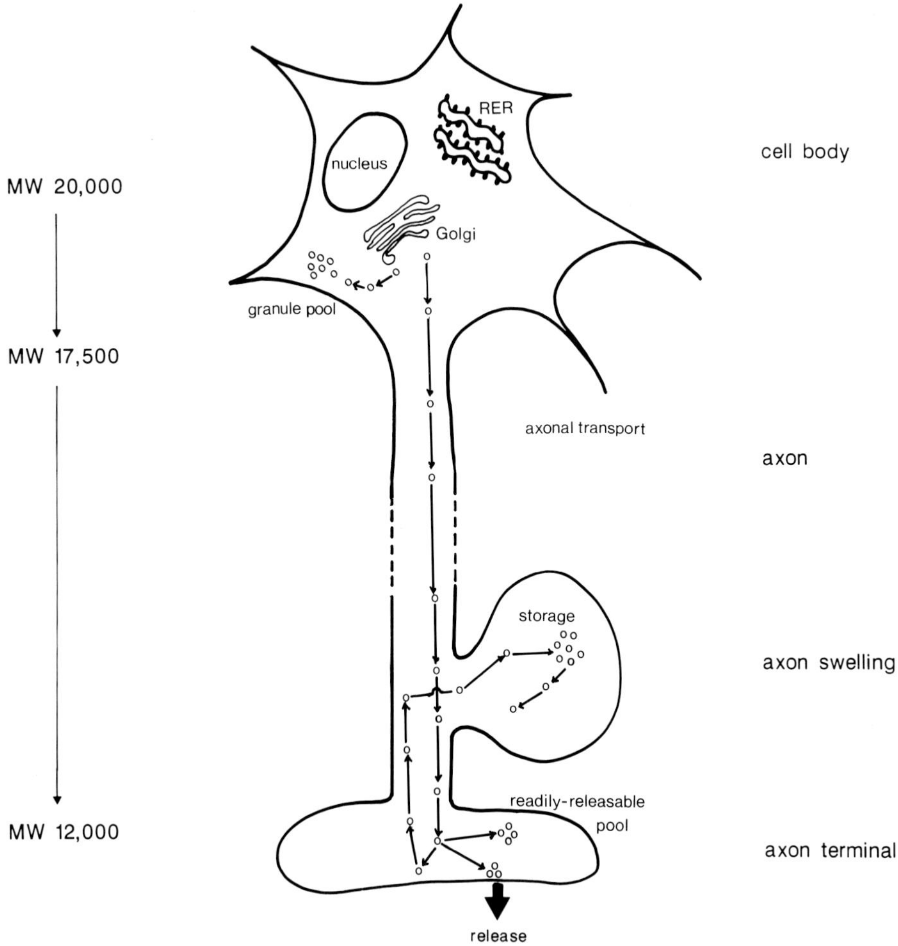

Fig. 2. Biosynthesis, transport, storage and release of hypothalamo-neurohypophysial hormone. Translation of mRNA occurs on the rough endoplasmic reticulum (*RER*) in the cell body which produces a large-molecular-weight (*MW*) preprohormone. The precursor is packaged in the Gogli, and granules are transported to the neural lobe for release from nerve terminals. During transport the precursor is processed into oxytocin and neurophysin I. (After Gainer et al. 1977a)

3. Amidation of the terminal glycine, which is common to other peptide processing (Bradbury et al. 1982; Amara et al. 1980; Mains et al. 1977; Suchanek et al. 1978).

These processes are illustrated in Fig. 2. It is important to point out that the passage through different intracellular environments per se is not essential for this intragranular processing. If the transport is arrested by treatment of the animal with small doses of colchicine then processing continues unhindered (Parish et al. 1981; Birkett 1983).

3 Anatomy of the Oxytocin System

3.1 Introduction

A series of now classic experiments established that the posterior pituitary gland was involved in the process of milk let-down. The phenomenon of milk ejection has been recognized for many centuries (Folley 1969), but its control has been discovered only comparatively recently. Scientific investigation of the milk-ejection reflex began in 1910 when Ott and Scott discovered that an intravenous injection of extract from the posterior pituitary caused a substantial increase in the flow of milk from a cannulated teat of a goat's udder. However, they did not appreciate the difference between an effect on milk ejection and on milk secretion. This distinction was made by Gaines (1915), who demonstrated that injection of an extract of posterior pituitary gland caused a rise in intramammary pressure; however he too failed to recognize the importance of these findings in relation to the control of milk ejection. In fact the modern concept of a neurohumoral reflex was not proposed until almost 30 years later, when Ely and Petersen (1941) showed that denervation of a cow udder did not affect the response of the mammary gland to the extract of pituitary. By this stage it had been shown that destruction of the posterior pituitary disrupted lactation (Gomez 1939), and further work confirming the involvement of components of the reflex quickly followed. A final common pathway was identified within the hypothalamus: Scharrer and Scharrer (1940, 1945) identified a microscopically distinct group of large cells, called magnocellular neurones, within the hypothalamus, and in 1951 Bargmann and Scharrer proposed that these magnocellular neurones synthesized the hormones vasopressin and oxytocin in their cell bodies. The products were transported, in mem-

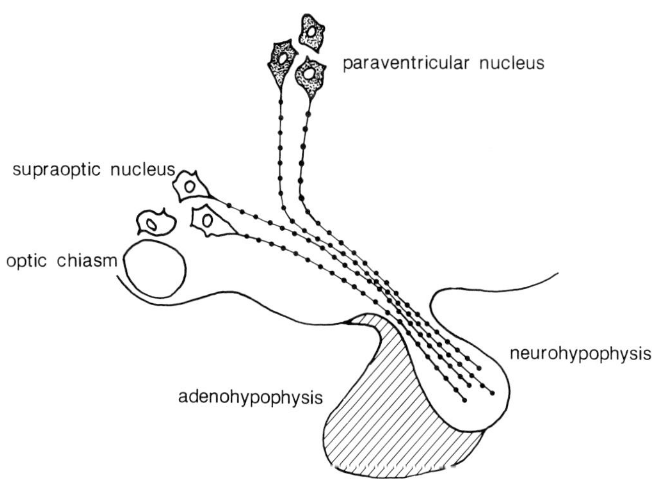

Fig. 3. The anatomy of the magnocellular neurosecretory system. Cell bodies aggregated in the paraventricular and supraoptic nuclei of the hypothalamus send hormone down their axons to terminals in the neurohypophysis on the ventral surface of the brain. (After Pickering 1978)

brane bound granules, to terminals in the posterior pituitary, where they awaited release into the systemic circulation (Fig. 3). Further support for this theory came from the demonstration of a milk-ejection factor in the blood during suckling (Peterson and Ludwick 1942), and myoepithelial cells of the mammary gland which were capable of responding to oxytocin, the active principle in the pituitary extract, were demonstrated in the mammary glands of several species (Richardson 1949; Linzell 1952).

3.2 Magnocellular Nuclei of the Hypothalamus

The cell bodies of the magnocellular neurones are found in two clearly defined hypothalamic nuclei, the supraoptic and the paraventricular. These nuclei are easily recognized in standard Nissl preparations as discrete aggregations of large intensely stained perikarya: the supraoptic nuclei, one on either side of the midline, appear as an homogeneous mass of cells straddling the lateral border of the optic chiasm. The paraventricular nuclei have often been thought of strictly as a compact group of magnocellular neurones. It is now conventional to view the nuclei as composed of distinct magnocellular and parvocellular divisions lying on either side of the dorsal third of the third ventricle. The presence of at least eight distinct cell layers which can be identified on the basis of cytoarchitectonics, and the connections and distribution of cells staining for oxytocin and vasopressin have been demonstrated (Swanson 1977; Swanson and Sawchenko 1980). Essentially the paraventricular nuclei comprise a magnocellular core embedded in a parvocellular matrix (Fig. 4). The magnocellular division contains three distinct elements and most of these neurones send their axonal projections to the neurohypophysis. The cells contain either oxytocin or vasopressin. The parvocellular division consists of five different regions, each of which contains some neurones that project

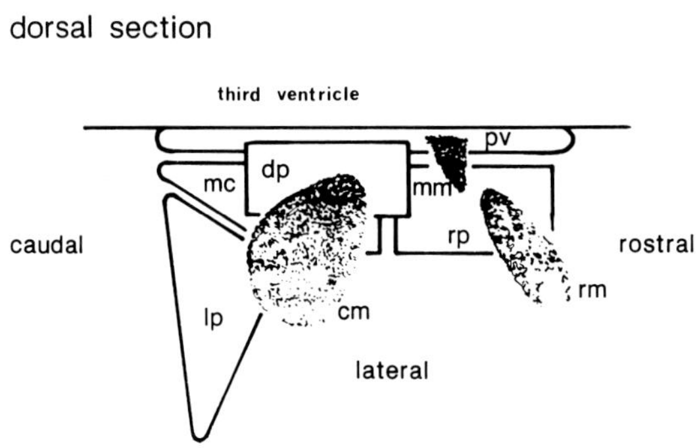

Fig. 4. Anatomy of the paraventricular magnocellular nucleus in a rat. The nucleus is divided into three magnocellular and five parvocellular compartments. *cm*, caudal magnocellular; *dp*, dorsal parvocellular; *mc*, medicaudal parvocellular; *mm*, medial magnocellular; *lp*, lateral parvocellular; *pv*, periventricular parvocellular; *rm*, rostral magnocellular; *rp*, rostral parvocellular. (Redrawn from Swanson and Sawchenko 1980)

to the neurohypophysis. Some of these parvocellular neurones stain for oxytocin and vasopressin. The majority of the cells, however, project to elsewhere in the brain (Swanson and Sawchenko 1980).

The two sets of nuclei are phylogenetically derived from the same hypothalamic nucleus (Lincoln and Russell 1986) so it is not surprising to find an intermingling of function between the nuclei. Before the application of immunohistochemical methods to the magnocellular neurosecretory system in the mid-1970s, it was not clear whether oxytocin and vasopressin were localized within the same or within separate populations of neurones, and whether or not there was preferential localization of these peptides in either the supraoptic or paraventricular nuclei. In fact, it was held for some time that oxytocin was primarily synthesized in the paraventricular nucleus and vasopressin in the supraoptic nucleus (Lederis 1961). However, the use of antisera against the two peptides has shown convincingly that the two hormones are produced in separate populations of cells in a variety of species, including the rat (Vandesande and Dierickx 1975; Vandesande et al. 1977). These observations are supported by the fact that the sum of the neurones staining for oxytocin and vasopressin in either the supraoptic or paraventricular nuclei correspond to the total number of magnocellular neurones counted (Sawchenko and Swanson 1982). In the supraoptic nucleus of the rat, a clear but incomplete topographic segregation of the cells staining for oxytocin and vasopressin has been found, with oxytocin neurones being concentrated rostrodorsally (Swaab et al. 1975b; Rhodes et al. 1981a; Swanson et al. 1981). Estimates of the ratio of vasopressin to oxytocin cells in the supraoptic nucleus of the rat range from about 1:1 (Vandesande and Dierickx 1975) to 1.6:1 (Swaab et al. 1975a, b). The organization of the oxytocin and vasopressin neurones in the paraventricular nucleus is no less distinctive. Two of the three magnocellular divisions of the nuclei are composed almost exclusively of some 400–600 oxytocin cells (Sawchenko and Swanson 1982). The third division of the nuclei consists of roughly equal proportions of oxytocin and vasopressin cells with about 1000 of each type (Swaab et al. 1975a, b; Sawchenko and Swanson 1982).

Despite the obvious morphological similarities between the magnocellular neurones of the supraoptic and paraventricular nuclei, there are substantial differences in their interconnections with the rest of the nervous system. Cajal (1911) first demonstrated that the neurones of the supraoptic nuclei projected to the neurohypophysis in the mouse. More recently, it has been shown using autoradiographic studies that the fibres from the nuclei course through the internal lamina of the median eminence and presumably end in the neural lobe (Saper et al. 1978; Dierickx 1980). Rasmussen (1940) reported that "practically all" the cells of the supraoptic nucleus disappear after extensive ablation of the pituitary and median eminence, suggesting not only that most of the cells project to the pituitary, but also that there are very few interneurones in the rat supraoptic nucleus. Léránth et al. (1975) confirmed the lack of interneurones in the supraoptic nuclei, but interneurones have been demonstrated in the monkey (Luiqi and Fox 1976) and rabbit (Felten and Cashner 1979). Fibres from the paraventricular nucleus project to the neurohypophysis and to a variety of sites associated primarily with the autonomic nervous system in the brain stem and spinal cord (Saper et al. 1976; Swanson and Sawchenko 1983; Sterba et al. 1979). Using retrogradely transported fluorescent dyes to analyse the projections from the paraventricular nuclei, it has been shown that in addition to the pathway to the neurohypophysis from the cells located within the core of the nucleus, 10%–15% of the parvocellular neurones send divergent axon collaterals to the dorsal vagal complex (Sterba et al. 1979) and to the marginal and intermediolateral zones of the spinal cord (Swanson and Sawchenko 1983). Other parvocellular projection sites include the median eminence (Vandesande et al. 1977), locus coeruleus (Swanson 1977) and parabrachial nucleus (Swanson 1977).

3.3 Accessory Magnocellular Nuclei

In addition to the oxytocin and vasopressin neurones located in the paraventricular and supraoptic nuclei, there are a considerable number of magnocellular neurones showing oxytocin- and vasopressin-like immunoreactivity scattered throughout the hypothalamus (Rhodes et al. 1981 b). Many of these dispersed magnocellular neurones are in fact gathered together into small aggregations, known as the accessory magnocellular nuclei. Axons from many of these cells project to the neurohypophysis and it has been reported that half the total number of fibres from hypothalamic neurones projecting to the neurohypophysis are located within the accessory nuclei (Fisher et al. 1979). However, the proportion of magnocellular neurones within each accessory nucleus is very small, so they present considerable difficulties of identification for systematic study of their electrophysiological responses. Clarke and Merrick (1985) have observed that neurones in the vicinity of the blood vessels that run between the supraoptic and paraventricular nuclei (Ambach and Palkovits 1979) show patterns of electrical activity similar to those of the oxytocin and vasopressin systems (see Sect. 4.4) in the rat, thereby inferring that these neurones function in the same manner as their counterparts in the main magnocellular nuclei. In fact it has been shown that milk ejection can continue in rats after ablation of the paraventricular nuclei (Voloschin and Tramezzani 1973).

3.4 Anatomy of the Oxytocin Terminals

The unmyelinated neurosecretory fibres from the magnocellular cells pass through the external layer of the median eminence and form the infundibulum (pituitary stalk) before terminating within the pars nervosa of the pituitary gland. Strictly, the term neurohypophysis refers to both the infundibulum and the pars nervosa, but it is often used loosely as a synonym for the posterior pituitary gland. Within the neural lobe the neurosecretory axons are characterized by numerous dilatations or swellings, the so-called Herring bodies (Dellmann and Rodriguez 1970). Each axon terminates in a large number of neurosecretory endings which make "synaptoid" contact with a basement membrane which lines a ramifying perivascular space (Livingston 1975). Running throughout this space are numerous fenestrated capillaries, so the neurosecretory terminals are effectively outside the blood-brain barrier. The terminals are further separated from the brain because the final parts of the axons and the terminals themselves are invested by specialized glial elements, the pituicytes (Tweedle and Hatton 1980a, b). The neurosecretory axons, terminals and Herring bodies are filled with numerous membrane-bound, dense-cored vesicles, the neurosecretory granules (Palay 1955; Morris 1976). These granules have a diameter of 150–200 nm and an electron-dense centre surrounded by a paler submembranous zone (Palay 1955). Each granule contains packaged neuropeptide and the appropriate neurophysin, and the solid contents of these dense-cored vesicles are thought to be material in a "steady state" in vivo (Bargmann and von Gaudecker 1969; Livingstone and Lederis 1971). Acute stimulation of the neural lobe, which results in the release of peptide, causes a loss of dense-cored vesicles from the nerve endings abutting the perivascular space (Sachs et al. 1971; Morris and Dyball 1974; Morris 1976). A shift towards an alkaline pH causes dissociation of the granule contents, an increase in osmotic pressure within the vesicle and an influx of water. This results in swelling of the vesicle, membrane distention and a loss of the electron-dense core (Cannata and Morris 1973; Morris and Cannata 1973; Dyer et al. 1973). In addition to the neurosecretory granules and the more conventional subcellular organelles such as microtubules and mitochondria, there are small electron-translucent microvesicles (40–60 nm in diameter) within the neurosecretory terminals (Smith 1970). These may be either dispersed throughout the ending or aggregated into clumps. At least some of these are thought to be involved in calcium homeostasis within the terminals (Nordmann and Chevallier 1980; see Sect. 5.4), whilst others may be the direct result of pinocytosis (Theodosis et al. 1977; see Sect. 5.4). The endings of the magnocellular cells also contain lysosomes, but these are found more densely in the Herring bodies (Dellmann and Rodriguez 1970). The Herring bodies are storage sites and contain 60% of all the dense-cored vesicles (Morris and Cannata 1973). Autoradiographic studies indicate that labelled material accumulates in the Herring bodies with time (Heap et al. 1975). This suggests that the Herring bodies are the end of the circulating pathway for granules that are not released. In fact there is a recognized and apparently prescribed pathway for neurosecretory granules produced in the magnocellular cell bodies (Fig. 5). The granules pass down the axons and arrive in the neurosecretory terminals. If they are not released, they are shipped to the Herring bodies, where they may either be recalled from storage during periods of particularly high peptide demand, or degraded.

The pituicytes provide a supportive matrix for the neurosecretory axons and terminals (Nordman 1977). Many of the axons are effectively wrapped in the cytoplasm of the pituicytes, as if the pituicytes provide a barrier between the neurosecretory terminals and the rest of the brain. These specialized glial cells send out processes among the neurosecretory axons and onto the basement membrane around the perivascular zone (Wittkowski and Brinkmann 1974). They contain abundant Golgi bodies, free ribosomes and, in the rat, characteristic lipid bodies. They are connected by prominent gap junctions (Hatton and Ellisman 1981), and it has been suggested that the pituicytes may regulate the extracellular environment of the neurosecretory terminals (Tweedle 1983). However, this may be a reciprocal arrangement, for some of the pituicytes receive synaptoid endings from the neurosecretory cells (Tweedle and Hatton 1980a, b). The pituicytes are

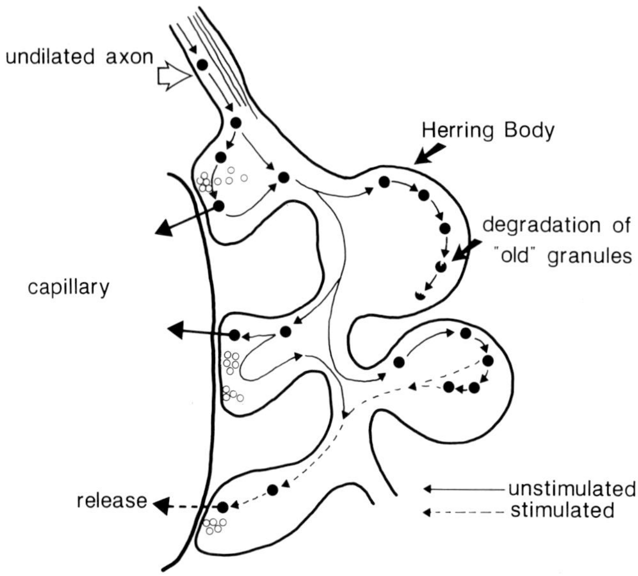

Fig. 5. Schematic illustration of the movement of neurosecretory granules through compartments of the hypothalamo-neurohypophysial nerve terminals in the neural lobe of the pituitary gland. (Redrawn from Heap et al. 1975)

dynamic cells, and during conditions of enhanced hormone release their processes retract and allow the neurosecretory terminals greater access to the basement membrane around the perivascular space (Tweedle and Hatton 1980a, b; Fig. 6, Table 1). Furthermore, at the onset of lactation, for example, the pituicytes appear to "unwrap" from the neurosecretory axons. There is a threefold decrease in the number of wrapped axons in lactation in the rat (Hatton et al. 1984). Presumably the unwrapping of the axons and the retraction of the pituicytes from the basement membrane affords greater access for hormone movement from the terminals into the neurohypophysial capillaries. It is important to realise that not only are there changes at the neurosecretory terminals at times of increased demand, there are also corresponding changes in the integrity of the magnocellular neurones themselves, for example during birth, lactation and dehydration. Briefly, the oxytocin neurones hypertrophy and there is an increase in the intracellular organelles associated with increased hormone synthesis (Kalimo 1975). There are also extensive structural reorganizations of the synaptic contacts and glial elements within the magnocellular nuclei (Hatton and Tweedle 1982; Theodosis et al. 1981; Theodosis and Poulain 1984). The mechanisms regulating these structural modifications are still uncertain, but oxytocin itself is implicated in at least initiating the changes (Theodosis et al. 1986a, b). However, the changes are not simply dependent on a continuation of a process started during pregnancy and labour, because other stimuli, such as dehydration, result in structural changes (Chapman et al. 1986). The mechanisms underlying the changes reported in the neural lobe, for example whether or not oxytocin is involved in initiating the changes in structure, are not known.

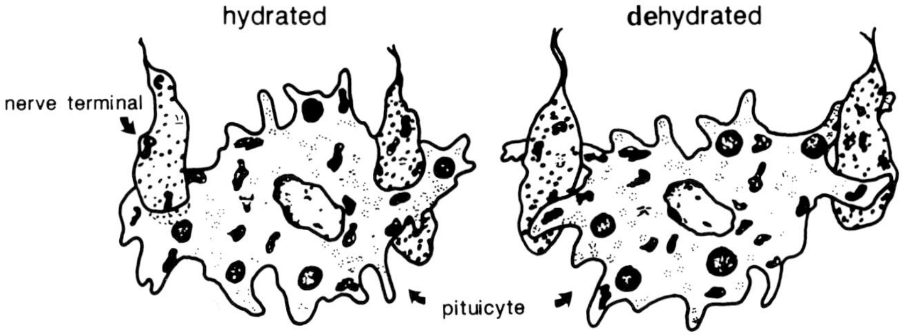

Fig. 6. An illustration of the possible relationships between neurosecretory nerve terminals and pituicytes in different states of hydration. In a well-hydrated animal, the terminals either end in the pituicyte cytoplasm or are wrapped in pituicyte cytoplasm. In cases of increased demand, e.g. dehydration, lactation and birth, the terminals are more exposed, as shown on the right. (Redrawn from Tweedle and Hatton 1980a)

Table 1. The number of neurosecretory axons enclosed by pituicyte cytoplasm during different treatments

Treatment	Axons/100 m^2 cytoplasm (mean ± SEM)
Normal male rats	2.1 ± 0.6
Water deprivation (24 h)	0.7 ± 0.2 [1]
Rehydrated	2.5 ± 0.6
Virgin female rats	1.7 ± 0.5
Prepartum female	1.6 ± 0.4
Postpartum female	0.6 ± 0.2 [1]
Lactating female	0.5 ± 0.1 [1]
Saline treatment (2%, 10 days)	0.1 ± 0.4 [1]

Data taken from Tweedle and Hatton (1980a, 1982)
[1] Significant at $p < 0.02$
Conditions of increased hormone demand, i.e. dehydration, birth and lactation, bring about decreased enclosure. This occurs rapidly (e.g. at parturition), is reversible (e.g. with rehydration) and reflects the severity of demand (e.g. 10-day saline treatment)

The neural lobe is not simply a mixture of neurosecretory terminals of the oxytocin and vasopressin magnocellular system and pituicytes. Other peptides, such as opioids, dopamine, noradrenaline and serotonin, are also found within the lobe (Sharman et al. 1982; Pittman et al. 1983). The sites of location of these additional compounds are in dispute. There are suggestions that they may be co-localized with oxytocin and vasopressin or may be found in presynaptic endings on the neurosecretory terminals. Whatever their origin, it is now recognized that these compounds may regulate the release of neuropeptides from the neural lobe (see Sect. 5.6).

4 Electrophysiology of the Oxytocin System

4.1 Introduction

Early experiments on the electrophysiological responses of neurosecretory cells were carried out by Cross and Green (1959). They recorded the electrical activity of hypothalamic neurones in anaesthetized rabbits and showed that hypothalamic cells in general display electrical activity similar to other nerve cells in the central nervous system. Attempts to identify recordings from magnocellular neurones in mammals relied on either histological verification of the recording site after completion of the experiment or identification by stimulating increased activity from the magnocellular neurones, e.g. their responses to osmotic stimuli. However, in 1964 Kandel introduced a technique which revolutionized the study of neurosecretion. He showed that electrical stimulation of the pituitary stalk evoked potentials which could be recorded at the level of the cell body of the magnocellular neurones. This original work was carried out on the neurosecretory cells of the preoptic nucleus of the goldfish, but Yagi et al. (1966) quickly employed the technique in mammals. Antidromic identification is now widely used in the study of both magnocellular neurones (see reviews: Poulain and Wakerley 1982; Clarke and Merrick 1985; Wakerley 1986) and for parvocellular neurones (see reviews: Yagi and Iwasaki 1977; Summerlee 1986).

4.2 Identification of Magnocellular Neurones

The magnocellular neurone system is particularly suited to the technique of antidromic identification by virtue of its anatomy; the pituitary stalk forms a discrete pathway on the ventral surface of the brain which can be specifically stimulated without activating nerve terminals in adjacent structures. Moreover, large numbers of neurones are aggregated in the supraoptic and paraventricular nuclei (Sofroniew 1983). The use of antidromic activation is important not only for identification of neurones but also for activating neurones that have no, or virtually no, spontaneous activity. Three standard tests are used to confirm that the evoked potentials are antidromically driven; constant latency, high-frequency following and collision-extinction (Fig. 7). These are described in detail elsewhere (see for example Dreifuss et al. 1981; Poulain and Wakerley 1982). Briefly, the latency of the antidromic response should be constant for any given cell, since it relies solely on the physical properties of the neurone, i.e. the conduction velocity of the axon (which will remain constant). Magnocellular neurones have relatively slow conduction speeds, 0.5–1 m/s, equivalent to the conduction velocity of unmyelinated C fibres (Poulain and Wakerley 1982). It should be noted that conduction velocities appear to be slightly higher in unanaesthetized animals than in anaesthetized animals. For example, the mean latency of the antidromic response of magnocellular neurones in anaestetized rats is about 14 ms (Clarke and Merrick 1985), whereas the latency in conscious rats is only about 8 ms (Summerlee and Lincoln 1981). This difference is perhaps not surprising, since it has been reported

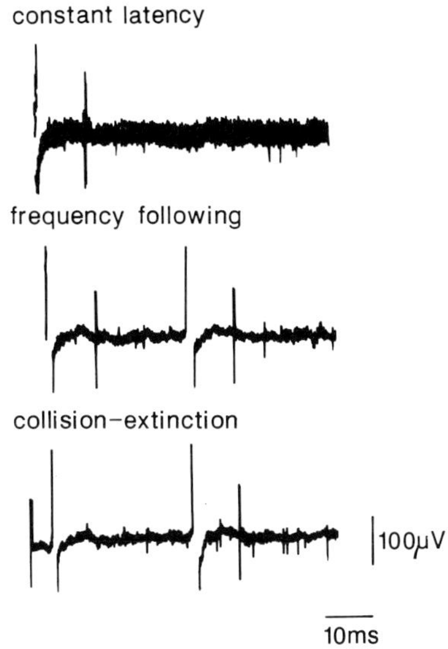

Fig. 7. An illustration of the three tests used for proof of antidromic activation of a single magnocellular neurone recorded in a conscious rabbit. Constant latency is shown where five stimulus-triggered sweeps of the oscilloscope have been superimposed: in each case a potential is recorded at the level of the cell body with an identical latency. High- frequency following shows the response to stimuli applied at 20 Hz or less. Collision-extinction shown the extinction of the antidromic potential when this is triggered by an orthodromic potential from the cell body

that conduction velocities of axons are affected by anaesthesia (Dyball and McPhaill 1974). The criterion of high-frequency following, that is the ability of the neurone to respond to every stimulus pulse with an antidromic potential, is based on the observation that synaptic transmission fails at a lower frequency than axonal conduction. This test is apparently not as reliable for magnocellular neurones, as they are not particularly "fail-safe" at high frequencies of stimulation (Clarke and Merrick 1985). Relatively frequently, such high-frequency stimulation leads to fractionation of the antidromic potential for magnocellular neurones (Wakerley and Lincoln 1973; Paisley and Summerlee 1984). The most reliable criterion is collision of an orthodromic and an antidromic potential, when the two potentials, travelling in opposite directions along the axon, collide and extinguish each other.

4.3 Patterns of Electrical Activity from Magnocellular Neurones

In the unstimulated, anaesthetized rat, the majority of antidromically identified neurones either show a slow irregular pattern of discharge fewer than three action potentials per second) or are completely silent. This slow rate of firing appears to be a feature of hypothalamic neurones in general (Lincoln 1969) but it is not attributable to the anaesthetic used, for similar low levels of activity are recorded in unanesthetized rats and rabbits (Summerlee and Lincoln 1981; Summerlee and Paisley 1982). It should be noted that this low level of activity remains remarkably constant in anaesthetized rats but shows dynamic changes closely related to the animal's level of arousal in unanaesthetized animals (Summerlee and Paisley 1982). A small number of neurones in the unstimulated anaesthetized rat discharge at higher frequencies. The best-documented are referred to as cells with phasic activity (for definition see Poulain et al. 1977). Phasic activity consists of periods of fairly steady discharge (usually in the range 5–15 action potentials per second) lasting several seconds or sometimes minutes, interspersed with periods of complete silence or a few intermittent potentials. These patterns of discharge are considered to be inherent and not externally driven. In rats in which the total afferent input has been removed (hypothalamic island preparations, Cross and Kitay 1967; Cross and Dyer 1971 a, b, 1972; Dyer et al. 1973), there is still some activity, albeit at a much lower mean rate of discharge (Dyball and Prilusky 1981). It may be of passing interest to comment that this depressed rate of firing from the isolated neurones could be a result of the acute damage that occurs following the isolation procedure. It has been shown in the cerebral cortex that neurological isolation of cortical neurones is followed by an initial depression of spontaneous activity (Burns et al. 1979). After about 1 week, the rate of discharge of these isolated neurones resembles those in cortical neurones in intact parts of the cortex of the same animal (Burns et al. 1979). Similarly, magnocellular neurones in an isolated slice of hypothalamic tissue maintained in vitro (Hatton et al. 1978; Wakerley and Noble 1982), and even cultured supraoptic neurones (Gähwiler and Dreifuss 1979), show low-level spontaneous activity.

The activity of magnocellular neurones can be enhanced by various stimuli, and the variation in response of the cells is used as a means of distinguishing between the oxytocin and the vasopressin neurones of the system.

4.4 Identification of Oxytocin Neurones by Patterns of Activity

The method for differentiating between the activitiy of the oxytocin and vasopressin neurones on the basis of their patterns of discharge originated from the observations of Wakerley and Lincoln in the 1970s. These workers noticed that anaesthetized rats would continue to eject milk in response to the sucking action of the young (Wakerley and Lincoln 1971; Lincoln et al. 1973). Each milk ejection was denoted by a transient rise in intramammary pressure and was accompanied by a behavioural response of the young. The authors demonstrated that each reflex milk ejection was mimicked by a bolus injection of 0.5–1 mU exogenous oxytocin. Moreover, this behavioural response and the transient rise in intramammary pressure were shown to be caused by the selective release of oxytocin (Wakerley et al. 1973). It is surprising that Vorherr et al. (1967), who published a method for a semiquantitative bioassay for oxytocin using the suckled, anaesthetized rat, did not observe reflex milk ejections in their preparations. Wakerley and Lincoln then studied the electrical activity of magnocellular neurones in the period during which a pulse of hormone was being released and found that neurones in the paraventricular nucleus could be divided into two populations on the basis of their activity (Wakerley and Lincoln 1973). One group of cells (just over 50%) showed a stereotyped burst of high-frequency activity 12–20 s before the rise in intramammary pressure and the behavioural response, while the activity of a second group of cells showed no correlation with milk ejection (Fig. 8). Similarly, antidromically identified neurones in the supraoptic nuclei could be divided into two groups according to the characteristic firing of half the neurones time-locked to milk ejection (Lincoln and Wakerley 1974). They concluded that those

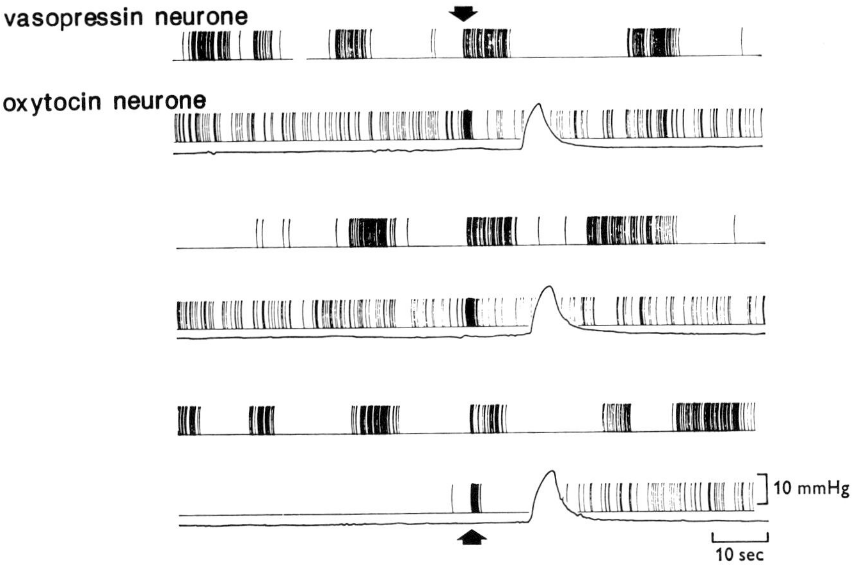

Fig. 8. Activity of a vasopressin and an oxytocin neurone recorded on the same electrode in an anaesthetized lactating rat. Each deflection of the pen recorder represents an action potential. Note the phasic pattern of discharge typical of vasopressin cell. The oxytocin neurones show a burst of high-frequency activity 10–12 s before the rise in intramammary pressure which is characteristic of milk ejection. (Data from Lincoln and Wakerley 1974)

neurones displaying a burst of potentials prior to milk ejection were oxytocin cells. Moreover, as the cells displayed remarkably constant responses in terms of duration, frequency and the latency from the onset of the burst to the pressure response, they concluded further that all oxytocin neurones are activated before every milk ejection in a synchronized manner. By implication, those neurones in lactating rats which did not show bursts of neurosecretory activity before milk ejection were classed as vasopressin cells.

Classification of vasopressin neurones by default has remained a problem in identification of magnocellular neurones. There is no specific stimulus for the release of vasopressin which is as selective as suckling is for oxytocin release. Although not strictly the subject of this chapter, it is pertinent to mention, briefly, the characteristics ascribed to the firing of vasopressin neurones, if only to highlight the caution still needed in distinguishing between these two populations of cells simply by electrophysiological characteristics. It is generally agreed that vasopressin neurones may, in part, be identified by their "phasic" pattern of discharge (see Poulain and Wakerley 1982). Wakerley and Lincoln (1971, 1973) noted that some of the non-responsive magnocellular neurones during milk ejection showed this on-off pattern of discharge. It was concluded that either phasic activity was an exclusive feature of vasopressin neurones, or oxytocin neurones which displayed phasic discharge were non-responsive at milk ejection. Subsequent experiments have supported the case for phasic activity being a key feature of vasopressin neurones (Wakerley et al. 1975; Dreifuss et al. 1976; Poulain et al. 1977). This classification is not absolute, and putative oxytocin neurones have been shown to display phasic patterns of discharge (Lincoln and Wakerley 1974; Summerlee 1982, 1983; Dyball and Leng 1986), with high-frequency bursts of activity, characteristic of pulsatile oxytocin release, superimposed on the phasic discharge. Perhaps this is not surprising bearing in mind the common nature of origin of the oxytocin and vasopressin neurones (Lincoln and Russell 1986). Only one set of experimental data supports the contention that phasic neurones are immunoreactive for vasopressin (Yamashita et al. 1983), and to date there has been no such positive identification of oxytocin neurones. Harris (1979) showed that chemoreceptor and baroreceptor stimulation differentially affects the discharge of oxytocin and vasopressin neurones. He reported that, in general, phasically active neurones were activated by stimulation of the carotid body chemoreceptors, whereas they were inhibited by baroreceptor stimulation. Neither method of stimulation had a consistent effect on the non-phasically discharging neurones. Dyball and Leng (1986) confirmed that the activity of oxytocin neurones in the anaesthetized rat is not affected by the α-receptor agonist, phenylephrine, whereas the putative vasopressin neurones are silenced. We have used this method for differentiating successfully between the activity of oxytocin and vasopressin neurones in the male and female rabbit (Summerlee 1987).

The distribution of oxytocin and vasopressin neurones determined by electrophysiological means is in good agreement with the disposition of oxytocin neurones identified by immunofluorescent techniques. It has been reported that there is a differential distribution of the two populations within the supraoptic nucleus of the rat. Clarke and Merrick (1985) comment that the majority of the oxytocin neurones were located in the dorsal half of the nucleus whereas the phasically discharging cells were predominantly recorded in the ventral part of the nucleus. These findings match the immunohistochemical localization by Rhodes et al. (1981 a, b). The distinction between predominantly oxytocin-neurone-containing and vasopressin-neurone-containing areas of the paraventricular nucleus are not so clear. Collating data from our studies on magnocellular neurone activity in the conscious rat and rabbit, the dorsal part of the paraventricular nucleus contains a greater proportion of antidromically-identified cells. Again, these findings correspond with the known anatomical arrangements of the nucleus (see Sect. 3.2). Furthermore, on occasions when one or more antidromically identified cells have been recorded on the same electrode, it is more common to record one oxytocin and one putative vasopressin neurone (Fig. 8, 9).

Irrespective of their position within or between the nuclei, all oxytocin neurones in the rat show a stereotyped and standard burst of high-frequency discharge (Wakerley and Lincoln 1973). During these bursts, which last 1–4 s, the frequency of firing reaches 80 or more action potentials per second. The peak rate of firing is usually attained in the first 0.5–1 s and the frequency tends to reduce across the remainder of the train of potentials. Most commonly, there is a reduction in the amplitude of successive potentials with, or shortly after attaining, the peak rate of firing (Poulain and Wakerley 1982; Dyball and Leng 1986). What is remarkable is the constancy of the response for an individual oxytocin neurone. Each neurone continues to respond before almost every milk ejection over very long periods. For instance, Summerlee (1983) reported that during continuous re-

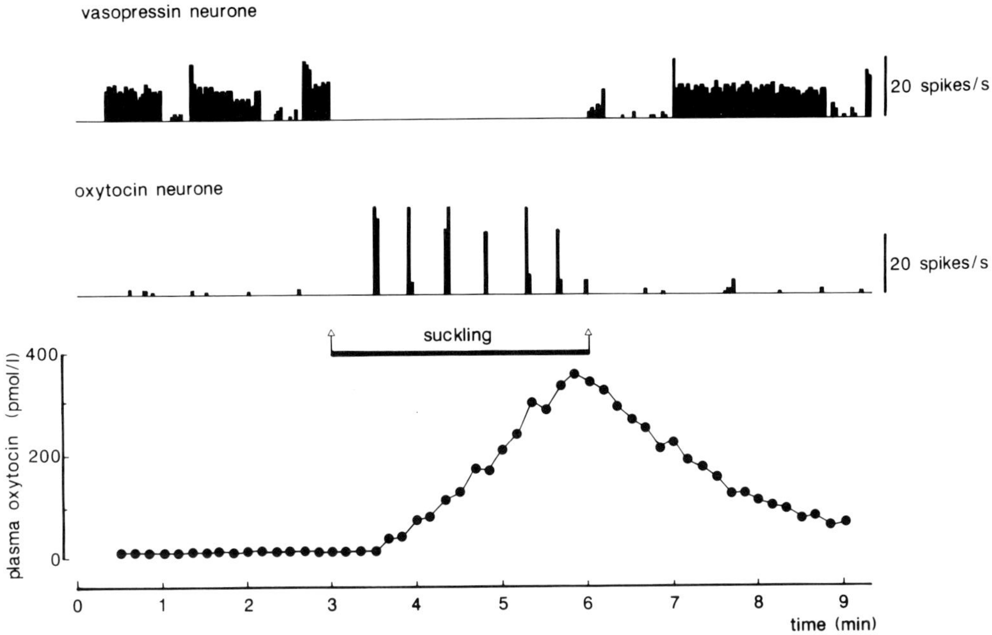

Fig. 9. The activity of a vasopressin and an oxytocin neurone recorded simultaneously on the same electrode in a conscious rabbit in association with suckling. At the same time plasma oxytocin was measured in the blood by radioimmunoassay. Occassionally vasopressin neurones in the rabbit show a "quasiphasic" pattern of discharge. The activity of the two types of cells is completely different during suckling. Vasopressin neurones are virtually silent for the duration of nursing; oxytocin neurones show discrete bursts of high-frequence discharge. The onset of this bursting pattern of firing is followed by a rise in plasma oxytocin

cordings from the same oxytocin neurones over several days, and associated with hundreds of milk ejections, the response of the neurone was relatively constant. More recently, Dyball and Leng (1986) have carried out an in-depth analysis of the response of oxytocin neurones during the milk-ejection bursts in anaesthetized rats. They showed that the number of action potentials per burst, the frequency of firing and the modal interspike interval remained constant for each paraventricular neurone (Fig. 10) during a short period of recording. However, there are modulations in the response of oxytocin neurones over the course of lactation in the rabbit (Summerlee et al. 1986). The characteristics of the bursts of neurosecretory activity during milk ejection in the rabbit change during lactation, but the number of bursts per nursing period remains constant for a particular neurone.

From the initial work of Wakerley and Lincoln (1973) it was proposed that oxytocin release was pulsatile. This concept was supported by the electrophysiological data in the rat and led to the idea that all the oxytocin neurones were activated simultaneously. Lincoln and Wakerley (1974) reported a series of single and multi-unit studies from the same nucleus in which activation of the oxytocin

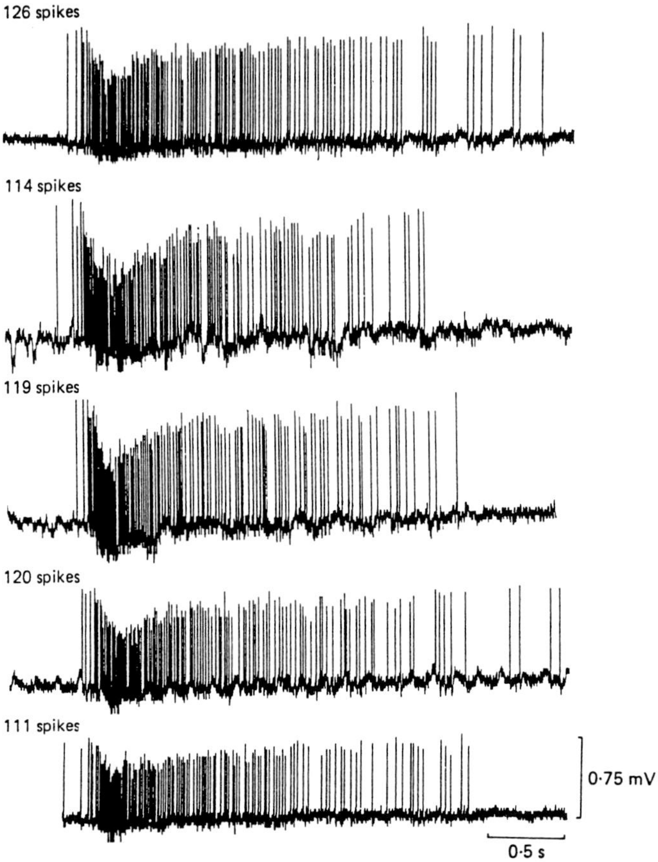

Fig. 10. Five of twelve milk-ejection bursts recorded over a 2-h period of one oxytocin cell in an anaesthetized rat. The pattern and duration of the milk-ejection bursts was remarkably constant over that time. The total number of spikes in each burst is given above each burst: throughout the recording period this varied between 111 and 126 spikes. (Data from Dyball and Leng 1986)

neurones appeared to occur together before milk ejection. But it was not until 1985 that Moos and colleagues (Belin and Moos 1986; Belin et al. 1985) demonstrated that oxytocin neurones within different sites of the same nucleus and in different nuclei showed simultaneous activation (Fig. 11). The debate about the origin of this stereotyped activation and how it might be synchronized across many neurones, not only in the same, but also in different magnocellular and accessory nuclei, is still raging. For example, is the burst of neurosecretory activity an inherent property of oxytocin neurones which are spontaneously excitable in a paroxysmal discharge? Or is the burst caused by an intense depolarizing stimulus from another site within the brain? Certainly one of the gaps in our understanding of the control of oxytocin secretion centres on the neural interpretation of the afferent stimulus. In the rat, at least, a continuous sucking stimulus from the young is somehow interpreted and transformed by the brain into a discrete

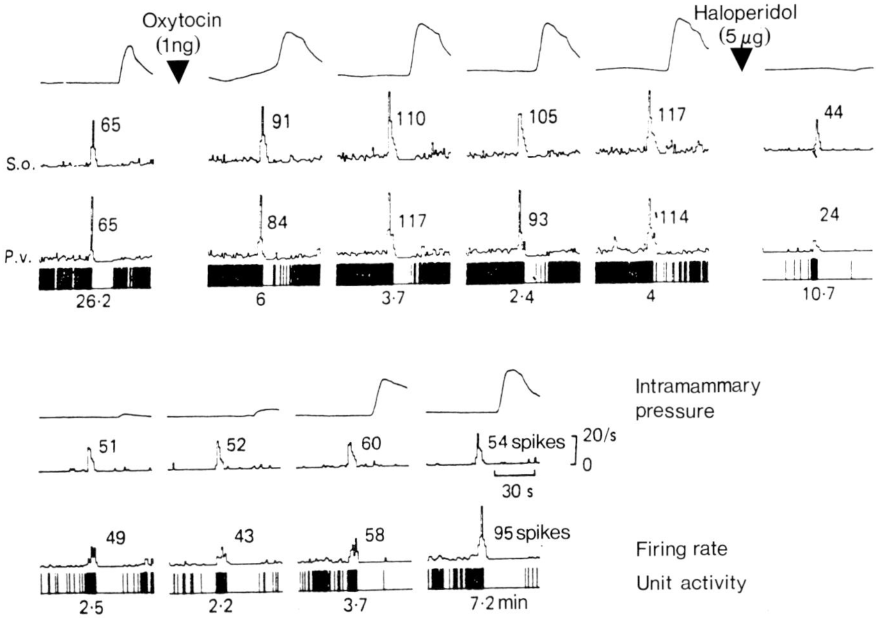

Fig. 11. Responses of a pair of paraventricular and supraoptic cells after i.c.v. injections of oxytocin and haloperidol 15 min later. Oxytocin increased the frequency and amplitude of the neurosecretory bursts in parallel in the two cells and the bursts occurred simultaneously. In contrast, haloperidol decreased the amplitude and frequency of milk ejection. The changes again occurred in parallel. (Data from Belin and Moos 1986)

and intermittent release of oxytocin. The route and mode of transfer of this sensory information from the nipple or teat to the oxytocin neurones is still not completely clear. The data concerning the afferent pathways of the milk-ejection reflex are discussed elsewhere (Juss and Wakerley 1981; Poulain and Wakerley 1982, 1986; Poulain and Dyer 1984). It seems unlikely that the oxytocin neurones are inherently hyperexcitable and the subject of almost continuous inhibition, as magnocellular neurones in culture (Gähwiler and Dreifuss 1979) and in tissue slices maintained in vitro (Hatton et al. 1978; Wakerley and Noble 1982; Andrew and Dudek 1983, 1984a, b) do not show paroxysmal or classic neurosecretory burst-like activity. The electrophysiological data favour the concept that the neurosecretory burst may be formulated by the arrival of a synchronized and/or snychronizing afferent barrage at the level of the nuclei.

Experiments to determine the generality of the findings in the rat have been carried out using a chronic recording technique in the unanaesthetized rabbit (Paisley and Summerlee 1984; Summerlee et al. 1986). The rabbit exhibits a completely different pattern of nursing from the rat: the rat suckles her young almost continuously for up to 18 h every day and milk ejection recurs every 4–6 min throughout that time (Lincoln et al. 1980), whereas the rabbit returns to her litter only once or twice every 24 h and then suckles for only 3–5 min (Zarrow et al. 1965). Despite the substantial differences, there are marked similarities in the operation of the milk-ejection reflex and its control. During nursing in the rabbit, the oxytocin neurones show several closely spaced bursts of high-frequency firing, superimposed on their background level of activity (Fig. 9). The bursts of firing are shorter than those recorded in the rat (1–2 s), as are the intervals between these bursts of neurosecretory activity (range 30–60 s). Cross-correlation analysis of simultaneous double recordings from two oxytocin neurones suggests that the response of the oxytocin neurones is synchronized in the rabbit (Paisley and Summerlee 1984). These closely spaced bursts of neurosecretory activity from the oxytocin neurones result in a complex profile of oxytocin in the plasma (Summerlee et al. 1986). Oxytocin levels rise shortly after the onset of the bursting discharge from the oxytocin neurones and are further elevated by each burst of firing.

Continuous recordings obtained from oxytocin neurones in conscious rats (Summerlee 1981, 1983) and rabbits (O'Byrne et al. 1986) during birth have shown that there is pulsatile release of oxytocin at that time (Fig. 12), as well as during lactation. During birth the oxytocin neurones show transient excitation with the expulsion of each fetus. The bursts are similar to those observed during reflex milk ejection but of greater magnitude (Fig. 13). Plasma oxytocin profiles during the expulsive phase of birth in the rabbit have shown that there is pulsatile release of oxytocin, and peak levels of hormone are an order of magnitude greater at this time than during suckling (O'Byrne et al. 1986). It is interesting to note that peak levels of oxytocin during birth in the rabbit are linearly related to the speed of delivery, which suggests that oxytocin facilitates birth in this species.

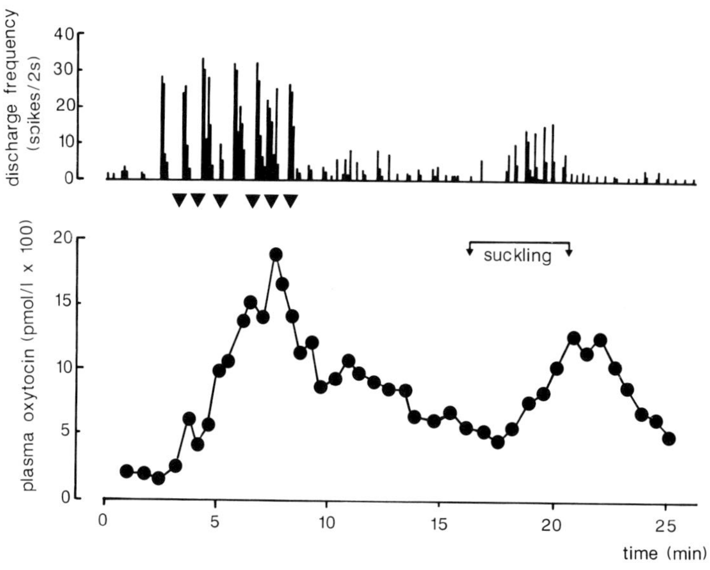

Fig. 12. The relationship between oxytocin neurone activity (*top*) and plasma oxytocin (*bottom*) during birth in a conscious rabbit. Onset of bursting discharge by the oxytocin neurone is followed by a rise in plasma oxytocin and delivery of fetuses (*solid triangles*). This rabbit suckled her young immediately after giving birth. Note the lower level of activation of the oxytocin neurone and the lower levels of plasma oxytocin

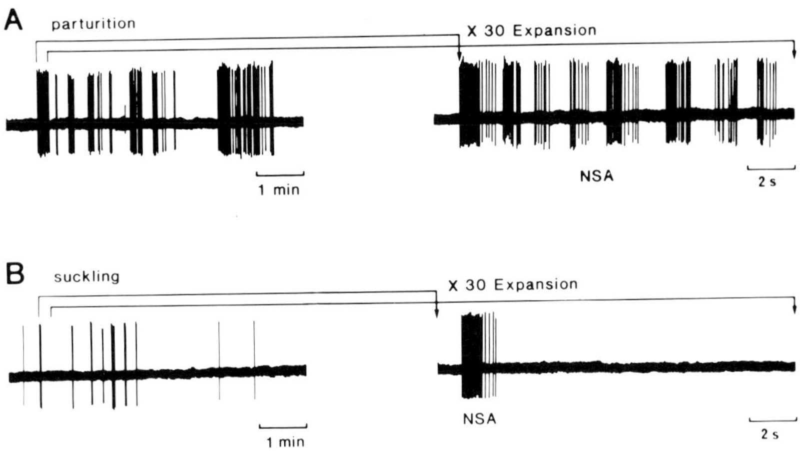

Fig. 13 A B. To illustrate the bursts of neurosecretory activity (*NSA*) from an oxytocin neurone during birth and postpartum suckling in a conscious rabbit. Note that the bursts in birth are considerably longer in duration compared with bursts in suckling. Moreover, each burst in birth is split into several smaller bursts of discharge which may be important for the facilitated release of oxytocin at the neural lobe. (From O'Byrne et al. 1986)

5 Stimulus-Secretion Coupling in the Oxytocin System

5.1 Introduction

The mechanism of stimulus-secretion coupling, originally proposed by Douglas and Rubin (1963) and Douglas and Poisner (1964 a, b), implies that electrical activity arriving at the nerve terminals causes depolarization of the endings and provokes a series of biochemical and morphological changes which result in the release of hormone. Depolarization causes an influx of calcium ions and the eventual movement of neurosecretory granules close to the cell membrane, fusion of the granule and terminal membranes and the final release of the graunlar content into the extracellular space by exocytosis (Morris et al. 1981; Nordmann 1983). The granule membrane is taken into the terminal (Theodosis 1982), and increased intracellular calcium is rapidly sequestered into microvesicles which may be released subsequently (Shaw and Morris 1980; Nordmann and Chevallier 1980: see Fig. 17).

It is generally assumed that action potentials arriving at the terminals cause the depolarization which triggers the rest of the events of stimulus-secretion coupling. Electrical stimulation of neurohypophyses incubated in vitro evokes the release of both oxytocin and vasopressin (Douglas and Poisner 1964 a, b; Haller et al. 1965; Nordmann and Dreifuss 1972), and this effect is dependent upon the generation of potentials (Dreifuss et al. 1971; Ishida 1970) which depolarize the neurosecretory terminals and activate the calcium-dependent process (Mikiten and Douglas 1965). High- frequency electrical stimulation has been shown to be more effective than low-frequency stimulation at stimulating hormone secretion

(Dreifuss et al. 1971; Haller et al. 1965; Cazalis et al. 1985). However, interpretation of this phenomenon, which is analogous to the process of facilitation at certain chemical synapses, is complicated by thc possible changes in action potential shape and membrane potential during and after tetanic stimulation (Nordmann and Dreifuss 1972; Nordmann and Stuenkel 1986). The arrival of action potentials may not be the only mechanism responsible for the secretion of hormone, as depolarization of the terminals in the absence of action potentials in the presence of potassium ions will cause the release of both oxytocin and vasopressin (Douglas and Poisner 1964a, b; Dreifuss et al. 1971).

5.2 Significance of Firing Patterns for Stimulus-Secretion Coupling

One of the most distinctive features of oxytocin neurones is their characteristic pattern of firing in high-frequency bursts during birth and suckling, although occasionally these neurones may exhibit phasic discharge (see Sects. 4.3, 4.4). Detailed study of these particular patterns of firing has revealed that it is not only the frequency but also the temporal organization of such firing which is important for secretion of hormone (Cazalis et al. 1985). The amount of hormone released is dependent on the frequency of potentials arriving at the terminals, but this is not a linear relationship: there is an increase in the quantity of hormone released if the number of depolarizations (stimuli) per unit time reaching the terminals is increased or if the stimulus duration is decreased whilst increasing the frequency of stimulation so the number of stimuli remains constant (Dreifuss et al. 1971). Lincoln et al. (1976) demonstrated that stimulation of the neural lobe in vivo at frequencies of 40–60 Hz for 2–4 s was the most effective stimulus parameter for oxytocin release in the lactating rat. This finding was supported by others (Dreifuss et al. 1971; Nordmann and Dreifuss 1972), and these parameters match those reported for the burst characteristics recorded from oxytocin neurones in the suckled rat at milk ejection (Wakerley and Lincoln 1973; Lincoln and Wakerley 1974). In general, the parameters of oxytocin neurone activation in birth in the rat are different from those during milk ejection (Summerlee 1981, 1983). The bursts during birth are longer (5–7 s) and occur at higher frequencies (60–80 Hz). Perhaps this is not surprising, as greater quantities of oxytocin appear to be released during birth in the rat than during suckling (Summerlee et al. 1988, in preparation). In a similar way, the optimal stimulus parameters for oxytocin release during milk ejection and birth in the rabbit are different. Electrical stimulation of the neural lobe in the rabbit in vivo has shown that very short (<2 s) bursts of stimulation at 100 Hz create the most effective release of oxytocin, judged by the transient rise in intramammary pressure. During reflex milk ejection in the conscious rabbit five to nine discrete bursts of high- frequency discharge (1–1.5 s at 80–100 Hz) are seen throughout the suckling period. Again, bursts of neurosecretory activity from putative oxytocin neurones during birth in the rabbit are longer than bursts during suckling, but the plasma oxytocin levels are an order of magnitude greater in birth (see Sect. 4.4).

Phasic discharge, the presumed prerogative of vasopressin cells (Poulain and Wakerley 1982) but also seen in some cases of stimulated oxytocin release (Dyball and Leng 1986; Summerlee 1982, 1983), is composed of a series of short (20–60 s) trains of action potentials at 5–15 Hz separated by silent periods of a similar duration (Wakerley et al. 1978). Bicknell et al. (1984) suggested that stimulation at 13 Hz of the isolated neural lobe caused a rapid diminution of the effectiveness of stimulating vasopressin release if continued beyond 18–36 s, whilst vasopressin release per train of potentials was increased as the interval between the trains was increased up to 20 s (Shaw et al. 1984). They concluded that a typical train of potentials from a phasically discharging neurone in vivo was close to the optimal duration for maintaining vasopressin release per burst. These data are supported by the work of Cazalis et al. (1985), who showed that prolonged stimulation of isolated neural lobes with patterns which resembled phasic discharge in vivo eventually reduced hormone release. Among the possible explanations for this mechanism is a putative change in the electrical properties of the neurones themselves and their terminals. Nordmann and Steunkel (1986) have produced evidence which strongly suggests that prolonged stimulation causes a change in the capacity of the axons and terminals to conduct compound action potentials. They recorded the compound potentials from isolated neural lobe tissue and showed that the latency of the compound action potential to stimulus of the lobe was not affected when the lobe was stimulated at a constant rate of <1 Hz, but at frequencies greater than 1 Hz the latency of the response increased and the amplitude of the compound action potential was reduced and in some cases completely vanished (Fig. 14). It should be emphasized that very few axons and terminals showed a rapid reduction in the magnitude of the response at stimuli as low as 5 Hz. In a similar way, stimulation in a pattern which mimicked phasic activity caused a

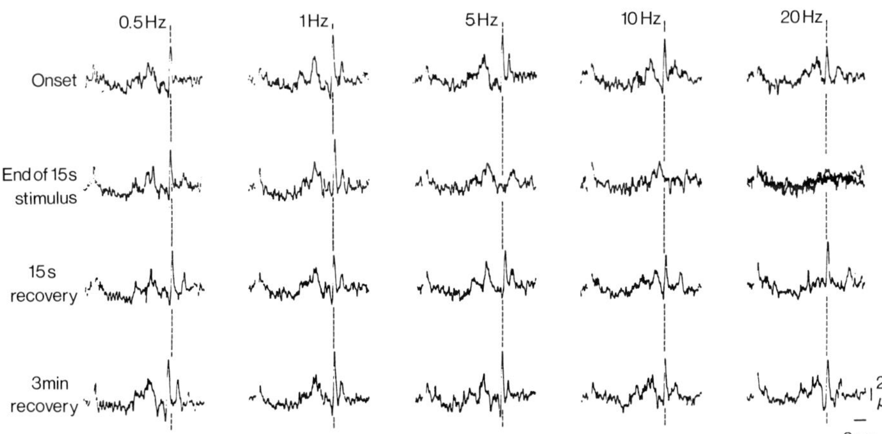

Fig. 14. Extracellular recordings of the compound action potential from neurosecretory nerve terminals stimulated, via the pituitary stalk, at different frequencies for a period of 15 s. A single stimulus applied for either 15 s or 3 min after the onset of the 15-s stimulation period provides a measure of recovery. The *dashed lines* provide a reference for the latency of the later response to that of the first stimulus. Note that for a particular ending an increased latency was observed after 15 s stimulation at 1 Hz. The superimposed traces at 20 Hz (*second from top*) were taken 4 and 15 s after the onset of stimulation. (Data from Nordmann and Steunkel 1986)

marked increase in the latency of the compound potential and a decrease in magnitude. Dreifuss et al. (1971) and Baertschi and Dreifuss (1979) described a similar effect in in vivo preparations where the amplitude of the antidromically driven compound action potential was reduced with low-frequency stimulation. Similarly, Pittman (1983) observed an increase in the antidromic latency of the compound action potential recorded from rat magnocellular neurones following stimulation of the pituitary stalk at different frequencies. Nordmann and Steunkel (1986) comment that these results indicate that the typical range of firing expected from hypothalamic neurones (0.5–2 potentials per second; Poulain and Wakerley 1982) is within the range where hormone release would be affected and hence plasma concentrations of oxytocin and vasopressin could be maintained.

The important factor differentiating the work of Nordmann and Steunkel (1986) from that of others studying the compound action potential is the size of the electrode they used; the electrode tip was 7–10 μm, which means that in theory they could be recording the activity from a single fibre and its terminations. If this is correct, the results have important implications for the functioning of the axons and terminals in cotrolling the release of oxytocin by controlling the degree of depolarization that will occur in response to an orthodromic potential from the cell body.

Oxytocin cells, in the rat, discharge at frequencies which can reach 80 potentials per second for a period of 0.5–4 s, and this activation occurs periodically throughout nursing (Wakerley and Lincoln 1973; see Sect. 4.4). Nordmann and Steunkel (1986) showed that stimulation of axons and their terminals at high frequency caused a large number of fibres to stop responding after only a few seconds. If the membrane properties of the cell bodies are similar to those reported for the terminals, this could explain the short duration of the neurosecretory burst seen at milk ejection. Moreover, it might explain the reported differences in the burst characteristics of oxytocin neurones in the rat and the rabbit (see above): oxytocin neurones in the rabbit discharge at even higher frequencies in milk ejection and birth than in the rat and consequently have shorter periods of high-frequency activation (Paisley and Summerlee 1984; Summerlee et al. 1986).

5.3 Calcium and Oxytocin Release

In 1971 it was established by Douglas and Sorimachi that the medium surrounding isolated rat neural lobes must contain calcium for either electrical or ionic stimulation of hormone release to occur. Electrical stimulation of isolated lobes did not evoke hormone release in the absence of calcium in the bathing medium, and, vice versa, addition of calcium in the absence of electrical stimulation did not provoke hormone release. These findings stress the importance of extracellular calcium for release. Moreover, during prolonged stimulation, a continual influx of calcium is essential for maintaining secretion (Russell and Thorn 1974).

It was also possible that calcium concentrations within the axon temrinal cytoplasm could rise following depolarization of the terminal membranes. Interesting data have been obtained from studies on the effects of calcium ionophores on calcium fluxes and hormone release. Most of the work has concentrated on the

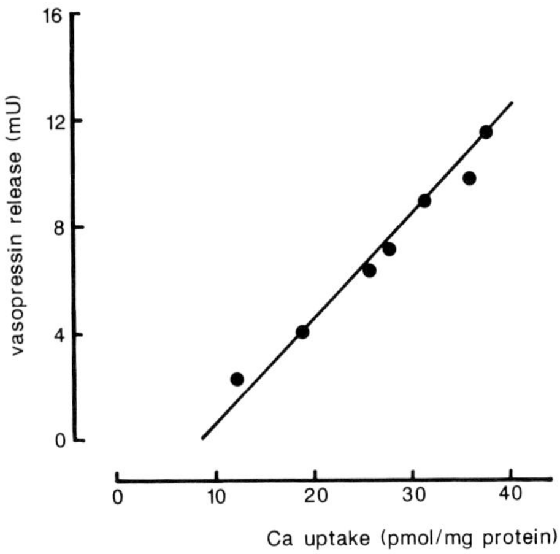

Fig. 15. The effect of external calcium concentration on vasopressin release. (Hormone data from Douglas and Poisner 1964 b)

release of vasopressin, but it seems reasonable to assume that the same principles apply to the release of oxytocin. Calcium ionophores are lipophilic substances which form reversible complexes with calcium and thus serve as carriers for calcium transport across biological membranes. Russell et al. (1974) applied the calcium ionophore in studies of vasopressin release from rat neurohypophyses. When isolated rat neural lobes were incubated in a calcium-free medium together with ionophore, the introduction of calcium to the medium caused a very large increase in hormone release. It would seem reasonable to hypothesize that the ionophore promoted the influx of calcium, increased the concentration of free calcium in the axoplasm and thereby increased release. This hormone release occurs in the absence of external calcium. Therefore the data suggest that a rise in axonal cytoplasmic calcium is sufficient to promote hormone release and that depolarization is not a prerequisite for secrction. This is supported by the findings of Douglas and Sorimachi (1971), who reported that removal of external sodium gives rise to a slow but significant increase in vasopressin release. This can be explained by an increase in intracellular calcium resulting from a blockage of the sodium- calcium exchange. Certainly neurohormone release and calcium uptake are closely linked. Plots of calcium uptake and vasopressin release as a function of external calcium show that the relationship is linear, and that one calcium ion can promote the release of one hormone unit or quantum (Douglas and Poisner 1964 b) (Fig. 15).

5.4 How Is Low Intracellular Free Calcium Established?

The intracellular resting level of free calcium in the neurohypophysis is probably in the same range reported for other neurones (50–150 n*M*). It now seems well established that upon stimulation of the neurosecretory cells, a trigger amount of calcium crosses the cell membrane, probably through special calcium channels. For this system to work, there must exist mechanisms which normalize the increased intracellular concentration of free calcium after stimulation. There are a

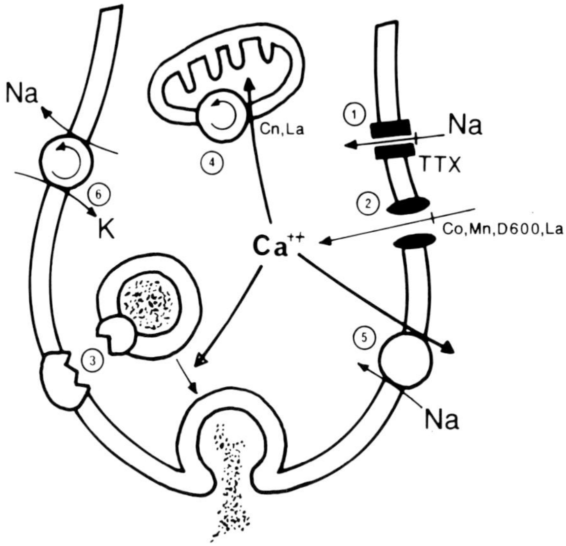

Fig. 16. Schematic illustration of calcium-dependent exocytosis and of processes that affect the axoplasmic calcium concentration. Sodium-dependent action potentials (*1*) depolarize the plasma membrane and turn on a calcium channel (*2*). The resulting rise in internal free calcium permits the interaction of plasma and granule membranes characteristic of exocytosis, involving specific membrane constituents (*3*). Following secretion, resting axoplasmic calcium is restored by sequestration into mitochondria (*4*), by sodium-calcium counterexchange (*5*) and possibly by other mechanisms; the counterexchange depends on the maintenance of a concentration gradient for sodium and therefore the integrity of the sodium pump (*6*). *TTX*, tetrodotoxin; *Co*, cobalt; *Mn*, manganese; *La*, lanthanum; *Cn*, cyanide. (Redrawn from Dreifuss 1975)

number of possible processes (Fig. 16): (1) binding of calcium to cytoplasmic molecules; (2) active sequestration of calcium inside the nerve terminals; (3) sodium-calcium exchange over the cell membrane:

1. Specific calcium-binding proteins have been identified in squid axoplasm (Baker and Schlaeffer 1978) and in the bovine neurohypophysis (Kretzinger 1976). Russell and Thorn (1977) isolated and purified these calcium-binding proteins. Their main finding was that in a soluble fraction of the terminals there was a protein which has an apparent dissociation constant for calcium of 1.1×10^{-5} *M*, which is high if one considers the internal calcium concentration. Therefore, it is possible that this protein might be important in controlling the low intracellular levels of free calcium.
2. Electron microscopy has revealed that there are at least three types of subcellular organelles in the neurohypophysial nerve terminal preparations – the mitochondria, neurosecretory granules and microvesicles (La Bella and Sanwal 1965) – and there is evidence to suggest that these subcellular organelles are involved in the sequestration of calcium inside the nerve terminals. In a variety of tissues, mitochondria have been implicated in the sequestration of intracellular calcium, but Russell and Thorn (1975) were the first to produce biochem-

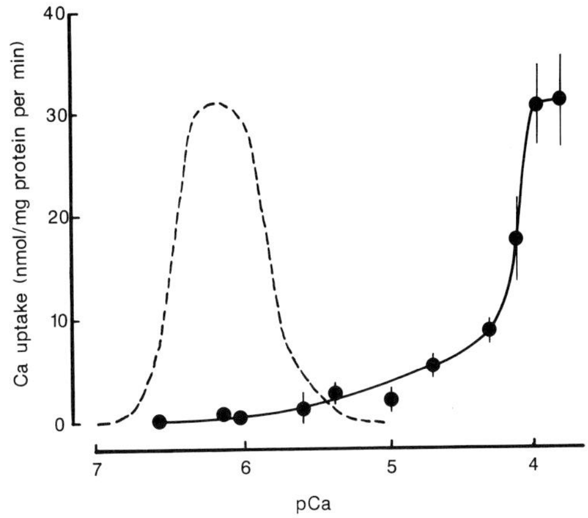

Fig. 17. Calcium uptake into isolated microvesicles (*dashed line*) and into mitochondria (*solid line*), as a function of external calcium concentration. (Redrawn from Nordmann 1983)

ical data to suggest that mitochondria in the neural lobe were able to take up calcium (Fig. 17). The uptake process was found to be adenosine triphosphate (ATP)-dependent and considerably reduced in the presence of an uncoupler of oxidative phosphorylation. Although the capacity of mitochondria to accumulate calcium has been shown to be high, the affinity constant of the sequestrating mechanism renders it unlikely that the mitochondria are the sole organelles for controlling cytoplasmic concentrations.

Thorn and his colleagues (Thorn et al. 1975) found that isolated neurosecretory granules contain comparatively high concentrations of calcium. They demonstrated that granules are able to take up a small amount of calcium over a short period. Following this uptake the granules burst. The process is thought to be ATP-α-dependent proton transport into the granules, which creates an osmotic gradient, followed by volume changes and passive movement of calcium into the granules (Casey et al. 1976). It should be noted that Kostron et al. (1977) have demonstrated that calcium uptake by chromaffin cells in the adrenal medulla in vitro is not dependent on ATP.

The role of microvesicles in the function of the neurosecretory terminals has been the subject of much debate. One of the most attractive hypotheses has been that these organelles represent the retrieved membrane of the granules after exocytosis (Nagasawa et al. 1970). However, following stimulation of the terminals, the number of microvesicles does not increase (Nordman and Morris 1976), which certainly implies that they are not involved in the endocytotic process. However, Morris and Nordmann (1980) observed a redistribution of the microvesicles towards the plasmalemma abutting the basement membrane of the secretory terminal in the area where the greatest depletion of neurosecretory granules occurs after stimulation of the terminals. Furthermore, Stoeckel et al. (1975) demonstrated that the microvesicles contain a calcium precipitate, and Nordmann and Chevallier (1980) showed that a microsomal fraction of terminals containing microvesicles accumulates large amounts of calcium by an ATP-dependent process.

The terminals cannot accumulate the calcium for long, and the ion has to be extruded. How the microvesicles release calcium is not known. Electron micrographs often show that these organelles fuse with the plasmalemma, so the calcium could be released by exocytosis (Nordmann and Chevallier 1980). Alternatively, calcium could be released slowly into the cytoplasm and long- term calcium homeostasis could be controlled by transporting systems located in the terminal membrane. However, such transport is against the electrochemical gradient so must involve active extrusion of calcium. There are three possible mechanisms:

1. External sodium ion concentration. Robinson et al. (1976) have demonstrated that concentrations of external sodium affect the efflux of calcium. When the concentration of sodium is low extrusion of calcium is low, and vice versa. This type of sodium-dependent calcium transport is advocated by Dreifuss and Nordmann (1974).
2. External calcium concentration. The efflux of calcium from the terminals is decreased by more than 30% after removal of external calcium (Nordmann 1983). Furthermore, the calcium-dependent calcium efflux is inhibited by sodium ions (Nordmann 1983). There is no evidence concerning the mechanism by which external calcium can modulate the extrusion of internal calcium, but it is possible that calcium activates the efflux of ionized cellular calcium at the external surface of the terminal membrane. The low affinity of external calcium for the transport system would render a countermechanism inefficient.
3. Calcium-dependent ATPase extrusion. Part of the uncoupled calcium efflux from isolated neural lobes is inhibited by a powerful inhibitor of calcium-stimulated ATPase (Nordmann 1983). It is possible that a large part of the total efflux is dependent on the cellular ATP level. However, a calcium ATP-dependent pump has not been identified, and the control of calcium efflux and ATP concentrations within the terminals has yet to be resolved.

5.5 How Does Calcium Induce Oxytocin Release?

The essential problem in the stimulus-secretion coupling concept is how an increase in intracellular free calcium concentration can induce oxytocin release. In studies by Russell and Thorn (1974) it has been demonstrated that, on stimulation, calcium ions in very small amounts are transported across the cell membranes of the nerve endings and that this process is essential for the release of neurohypophysial hormones. It appears that movement of calcium is the trigger for release, so activation of membrane calcium channels is necessary for normal hormone release.

Recently, the use of voltage-sensitive dyes has confirmed directly that potassium depolarizes neurosecretory nerve terminals in the neural lobe (Nordmann et al. 1982). However, whereas depolarization is a linear function of external potassium, hormone release is not. Although changes of external potassium might give rise to changes in the ionic composition of the nerve endings, there is little doubt that in the presence of external calcium ions, an increase in hormone release is induced by the depolarizing effects of the potassium. Nordmann and coworkers (Dyball and Nordmann 1977; Nordmann et al. 1982) looked for evidence to demonstrate a depolarizing-induced entry of calcium into the nerve terminals.

They showed that removal of external sodium increases calcium uptake but considerably reduces calcium efflux from the neural lobe, and that potassium depolarization increases hormone release and calcium uptake for prolonged periods but has only a very transient effect on calcium efflux. These data strongly suggest that the increase in calcium entry may be due to the depolarization of the nerve terminals. It is likely that in the neurohypophysis, as in other excitable systems, the major entry of calcium during depolarization is by a voltage-sensitive mechanism. Experiments have shown that tetrodotoxin (TTX) which specifically blocks sodium channels, blocks the release of hormone (Ishida 1967). Although this could indicate a common route for sodium and calcium ions, other experiments have shown that this is not the case (Nordmann and Dreifuss 1972). Potassium-induced calcium uptake and hormone release are not blocked by TTX. It seems that electrically induced depolarization is sufficiently large to increase calcium permeability directly or, if smaller, via activation of sodium channels. It has been shown that stimulation of neurosecretory tissue increases the passive permeability for sodium ions followed by an increase in permeability to calcium through specific "late" or "slow" calcium channels (Nordmann and Dreifuss 1972). The terms "late" or "slow" are derived from work on giant squid axon, where it has been shown that calcium entry definitely occurs in two phases, an early phase which is parallel to the increase in sodium permeability and a following late phase (Baker et al. 1973).

The intracellular action of calcium in triggering secretion is still the subject of debate. The available evidence appears to rule out the possibility of a direct and functionally important role in organization of microtubules for release, since colchicine does not depress vasopressin secretion from isolated rat neurohypophyses (Russell and Thorn 1973). Cytocholasin B, on the other hand, does depress secretion; however, since this substance is also known to interfere with glucose uptake and utilization, its inhibitory action on neurohypophysial secretion cannot be taken as support for a direct involvement of microfilaments in the release process. Dreifuss and colleagues (Dreifuss et al. 1973) found no convincing evidence in support of a major role of cyclic AMP in hormone secretion from the isolated rat neurohypophysis.

Interest turned to the neurosecretory granules containing the hormone. The granules are known to be negatively charged (Vilhardt and Jorgensen 1972), since they move towards the anode in an electric field. It has been proposed that calcium decreases the negative charge of the neurosecretory granules whilst at the same time reducing the viscosity of the axoplasm (Hodgkin and Katz 1949). It is also possible that absorption of calcium to the cytoplasmic surfaces of plasma granule membranes, and the resulting reduction of the potential barrier of repulsive electrostatic forces, might conceivably allow granules located in close proximity to the plasma membrane to approach it more effectively.

5.6 Control of Oxytocinergic Terminals at the Level of the Neurohypophysis

Depolarization of the neurosecretory terminals in the neural lobe causes the discharge of neurosecretory granules by exocytosis (Poulain and Wakerley 1982: see

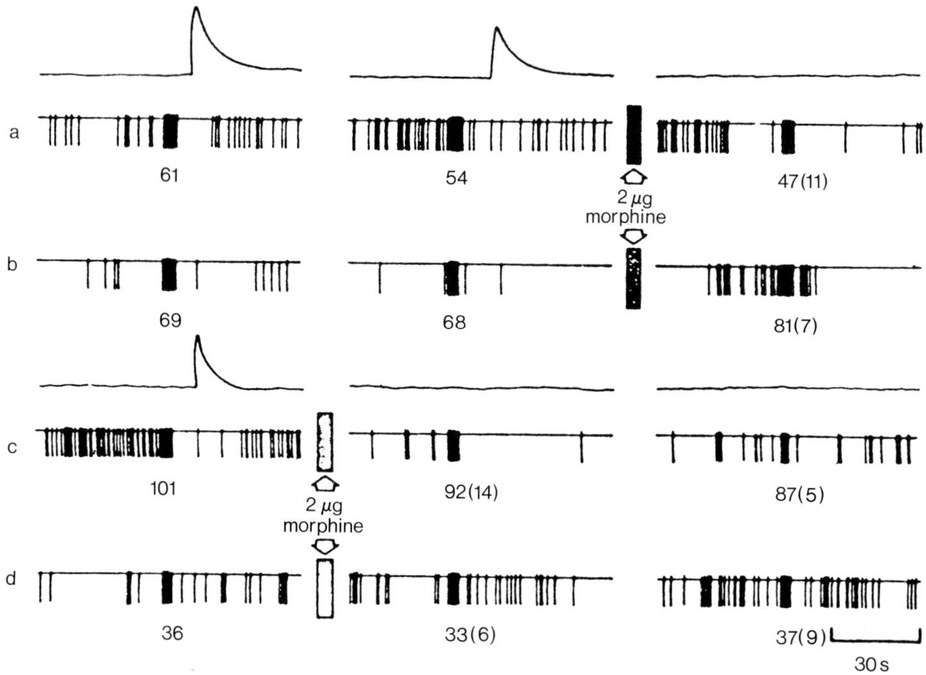

Fig. 18 a–d. Effects of i.c.v. morphine on oxytocin release in anaesthetized lactating rats. Four separate records are shown from different animals. Activation of the oxytocin neurones is followed by a rise in intramammary pressure at reflex milk ejection. (Numbers under the bursts show the number of spikes in each burst). After treatment with morphine, release of oxytocin is blocked but the activation of the neurones is still seen. It is suggested that the opioid acts at the nerve terminal to "dissociate" electrical activity from release of hormone. (Data from Clarke et al. 1979)

Sect. 5) and it has been suggested that there are mechanisms present within the lobe itself for controlling the release of oxytocin, particularly since the discovery of opioid peptides within the neurohypophysis (Cox 1982; Akil et al. 1984). The idea that opioids may play a part in regulating the oxytocinergic terminals stemmed from the finding that exogenous morphine suppressed the rise in intramammary pressure which usually follows electrical stimulation of the neural stalk, even though the response of the mammary gland to exogenous oxytocin was unaffected (Clarke et al. 1979). It was suggested that morphine uncoupled the depolarization caused by the electrical activity from the hormone release at the terminals, and this was supported by the demonstration that oxytocin neurones continued to show bursts of neurosecretory activity in response to the sucking action of the young but these bursts were no longer followed by the expected rise in intramammary pressure (Fig. 18). Moreover, morphine and other opioid peptides inhibited release of oxytocin from the isolated neurohypophysis in vitro (Bicknell and Leng 1982; Clarke and Patrick 1983), and these effects could be reversed by the opiate antagonist, naloxone. In fact, electrical stimulation of oxytocin release, both in vivo and in vitro, was potentiated by naloxone alone (Bicknell and Leng 1982; Bicknell et al. 1985), indicating that endogenous opioids were active. Furthermore, as naloxone enhanced sucking-induced release of oxytocin in some rats (Clarke et al. 1979), the endogenous opioids might have a physiological role in controlling milk ejection. It has recently been suggested that endogenous opioids might have a direct role in the control of labour (Bicknell 1985; Leng et al. 1985). Certainly the neural lobe contains a variety of opioid peptides such as enkephalin (Kumar et al. 1979; Rossier et al. 1977; 1979), dynorphin (Goldstein and Ghazarossian 1980; Hollt et al. 1980; Nakao et al. 1981; Giraud et al. 1983) and α-neo-endorphin (Ito et al. 1981; Weber et al. 1982).

There are several possible ways in which these endogenous opioids might have access to the oxytocinergic terminals of the posterior pituitary. Rossier et al. (1979) identified an enkephalin pathway to the neurohypophysis originating from the supraoptic and paraventricular nuclei, and it was proposed that enkephalin might coexist with the oxytocin (and vasopressin) and be co-located in the neurosecretory terminals (Martin and Voigt 1981). These findings have been substantiated in the rat (Watson et al. 1982; van Leeuwen 1982) and demonstrated in the cat (Micevych and Elde 1980), monkey (Haber and Elde 1982) and fish (Reaves and Hayward 1979). Ultrastructural studies of the neurohypophysis have suggested that enkephalin and neurophysin coexist in the same terminals and even in the same granules within those terminals (Coulter et al. 1981). There has been debate about whether or not there is coexistence of enkephalins and the posterior pituitary peptides, but Martin et al. (1983) claim that met-enkephalin and cholecystokinin coexist with oxytocin and leu-enkephalin with vasopressin. However, van Leeuwen (van Leeuwen 1981; van Leeuwen and De Vreis 1983) has demonstrated the presence of separate enkephalinergic immunoreactive fibres in the perimeter and the centre of the neural lobe. No conlcusions were drawn about the possible endings of these fibres, but synaptoid contacts have been shown between leu-enkephalin terminals and pituicytes (van Leeuwen et al. 1983). It has been demonstrated that pro-opiomelanocortin is present in some of the terminals of the median eminence and pituitary, although it is recognized that most of this opioid originates from the arcuate nucleus. Pro-opiomelanocortin gives rise to the opioid β-endorphin, which is present within the melanotrophs of the intermediate lobe of the pituitary. O'Donohue and Dorsa (1982) suggested that β-endorphin could diffuse from the intermediate lobe into the neurohypophysis. Originally it was suggested that the opioids might act directly on the terminals of the oxytocin cells to suppress release (Clarke et al. 1979), akin to the presynaptic inhibition reported for spinal neurones (Iversen et al. 1980). Perhaps the opioid affected calcium flux across the terminal membrane, but Nordmann et al. (1986) have shwon that oxytocin release and calcium uptake in either the isolated neurohypophysis or in isolated neurosecretory terminals (neurosecretosomes) is not affected by the presence of enkephalins or naloxone. In fact, they have recently provided evidence to suggest that relaxin, a peptide hormone produced primarily by the ovary (Porter 1979), might be important, in vitro, in gating the calcium influx into the neurosecretory elements (Dayanithi et al. 1987). An alternative mechanism for the opioid control of oxytocin release has been postulated following the discovery that the majority of the opioid binding sites are located on the pituicytes and not on the peptidergic terminals (van Leeuwen et al. 1983). However, this putative site of action does not provide the complete answer, because the opioid binding sites on pituicytes are K-receptors (Bunn et al. 1985) and K-selective opiates do not inhibit oxytocin release (Bicknell et al. 1985). Therefore, neither the mechanism nor the site of action of the opioid control of neurosecretion from the neural lobe is entirely understood.

There are several other compounds which may modulate the release of oxytocin at the level of the neurosecretory nerve terminals. Dopamine has a powerful inhibitory effect on oxytocin release, at least in vitro, and is present within the nerve terminals of the neurointermediate lobe (Saavedra et al. 1975). There have been several investigations of the effects of dopamine on both oxytocin and vasopressin release. Bridges et al. (1976) reported that dopamine stimulated the release of both peptides from the isolated neural lobe but high doses of dopamine were required. In contrast, others have reported a suppression of oxytocin release (Vizi and Volbekas 1980) and vasopressin release (Lightman et al. 1982). These differences may be expressions of the differential effects on the D1 and D2 receptors. Racke et al. (1982a) demonstrated that facilitation was mediated through D1 receptors and blocked by cis-flupenthixol, whereas the inhibitory action was mediated by D2 receptors and blocked by sulpiride. Certainly, it has been reported that vasopressin release is associated with increased levels of cyclic nucleotides in the neural lobe, which would be consistent with an action through the D1 receptors (Vale and Hope 1982). Clarke and Merrick (1985) showed that haloperidol, a D1 antagonist, causes a short-lived suppression of oxytocin release evoked by electrical stimulation of the neural lobe in vivo, and this finding would fit with the concept that the D1 receptors are linked with facilitation of release in the lobe. However, it is equally possible that haloperidol might cause a transient change in blood flow through the lobe, which would have an indirect effect on release. It has been demonstrated that the dopamine content of the lobe parallels the physiological demands for oxytocin release (Alper and Moore 1982; Holzbauer et al. 1978, 1983) and that dopamine levels within the lobe have a diurnal variation (Barden et al. 1982).

Noradrenaline is also present in the neural lobe and is released with dopamine upon depolarization of the terminals (Sharman et al. 1982). It is mainly, but not completely, accounted for by sympathetic fibres from the rostral cervical ganglion, and may be involved in the control of blood flow through the gland (Baumgarten et al. 1972). Stimulation of the rostral cervical ganglion causes the release of both neurohypophysial peptides (Karasek et al. 1980). Furthermore, the β- adrenergic agonist, isoprenaline, has been reported to stimulate the release of vasopressin via an adenylate cyclase system which is distinct from the dopamine-linked system (Racke et al. 1982b). β-Adrenoceptor agonists which do not cross the blood-brain barrier inhibit reflex milk ejection when injected peripherally (Tribollet et al. 1978), whereas propranolol, a β- adrenoceptor antagonist, enhances oxytocin release evoked by electrical stimulation of the infundibulum in vivo (Poulain and Dyer 1984). This supports the existence of a β-adrenergic inhibitory mechanism within the neurohypophysis, originally suggested by Tribollet et al. (1978).

It has also been shown that γ-aminobutyric acid (GABA) is present in the posterior pituitary of goat (Anderson et al. 1961), cow (La Bella et al. 1968) and rat (Beart et al. 1974), as well as its synthetic enzyme glutamic acid decarboxylase

(Kanazawa et al. 1976; Minchin and Beart 1975). In the isolated neurohypophysis GABA is synthesized from radioactive glucose or acetate (Iversen and Kelly 1975). This seems to be related to the production and transport of oxytocin or vasopressin, and the pituicytes appear to accumulate radioactively labelled GABA or its precursors (Schon and Iversen 1974). Zing et al. (1979) showed that the neurosecretory axons and terminals possess GABA receptors and proposed that the pituicytes synthesize and release GABA to control release from the nerve terminals.

6 Concluding Remarks

Our understanding of the principles of stimulus-secretion coupling has been significantly advanced by study of the oxytocin system, and at the same time we have learnt a great deal about the relationships between stimuli that cause the release of oxytocin, activation of the oxytocin neurones and the appearance of hormone in the circulation. However, there are still important questions to be answered about the secretion of oxytocin, for example the following: (1) the role and site of action of endogenous opioids on the axon terminals; (2) the problems of coexistence of opioids with neurohypophysial hormones and the possible importance of co-release; (3) the mechanism(s) of gating the calcium influx into the terminals which triggers secretion; (4) the relevance of the apparent fatigue shown by axon terminals in response to the arrival of action potentials in the neural lobe.

Acknowledgments. The authors would like to thank David Barrett and Brian Pickering for their help and support and Miss B. Phelps for typing this manuscript.

References

Akil H, Watson SJ, Young E, Lewis ME, Khachaturian H, Walker JM (1984) Endogenous opioids: biology and function. Annu Rev Neurosci 7:223–225

Alper RH, Moore KE (1982) Injection of hypertonic saline or mannitol accelerates the dehydration-induced activation of dopamine synthesis in the neurointermediate lobe of the rat hypophysis. Neuroendocrinology 35:469–474

Amara SG, David DN, Rosenfeld MG, Roos BA, Evans RM (1980) Characterization of rat calcitonin mRNA. Proc Natl Acad Sci USA 77:4444–4448

Ambach G, Palkovits M (1979) The blood supply of the hypothalamus of the rat. In: Anatomy of the hypothalamus. Dekker, New York

Anderson B, Larsson S, Pocchiari F (1961) Aspects on the glucose metabolism of the hypothalamus and the pituitary in goats. Acta Physiol Scand 51:314–324

Andrew RD, Dudek FE (1983) Burst discharge in mammalian neuroendocrine cells involves an intrinsic regenerative mechanism. Science 221:1050–1052

Andrew RD, Dudek FE (1984a) Analysis of intracellular recorded phasic bursting by mammalian neuroendocrine cells. J Neurophysiol 51:552–566

Andrew RD, Dudek FE (1984b) Intrinsic inhibition in magnocellular neuroendocrine cells of rat hypothalamus. J Physiol (Lond) 353:171–185

Baertschi AJ, Dreifuss JJ (1979) The antidromic compound action potential of the hypothalamo-neurohypophysial tract, a tool for assessing posterior pituitary activity in vivo. Brain Res 171:437–451

Baker PF, Schlaeffer WW (1978) Uptake and binding of calcium by axoplasm isolated from giant axons of *Loligo* and *Myxicola*. J Physiol (Lond) 276:103–125
Baker PF, Meves H, Ridgway EB (1973) Calcium entry in response to maintained depolarization of squid axons. J Physiol (Lond) 231:527–548
Barden N, Chevillard C, Saavedra JM (1982) Diurnal variations in rat posterior pituitary catecholamine levels. Neuroendocrinology 34:148–150
Bargmann W, Scharrer E (1951) The site of origin of the hormones of the posterior pituitary. Am Sci 39:255–259
Bargmann W, von Gaudecker B (1969) Über die Ultrastruktur sekretorischer Elementargranula. Z Zellforsch Mikrosk Anat 96:495–504
Baumgarten HG, Bjorklund A, Holstein AF, Nobin A (1972) Organization and ultrastructural identification of the catecholamine nerve terminals in the neural lobe and pars intermedia of the rat pituitary. Z Zellforsch Mikrosk Anat 126:483–517
Beart PM, Kelly JS, Schon F (1974) γ-Aminobutyric acid in the rat peripheral nervous system pineal and posterior pituitary. Biochem Soc Trans 2:266–268
Belin V, Moos F (1986) Paired recordings from supraoptic and paraventricular oxytocin cells in suckled rats: recruitment and synchronization. J Physiol (Lond) 377:369–390
Belin V, Moos F, Richard P (1985) Synchronization of oxytocin cells in the hypothalamic and supraoptic nuclei in suckled rats: direct proof with paired extracellular recordings. Exp Brain Res 57:201–203
Bicknell RJ (1985) Endogenous opioid peptides and hypothalamic neuroendocrine neurones. J Endocrinol 107:437–446
Bicknell RJ, Leng G (1982) Endogenous opiates regulate oxytocin but not vasopressin secretion from the neurohypophysis. Nature 298:161–162
Bicknell RJ, Brown D, Chapman C, Hancock PD, Leng G (1984) Reversible fatigue of stimulus-secretion coupling in the rat neurohypophysis. J Physiol (Lond) 348:601–613
Bicknell RJ, Chapman C, Leng G (1985) Effects of opioid agonists on oxytocin and vasopressin release in vitro. Neuroendocrinology 41:142–148
Birkett SD, Swann RW, Gonzalez CB, Pickering BT (1983) Analysis of the neurohypophysial components accumulating in the supraoptic nucleus of the rat after injection of colchicine. Arch Biochem Biophys 225[2]:430–435
Bradbury AF, Finnie MDA, Smyth DG (1982) Mechanism of C-terminal amide formation by pituitary enzymes. Nature 298:686–688
Bridges TE, Hillhouse EW, Jones MT (1976) The effect of dopamine on neurohypophysial hormone release in vivo and from the rat neural lobe and hypothalamus in vitro. J Physiol (Lond) 260:647–666
Brownstein MJ (1983) Biosynthesis of vasopressin and oxytocin. Annu Rev Physiol 45:129–135
Bunn SJ, Hanley MR, Wilkin GP (1985) Evidence for a kappa-opioid receptor on pituitary astrocytes: an autoradiographic study. Neurosci Lett 55:317–323
Burns BD, Stean JPB, Webb AC (1979) The effects of sleep on neurones in isolated cerebral cortex. Proc R Soc London [Biol] 206:281–291
Cajal Ramon y S (1911) Histologie due système nerveux de l'homme et des vertébrés, vol II Maloine, Paris
Cannata MA, Morris JF (1973) Changes in the appearance of hypothalamo-neurohypophysial neurosecretory granules associated with their maturation. J Endocrinol 57:531–538
Casey RP, Njus D, Raooa GR, Sehr PA (1976) Adenosine triphosphate-evoked catecholamine release in chromaffin granules. Biochem J 158:583–588
Cazalis M, Dayanithi G, Nordmann JJ (1985) The role of patterned burst and interburst interval on the excitation-coupling mechanism in the isolated rat neural lobe. J Physiol (Lond) 369:45–60
Chapman DB, Theodosis DT, Montagnese C, Poulain DA, Morris JF (1986) Osmotic stimulation causes structural plasticity of neurone-glia relationship of the oxytocin- but not vasopressin-secreting neurones in the hypothalamic supraoptic nucleus. Neuroscience 17:679–686

Clarke G, Merrick LP (1985) Electrophysiological studies of magnocellular neurones. In: Ganten D, Pfaff DW (eds) Current topics in neuroendocrinology, vol 4. Springer, Berlin Heidelberg New York, pp 17–59
Clarke G, Patrick G (1983) Differential inhibitory action by morphine on the release of oxytocin and vasopressin from isolated neural lobe. Neurosci Lett 39:175–180
Clarke G, Wood P, Merrick LP, Lincoln DW (1979) Opiate inhibition of peptide release from the neurohumoral terminals of hypothalamic neurones. Nature 282:746–748
Coghlan JP, Aldred P, Butkus A, Crawford RJ, Darby IA, Fernley RT, Haralambidis J, Hudson PJ, Mitri R, Niall HD, Penschow JD, Roche PJ, Scalon DB, Tregear GW (1984) Hybridization histochemistry. Excerpta Medical, vol 18. Elsevier, Amsterdam
Coulter HD, Elde RP, Unverzagt SL (1981) Co-localization of neurophysin- and enkephalin-like immunoreactivity in cat pituitary. Peptides (Fayetteville) 2:51–55
Cox BM (1982) Mini review. Endogenous opioid peptides: a guide to structures and terminology. Life Sci 31:1645–1658
Cross BA, Dyer RG (1971 a) Unit activity in diencephalic islands – the effects of anaesthetics. J Physiol (Lond) 212:467–481
Cross BA, Dyer RG (1971 b) Cyclic changes in neurones of the anterior hypothalamus during the estrous cycle and the effects of anaesthetics. In: Gorski R, Sawyer CH (eds) Steroid hormones and brain function. University of California Press, Los Angeles, pp 95–102
Cross BA, Dyer RG (1972) Ovarian modulation of unit activity in the anterior hypothalamus of the cyclic rat. J Physiol (Lond) 222:5P
Cross BA, Green JD (1959) Activity of single neurones in the hypothalamus: effect of osmotic and other stimuli. J Physiol (Lond) 148:554–569
Cross BA, Kitay JI (1967) Unit activity in diencephalic islands. Exp Neurol 19:316–330
Dayanithi G, Cazalis M, Nordmann JJ (1987) Relaxin affects the release of oxytocin and vasopressin from the neurohypophysis. Nature 325:813–816
Dellmann HD, Rodriguez EM (1970) Herring bodies: an electron microscopic study of local degeneration and regeneration of neurosecretory axons. Z Zellforsch Mikrosk Anat 111:293–315
Dierickx K (1980) Immunocytochemical localization of the vertebrate cyclic nonapeptide neurohypophyseal hormones and neurophysins. Int Rev Cytol 62:119–185
Douglas WW, Poisner AM (1964 a) Stimulus-secretion coupling in a neurosecretory organ: the role of calcium in the release of vasopressin from the neurohypophysis. J Physiol (Lond) 172:1–18
Douglas WW, Poisner AM (1964 b) Calcium movements in the neurohypophysis of the rat and its relation to the release of vasopressin. J Physiol (Lond) 172:19–30
Douglas WW, Rubin RP (1963) The mechanism of catecholamine release from the adrenal medulla and the role of calcium in stimulus-secretion coupling. J Physiol (Lond) 167:288–310
Douglas WW, Sorimachi M (1971) Electrically evoked release of vasopressin from isolated neurohypophyses in sodium-free media. Br J Pharmacol 42:647P
Dreifuss JJ (1975) A review on neurosecretory granules: their contents and mechanisms of release. Ann NY Acad Sci 248:184–201
Dreifuss JJ, Nordmann JJ (1974) Sodium dependent calcium efflux from the rat neurohypophysis. J Physiol (Lond) 240:46–47P
Dreifuss JJ, Kalnins I, Kelly JS, Ruf KB (1971) Action potentials and release of neurohypophysial hormones in vitro. J Physiol (Lond) 215:805–817
Dreifuss JJ, Grau JD, Nordmann JJ (1973) Effects on isolated neurohypophysis of agents which affect the membrane permeability to calcium. J Physiol (Lond) 215:805–817
Dreifuss JJ, Tribollet E, Baertschi AJ (1976) Excitation of supraoptic neurones by vaginal distention in lactating rats: correlation with neurohypophysial hormone release. Brain Res 113:600–605
Dreifuss JJ, Tribollet E, Muhlethaler M (1981) Temporal patterns of neural activity and their relation to the secretion of posterior pituitary hormones. Biol Reprod 24:51–72
Dyball REJ, Leng G (1986) Regulation of the milk ejection reflex in the rat. J Physiol (Lond) 380:239–256

Dyball REJ, McPhaill CI (1974) Unit activity in the supraoptic and paraventricular nuclei – the effects of anaesthetics. Brain Res 67:43–50

Dyball REJ, Nordmann JJ (1977) Reactivation by veratridine of hormone release from K^+-depolarized rat neurohypophysis. J Physiol (Lond) 269:65–66P

Dyball REJ, Prilusky J (1981) Responses of supraoptic neurones in the intact and deafferented rat hypothalamus to injections of hypertonic sodium chloride. J Physiol (Lond) 311:443–452

Dyer RG, Dyball REJ, Morris JF (1973) The effect of hypothalamic deafferentation upon the ultrastructure and hormone content of the paraventricular nucleus. J Endocrinol 57:509–516

Ely F, Petersen WE (1941) Factors involved in the ejection of milk. J Dairy Sci 24:211–223

Folley SJ (1969) The milk ejection reflex: a neuroendocrine theme in biology, myth and art. J Endocrinol 44:IX–XX

Felten DL, Cashner KA (1979) Cytoarchitecture of the supraoptic nucleus: a Golgi study. Neuroendocrinology 29:221–230

Fisher AWF, Price PG, Burford GD, Lederis K (1979) A 3-dimensional reconstruction of the hypothalamo-neurohypophysial system of the rat. Cell Tissue Res 204:343–354

Furutani Y, Morimoto Y, Shibahara S, Noda M, Takahashi H, Hirose T, Asai M, Inayama S, Hayashida H, Miyata T, Numa S (1983) Cloning a sequence analysis of cDNA for ovine corticotropin-releasing factor precursor. Nature 301:537–540

Gähweiler BH, Dreifuss JJ (1979) Phasically firing neurones in long-term cultures of the rat hypothalamic supraoptic area: pacemaker and follower cells. Brain Res 177:95–103

Gainer H, Brownstein MJ (1978) Identification of the precursors of rat neurophysins. In: Vincent JD (ed) Biologie cellulaire des processus neurosecretoires hypothalamique.

Gainer H, Sarne Y, Brownstein MJ (1977a) Neurophysin biosynthesis: conversion of a putative precursor during axonal transport. Science 195:1354–1356

Gainer H, Sarne Y, Brownstein MJ (1977b) Biosynthesis and axonal transport of rat neurohypophysial proteins and peptides. J Cell Biol 73:366–381

Gaines WL (1915) A contribution to the physiology of lactation. Am J Physiol 38:285–312

Giraud P, Castanas E, Patey G, Oliver C, Rossier J (1983) Regional distribution of methionine-enkephalin-Arg^6-Phe^7 in the rat brain: comparative study with the distribution of other opioid peptides. J Neurochem 41:154–160

Goldstein A, Ghazarossian VE (1980) Immunoreactive dynorphin in pituitary and brain. Proc Natl Acad Sci USA 77:6207–6210

Gomez ET (1939) The relation of the posterior hypophysis in the maintenance of lactation in hypophysectomised rats. J Dairy Sci 22:488

Gubler U, Monahan JJ, Lomedico PT, Bhatt RS, Collier KJ, Hoffman BJ, Bohlen P, Esch F, Ling N, Zeytin F, Brazeau P, Poonian MS, Gage LP (1983) Cloning and sequence analysis of cDNA for the precursor of human growth hormone-releasing factor somatocrinin. Proc Natl Acad Sci USA 80:4311–4314

Haber S, Elde R (1981) The distribution of enkephalin immunoreactive fibers and terminals in the monkey central nervous system: an immunohistochemical study. Neuroscience 7:1049–1095

Haller EW, Sachs H, Sperelaks H, Share L (1965) Release of vasopressin from isolated guinea-pig pituitaries. Am J Physiol 209:79–83

Harris MC (1979) Effects of chemoreceptor and baroreceptor stimulation on the discharge of hypothalamic supraoptic neurones in rats. J Endocrinol 82:115–125

Hatton JD, Ellisman MH (1981) Distribution of orthogonal arrays and their relationship to intercellular functions in neuroglia of the freeze-fractured hypothalamo-neurohypophyseal system. Cell Tissue Res 215:308–323

Hatton GI, Tweedle CD (1982) Magnocellular neuropeptidergic neurons in hypothalamus: increases in membrane apposition and number of specialized synapses from pregnancy to lactation. Brain Res Bull 8:197–204

Hatton GI, Armstrong WE, Gregory WA (1978) Spontaneous and osmotically stimulated activity in slices of rat hypothalamus. Brain Res Bull 3:497–508

Hatton GI, Perlmutter LS, Salm AK, Tweedle CD (1984) Dynamic neuronal-glial interactions in hypothalamus and pituitary: implications for control of hormone synthesis and release. Peptides 5[Suppl 1]:121–138

Heap PF, Jones CW, Morris JF, Pickering BT (1975) Movement of neurosecretory product through the anatomical compartments of the rat neural lobe. Cell Tissue Res 156:483–492

Hodgkin AL, Katz B (1949) The effect of calcium on the axoplasm of giant nerve fibres. Brain Res 79:397–403

Hollt V, Haarmann I, Bovermann K, Jerlicz M, Herz A (1980) Dynorphin-related immunoreactive peptides in rat brain and pituitary. Neurosci Lett 18:149–153

Holzbauer M, Sharman DF, Godden U (1978) Observations on the function of the dopaminergic nerves innervating the pituitary gland. Neuroscience 3:1251–1262

Holzbauer M, Muscholl E, Racke K, Sharman DF (1983) Evidence that dopamine is a neurotransmitter in the neurointermediate lobe of the hypophysis. In: Cross BA, Leng G (eds) The neurohypophysis: structure, function and control. Elsevier, Amsterdam, pp 357–364 (Progress in brain research, vol 68)

Ishida A (1967) The effect of tetrodotoxin on calcium-dependent link in stimulus-secretion coupling in neurohypophysis. Jpn J Physiol 17:308–320

Ishida A (1970) The oxytocin release and the compound action potential evoked by electrical stimulation of the isolated neurohypophysis of the rat. Jpn J Physiol 20:84–96

Ito S, Iwanaga T, Yui R, Yamaguchi K, Hama H, Kamoi K, Shibata A (1981) Presence of α-neo- endorphin-like immunoreactivity in the posterior lobe of the pituitary gland. Life Sci 29:1457–1461

Ivell R, Richter D (1984) Structure and comparison of the oxytocin and vasopressin genes from rat. Proc Natl Acad Sci USA 81:2006– 2010

Iversen LL, Kelly JS (1975) Uptake and metabolism of GABA by neurones and glial cells. Biochem Pharmacol 24:933–958

Iversen LL, Iversen SD, Bloom FE (1980) Opiate receptors influence vasopressin release from nerve terminals in rat neurohypophysis. Nature 284:350–351

Jones CW, Pickering BT (1970) Rapid transport of neurohypophysial hormones in the hypothalamo-neurohypophysial tract. J Physiol (Lond) 208:73–74P

Juss TS, Wakerley JB (1981) Mesencephalic areas controlling pulsatile oxytocin release in the suckled rat. J Endocrinol 91:233–244

Kalimo H (1975) Ultrastructural studies on the hypothalamic neurosecretory neurones of the rat: III. Parventricular and supraoptic neurones during lactation and dehydration. Cell Tissue Res 163:151–168

Kanazawa I, Iversen LL, Kelly JS (1976) Glutamate decarboxylase activity in the rat posterior pituitary, pineal gland, dorsal root ganglion and superior cervial ganglion. J Neurochem 27:1267–1269

Kandel ER (1964) Electrical properties of hypothalamic neuroendocrine cells. J Gen Physiol 47:691–717

Karasek M, Traczyk WZ, Orlowska-Majdak M, Rubacha G (1980) Quantitative changes of the neurosecretory granules in the rat neurohypophysis after preganglionic stimulation of the superior cervical ganglion. Acta Med Pol 21:351–352

Kostron J, Winkler H, Geissler D, König P (1977) Uptake of calcium by chromaffin granules in vitro. J Neurochem 28:487–493

Kretzinger RH (1976) Calcium-binding proteins. Annu Rev Biochem 45:239– 266

Kumar MSA, Chen CL, Muther TF (1979) Changes in the pituitary and hypothalamic content of methionine enkephalin during estrous cycle in rats. Life Sci 25:1687–1696

La Bella FS, Sanwal M (1965) Isolation of nerve endings from the posterior pituitary gland. J Cell Biol 25:179–191

La Bella F, Vivian S, Queen G (1968) Abundance of cystathionine in the pinal body. Free amino acids and related compounds of bovine pineal, anterior and posterior pituitary and brain. Biochem Biophys Acta 158:286–288

Land H, Schutz G, Schmale H, Richter D (1982) Nucleotide sequence of cloned cDNA encoding bovine arginine vasopressin-neurophysin II precursor. Nature 295:299–303

Lederis K (1961) Vasopressin and oxytocin in the mammalian hypothalamus. Gen Comp Endocrinol 1:80–89

Leng G, Mansfield S, Bicknell RJ, Dean ADP, Ingram CD, Marsh MIC, Yates JO, Dyer RG (1985) Central opioids: a possible role in parturition? J Endocrinol 106:219–224

Léránth CS, Zaborszky L, Marton J, Palkovits M (1975) Quantitative studies on the supraoptic nucleus in the rat: I. Synaptic organization. Exp Brain Res 22:509–523

Lightman SL, Iversen LL, Forsling MI (1982) Dopamine and (D-Ala, D-Leu) enkephalin inhibit the electrically stimulated neurohypophyseal release of vasopressin in vitro: evidence for calcium-dependent opiate action. J Neurosci 2:78–81

Lincoln DW (1969) Correlation of unit activity in the hypothalamus with EEG patterns associated with the sleep cycle. Exp Neurol 24:1–18

Lincoln DW, Russell JA (1986) Oxytocin and vasopressin secretion: new perspectives. In: Fink G, Harmar AJ, McKerns KW (eds) Neuroendocrine molecular biology. Plenum, New York, pp 185–209

Lincoln DW, Wakerley JB (1974) Electrophysiological evidence for the activation of supraoptic neurones during the release of oxytocin. J Physiol (Lond) 242:533–554

Lincoln DW, Hill A, Wakerley JB (1973) The milk-ejection reflex of the rat: an intermittent function not abolished by surgical levels of anaesthesia. J Endocrinol 57:459–476

Lincoln DW, Clarke G, Mason CA, Dreifuss JJ (1976) Physiological mechanisms determining the release of oxytocin in milk ejection and labour. In: The Neurohypophysis. Karger, Basel

Lincoln DW, Hentzen K, Hin HT, van der Schoot P, Clarke G, Summerlee AJS (1980) Sleep: a prerequisite for reflex milk ejection in the rat. Exp Brain Res 38:151–162

Linzell JL (1952) The silver staining of myoepithelial cells, particularly in the mammary gland, and their relation to the ejection of milk. J Anat 86:49–57

Livingston A (1975) Morphology of the perivascular regions of the rat neural lobe in relation to hormone release. Cell Tissue Res 159:551–561

Livingston A, Lederis K (1971) Functional ultrastructure of the neurohypophysis. Mem Soc Endocrinol 19:233

Luqui IJ, Fox CA (1976) The supraoptic nucleus and the supraoptico-neurohypophyseal tract in the monkey (*Macaca mulatta*). J Comp Neurol 168:7–40

Mains RD, Eipper BA, Ling N (1977) Common precursor to corticotropins and endorphins. Proc Natl Acad Sci USA 74:3014–3018

Martin R, Voigt KH (1981) Enkephalins co-exist with oxytocin and vasopressin in nerve terminals of rat neurohypophysis. Nature 289:502–504

Martin R, Geis R, Holl R, Schäffer M, Voigt KH (1983) Co-existence of unrelated peptides in oxytocin and vasopressin terminals of rat neurohypophyses: immunoreactive methionine^5- enkephalin-, leucine^5-enkephalin- and cholecystokinin-like substances. Neuroscience 8:213–227

Micevych P, Elde R (1980) Relationship between enkephalinergic neurons and the vasopressin-oxytocin neuroendocrine system of the cat: an immunohistochemical study. J Comp Neurol 190:135–146

Mikiten TM, Douglas WW (1965) Effect of calcium and other ions on vasopressin release from rat neurohypophyses stimulated electrically in vitro. Nature 207:302

Minchin MCW, Beart PM (1975) Compartmentation of amino acid metabolism in the rat posterior pituitary. J Neurochem 24:881–884

Morris JF (1976) Distribution of neurosecretory granules among the anatomical compartments of the neurosecretory processes of the pituitary gland: a quantitative ultrastructural approach to hormone storage in the neural lobe. J Endocrinol 68:225–234

Morris JF, Cannata MA (1973) Ultrastructural preservation of the dense core of the posterior pituitary granules and its implications for hormone release. J Endocrinol 57:517–529

Morris JF, Dyball REJ (1974) A quantitative study of ultrastructural changes in the hypothalamo- neurohypophysial system during and after experimentally induced hypersecretion. Cell Tissue Res 149:525–535

Morris JF, Nordmann JJ (1980) Membrane recapture after hormone release from nerve endings in the neural lobe of the rat pituitary gland. Neurscience 5:639–649

Morris JF, Nordmann JJ, Shaw FP (1981) Granules, microvesicles, and vacuoles – their roles in the functional compartments of the neural lobe. In: Neurosecretion. Plenum, New York

Nagasawa J, Douglas WW, Schultz RA (1970) Micropinocytotic origin of coated and smooth microvesicles ("synaptic vesicles") in neurosecretory terminals of posterior pituitary glands demonstrated by incorporation of horseradhish peroxidase. Nature 332:341–342

Nakao K, Yoshimasa T, Oki S, Tanaka I, Nakai Y, Wakimasu M, Fujino M, Imura H (1981) Presence of dynorphin-like immunoreactivity in rat pituitary gland and hypothalamus. Regul Pept 2:201–208

Nordmann JJ (1977) Ultrastructural morphometry of the rat neurohypophysis. J Anat 123:213–218

Nordmann JJ (1983) Stimulus-secretion coupling. In: Cross BA, Leng G (eds) The neurohypophysis: structure, function and control. Elsevier, Amsterdam, pp 281–304 (Progres in Brain Research, vol 60)

Nordmann JJ, Chevallier J (1980) The role of microvesicles in buffering (Ca) in the neurohypophysis. Nature 287:54–56

Nordmann JJ, Dreifuss JJ (1972) Hormone release evoked by electrical stimulation of rat neurohypophyses in the absence of action potentials. Brain Res 45:604–607

Nordmann JJ, Morris JF (1976) Membrane retrieval at neurosecretory axon endings. Nature 261:723–725

Nordmann JJ, Stuenkel EL (1986) Electrical properties of axons and neurohypophysial nerve terminals and their relationship to secretion in the rat. J Physiol 380:521–539

Nordmann JJ, Desmazes JP, Georgescault D (1982) The relationship between the membrane potential of neurosecretory nerve endings, as measured by voltage-sensitive dye, and the release of neurohypophysial hormones. Neuroscience 7:731–737

Nordmann JJ, Dayanithi G, Cazalis M (1986) Do opioid peptides modulate, at the level of the nerve endings, the release of neurohypophysial hormones? Exp Brain Res 61:560–566

O'Byrne KT, Ring JPG, Summerlee AJS (1986) Plasma oxytocin and oxytocin neurone activity during delivery in rabbits. J Physiol (Lond) 370:501–513

O'Donohue TL, Dorsa DM (1982) The opiomelanotropinergic neuronal and endocrine system. Peptides (Fayetteville) 3:353–395

Ott T, Scott JC (1910) The action of infundibulum upon the mammary secretions. Proc Soc Exp Biol Med 8:48

Paisley AC, Summerlee AJS (1984) Activity of putative oxytocin neurones during reflex milk ejection in conscious rabbit. J Physiol (Lond) 347:465–478

Palay SL (1955) An electron microscope study of the neurohypophysis in normal, hydrated and dehydrated rats. Anat Rec 121:348–360

Parish DC, Rodriguez EM, Birkett SD, Pickering BT (1981) Effects of small doses of colchicine on the components of the hypothalamo-neurohypophysial system of the rat. Cell Tissue Res 220:809–827

Perlman D, Halvorson HO (1983) A putative signal peptidase recognition site and sequence in eukaryotic and prokaryotic signal peptides. J Mol Biol 167:391–409

Petersen WE, Ludwick TM (1942) The humoral nature of the factor causing the let-down of milk. Fed Proc 1:66–67

Pickering BT (1978) The neurohypophysial neurone: a model for the study of secretion. Essays Biochem 14:45–81

Pickering BT, Jones CW (1971) The biosynthesis and intraneuronal transport of neurohypophysial hormones. Preliminary studies in the rat. In: Heler H, Lederis K (eds) Subcellular organization and function in endocrine tissues. Cambridge University Press, Cambridge, pp 337–357

Pickering BT, Swann RW, Gonzalez CB (1983) Biosynthesis and processing of neurohypophysial hormones. Pharmacol Ther 22:143–161

Pittman QJ (1983) Increase in antidromic latency of neurohypophysial neurons during sustained activation. Neurosci Lett 7:773–808

Pittman QJ, Lawrence D, Lederis K (1983) Presynaptic interactions in the neurohypophysis: endogenous modulators of release. In: Cross BA, Leng G (eds) The neurohypophysis: structure, function and control. Elsevier, Amsterdam, pp 319–332 (Progress in Brain Research, vol 60)

Porter DG (1979) Relaxin: old hormone, new prospects. Oxf Rev Reprod Biol 1:1–67

Poulain DA, Dyer RG (1984) Reproducible increases in intramammary pressure after spinal cord stimulation in lactating rats. Exp Brain Res 55:313–316

Poulain DA, Wakerley JB (1982) Electrophysiology of hypothalamic magnocellular neurones secreting oxytocin and vasopressin. Neuroscience 7:773–808

Poulain DA, Wakerley JB (1986) Afferent projections from the mammary glands to the spinal cord in the lactating rat: II. Electrophysiological responses of spinal neurons during stimulation of the nipples, including suckling. Neuroscience 19:511–521

Poulain DA, Wakerley JB, Dyball REJ (1977) Electrophysiological differentiation of oxytocin and vasopressin-secreting neurones. Proc R Soc Lond [Biol] 196:367–384

Racke K, Ritzel H, Trapp B, Muscholl E (1982 a) Dopaminergic modulation evoked vasopressin release from the isolated neurohypophysis of the rat. Naunyn Schmiedebergs Arch Pharmacol 319:56–65

Racke K, Rothländer M, Muscholl E (1982 b) Ioprenaline and forskolin increase evoked vasopressin release from rat pituitary. Eur J Pharmacol 82:97–100

Rasmussen AT (1940) Effects of hypophysectomy and hypophysial stalk resection on the hypothalamic nuclei of animals and man. Res Publ Assoc Res Nerv Ment Dis 20:245–269

Reaves TA, Hayward JN (1979) Immunocytochemical identification of enkephalinergic neurons in the hypothalamic magnocellular preoptic nucleus of the goldfish *Carassius auratus*. Cell Tissue Res 200:147

Rhodes CH, Morrell JI, Pfaff DW (1981 a) Immunohistochemical analysis of magnocellular elements in rat hypothalamus: distribution and numbers of cells containing neurophysin, oxytocin and vasopressin. J Comp Neurol 198:45–64

Rhodes CH, Morrell JI, Pfaff DW (1981 b) Distribution of estrogen-concentrating, neurophysin-containing, magnocellular neurones in the rat hypothalamus as demonstrated by a technique combining steroid autoradiography and immunohistology in the same tissue. Neuroendocrinology 33:18–23

Richardson KC (1949) Contractile tissue in the mammary gland, with specific reference to myoepithelium in the goat. Proc R Soc Lond [Biol] 136:30–45

Richter D (1983) Synthesis, processing and gene structure of vasopressin and oxytocin. Prog Nuclei Acid Res Mol Biol 30:245–266

Richter D, Schmale H (1984) Vasopressin expression in normal and diabetes insipidus (Brattleboro) rats. TINS 7:317–319

Robinson ICAF, Russell JT, Thorn NA (1976) Calcium and stimulus-secretion coupling in the neurohypophysis. V. The effects of the Ca^{2+} ionophores A23187 and X537A on vasopressin release and $^{45}Ca^{2+}$ efflux: interactions with sodium and a verapamil analogue (D600). Acta Endocrinol (Copenh) 83:36–49

Rossier J, Vargo TM, Minick S, Ling L, Bloom F, Guillemin R (1977) Regional dissociation of β-endorphin and enkephalin contents in rat brain and pituitary. Proc Natl Acad Sci USA 74:5162–5165

Rossier J, Battenberg E, Pittman Q, Bayon A, Koda L, Miller R, Guillemin R, Bloom F (1979) Hypothalamic enkephalin neurones may regulate the neurohypophysis. Nature 277:653–655

Ruppert S, Scherer G, Schutz G (1984) Recent gene conversion involving bovine vasopressin and oxytocin precursor genes suggested by nucleotide sequence. Nature 308:554–556

Russell JT, Thorn NA (1973) Lack of inhibition by colchicine and vinblastine of vasopressin release and calcium efflux from isolated rat neurohypophyses. Acta Physiol Scand 87:20–21A

Russell JT, Thorn NA (1974) Calcium and stimulus-secretion coupling in the neurohypophysis: I. 4S-calcium transport and vasopressin release in slices from ox neurohypophyses stimulated electrically or by a high potassium concentration. Acta Endocrinol (Copenh) 76:449–470

Russell JT, Thorn NA (1975) Adenosine triphosphate dependent calcium uptake by subcellular fractions from bovine neurohypophyses. Acta Physiol Scand 93:364–377

Russell JT, Thorn NA (1977) Isolation and purification of calcium-binding proteins from the bovine neurohypophysis. Biochim Biophys Acta 491:398–408

Russell JT, Hansen EL, Thorn NA (1974) Calcium and stimulus- secretion coupling in the neurohypophysis. III. Ca^{2+} ionophore (A-23187)-induced release of vasopressin from isolated rat neurohypophyses. Acta Endocrinol (Copenh) 77:443–450

Saavedra JM, Palkovits M, Kizer JS, Brownstein M, Zivin JA (1975) Distribution of biogenic amines and related enzymes in the rat pituitary gland. J Neurochem 25:257–260

Sachs H, Takabatake Y (1964) Evidence for a precursor in vasopressin biosynthesis. Endocrinology 75:943–948

Sachs H, Saito S, Sunde D (1971) Biochemical studies on the neurosecretory and neuroglial cells of the hypothalamo-neurohypophysial complex. Mem Soc Endocrinol 19:325–336

Saper CB, Loewy AB, Swanson LW, Cowan WM (1976) Direct hypothalamo-autonomic connections. Brain Res 117:305–312

Saper CB, Swanson LW, Cowan WM (1978) The efferent connections of the anterior hypothalamic area of the rat, cat and monkey. J Comp Neurol 182:575–600

Sawchenko PE, Swanson LW (1982) Immunohistochemical identification of neurons in the paraventricular nucleus of the hypothalamus that project to the medulla or to the spinal cord in the rat. J Comp Neurol 205:260–272

Scharrer E, Scharrer B (1940) Secretory cells within the hypothalamus. Res Publ Assoc Res Nerv Ment Dis 20:170–194

Scharrer E, Scharrer B (1945) Neurosecretion. Physiol Rev 25:171–181

Schmale H, Heinsohn S, Richter D (1983) Structural organisation of the rat gene for the arginine vasopressin-neurophysin precursor. EMBO J 2:763–767

Schon F, Iversen LL (1974) The use of autoradiographic techniques for the identification and mapping of transmitter specific neurones in the brain. Life Sci 15:157–175

Seeburg PH, Adelman JP (1984) Characterization of cDNA for precursor of human luteinizing hormone releasing hormone. Nature 311:666–668

Sharman DC, Holzer P, Holzbauer M (1982) In vitro release of endogenous catecholamines from the neural and intermediate lobe of the hypophysis. Neuroendocrinology 34:175–179

Shaw FD, Morris JF (1980) Calcium localization in the rat neurohypophysis. Nature 287:56–58

Shaw FJ, Bicknell RJ, Dyball REJ (1984) Facilitation of vasopressin release from the neurohypophysis by application of electrical stimuli in bursts. Neuroendocrinology 39:371–376

Shen LP, Pictet RL, Rutter WJ (1982) Human somatostatin: I. Sequence of cDNA. Proc Natl Acad Sci USA 79:4575–4579

Smith V (1970) The origin of small vesicles in neurosecretory axons. Tissue Cell 2:427–433

Sofroniew MV (1983) Morphology of vasopressin and oxytocin neurones and their central and vascular projections. In: Cross BA, Leng G (eds) The neurohypophysis: structure, function and control. p 101–114 (Progress in Brain Research, vol 60)

Steiner DF, Quinn PS, Chan SJ, Marsh J, Tager HS (1980) Processing mechanisms in the biosynthesis of proteins. Ann NY Acad Sci 343:1–16

Sterba G, Hoffman F, Solecki R, Naumann W, Hoheisel G, Schober F (1979) The neurosecretory hypothalamo-hindbrain pathway and its possible significance for the regulation of blood pressure and the milk-ejection reflex. Cell Tissue Res 196:321–336

Stoeckel ME, Hindelang-Gertner C, Dellmann HD, Parte A, Stutinsky F (1975) Subcellular localization of calcium in the mouse hyophysis: I. Calcium distribution in the adeno- and neurohypophysis under normal conditions. Cell Tissue Res 157:307– 322

Suchanek G, Kreil G, Hermodson MA (1978) Amino acid sequence of honey bee prepromelittin synthesized in vitro. Proc Natl Acad Sci USA 75:701–704
Summerlee AJS (1981) Extracellular recordings from oxytocin neurones during the expulsive phase of birth in unanaesthetized rats. J Physiol (Lond) 321:1–9
Summerlee AJS (1982) Phasic patterns of discharge from putative oxytocin neurones in unanaesthetized rats. J Physiol (Lond) 327:43P
Summerlee AJS (1983) Hypothalamic neurone activity: hormone release and behaviour in freely moving rats. Q J Exp Physiol 68:505–515
Summerlee AJS (1986) The neural control of luteinizing hormone release. Prog Neurobiol 26:147–178
Summerlee AJS (1988) Response of putative vasopressin neurones to phenylephrine in male and female rabbits. J Physiol (in press)
Summerlee AJS, Lincoln DW (1981) Electrophysiological recordings from oxytocinergic neurones during suckling in the unanaesthetized lactating rat. J Endocrinol 90:255–265
Summerlee AJS, Paisley AC (1982) The effects of behavioural arousal on the activity of hypothalamic neurons in unanaesthetized, freely moving rats and rabbits. Proc R Soc Lond [Biol] 214:263–272
Summerlee AJS, Paisley AC, O'Byrne KT, Fairhall KM, Robinson ICAF, Fletcher J (1986) Aspects of neuronal and endocrine components of reflex milk ejection in conscious rabbits. J Endocrinol 108:143–149
Swaab DF, Nijveldt F, Pool CW (1975a) Distribution of oxytocin and vasopressin cells in the rat supraoptic and paraventricular nucleus. J Endocrinol 67:461–462
Swaab DF, Pool CW, Nijveldt F (1975b) Immunofluorescence of vasopressin and oxytocin in the rat hypothalamo-neurohypophyseal system. J Neural Transm 36:195–215
Swanson LW (1977) Immunohistochemical evidence for a neurophysin-containing autonomic pathway arising in the paraventricular nucleus of the hypothalamus. Brain Res 128:356–363
Swanson LW, Sawchenko PE (1980) Paraventricular nucleus: a site for the integration of neuroendocrine and autonomic mechanisms. Neuroendocrinology 31:410–417
Swanson LW, Sawchenko PE (1983) Hypothalamic integration: organization of the paraventricular and supraoptic nuclei. Annu Rev Neurosci 6:269–324
Swanson LW, Sawchenko PE, Bérod A, Hartman BK, Helle KB, van Orden DE (1981) An immunohistochemical study of the organization of catecholaminergic cells and terminal fields in the paraventricular and supraoptic nuclei of the hypothalamus. J Comp Neurol 196:271–285
Takabatake Y, Sachs H (1964) Vasopressin biosynthesis: III. In vitro studies. Endocrinology 75:934–942
Theodosis DT (1982) Secretion-related accumulation of horseradish peroxidase in magnocellular cell bodies of the rat supraoptic nucleus. Brain Res 233:3–16
Theodosis DT, Poulain DA (1984) Evidence for structural plasticity in the supraoptic nucleus of the rat hypothalamus in relation to gestation and lactation. Neuroscience 11:183–193
Theodosis DT, Dreifuss JJ, Orci L (1977) Two classes of microvesicles in the neurohypophysis. Brain Res 123:159–163
Theodosis DT, Poulain DA, Vincent JD (1981) Possible morphological bases for synchronization of neuronal firing in the rat supraoptic nucleus during lactation. Neuroscience 6:919–929
Theodosis DT, Chapman DB, Motagnese C, Poulain DA, Morris JF (1986a) Structural plasticity in the hypothalamic supraoptic nucleus at lactation affects oxytocin-, but not vasopressin-secreting neurones. Neuroscience 17:661–677
Theodosis DT, Montagnese C, Rodriguez F, Vincent JD, Poulain DA (1986b) Oxytocin induces morphological plasticity in the adult hypothalamo-neurohypophysial system. Nature 322:738–740
Thorn NA, Russell JT, Vilhardt H (1975) Hexosamine, calcium and neurophysin in secretory granules and the role of calcium in hormone release. Ann NY Acad Sci 248:202–217

Tribollet E, Clarke G, Dreifuss JJ, Lincoln DW (1978) The role of central adrenergic receptors in the reflex release of oxytocin. Brain Res 142:69–84

Tweedle CD (1983) Ultrastructural manifestations of increased hormone release in the neurohypophysis. In: Cross BA, Leng G (eds) The neurohypophysis: structure, function and control. Elsevier, Amsterdam, pp 259–272 (Progress in Brain Research, vol 60)

Tweedle CD, Hatton GI (1980a) Evidence for dynamic interactions between pituicytes and neurosecretory endings in the neurohypophysis of the rat. Neuroscience 5:661–667

Tweedle CD, Hatton GI (1980b) Glial cell enclosure of neurosecretory endings in the rat. Brain Res 192:555–559

Tweedle CD, Hatton GI (1982) Magnocellular neuropeptidergic terminals in neurohypophysis: rapid glial release of enclosed axons during parturition. Brain Res Bull 8:205–209

Vale MR, Hope DB (1982) Cyclic nucleotides and the release of vasopressin from the rat posterior pituitary gland. J Neurochem 39:569–573

Vandesande F, Dierickx K (1975) Identification of the vasopressin producing and oxytocin producing neurons in the hypothalamic magnocellular neurosecretory system of the rat. Cell Tissue Res 164:153–162

Vandesande F, Dierickx K, de Mey J (1977) The origin of the vasopressinergic and oxytocinergic fibers of the external region of the median eminence of the rat hypophysis. Cell Tissue Res 180:443–452

van Leeuwen FW (1981) Light- and electron-microscopical demonstration of Leu-enkephalin immunoreactivity in the rat neural lobe. Neurosci Lett [Suppl] 7:182

van Leeuwen FW (1982) Enkephalin immunoreactivity in fibers terminating in a synaptoid fashion on pituicytes in the rat neural lobe. In: Costa E, Trabacchi M (eds) Regulatory peptides: from molecular biology to function. Raven, New York, pp 203–208

van Leeuwen FW, de Vries GJ (1983) Enkephalin-glial interaction and its consequence for vasopressin and oxytocin release from the rat neural lobe. Prog Brain Res 60:343–350

van Leeuwen FW, Pool CW, Sluiter A (1983) Enkephalin immunoreactivity in synaptoid elements in glial cells in the rat neural lobe. Neuroscience 8:229–241

Vilhardt H, Jørgensen O (1972) Free flow electrophoresis of isolated secretory granules from bovine neurohypophyses. Experientia 28:852

Vizi ES, Volbekas V (1980) Inhibition by dopamine of oxytocin release from isolated posterior lobe of the hypophysis of the rat; disinhibitory effect of β-endorphin/enkephalin. Neuroendocrinology 31:46–52

Vogt M (1953) Vasopressor, antidiuretic and oxytocic activities of extracts of dog's hypothalamus. Br J Pharmacol 8:193–196

Voloschin LM, Tramezzani JH (1973) The neural input of the milk ejection reflex in the hypothalamus. Endocrinology 92:973–983

Vorherr H, Kleeman CR, Lehman E (1967) Oxytocin induced stretch reaction in suckling mice and rats: a semi-quantitative bioassay for oxytocin. Endocrinology 81:711–715

Wakerley JB (1986) Electrophysiology of the central vasopressin system. In: Gash DM, Boer GJ (eds) Vasopressin: principles and properties. Plenum, New York

Wakerley JB, Lincoln DW (1971) Phasic discharge of antidromically identified units in the paraventricular nucleus of the hypothalamus. Brain Res 25:192–194

Wakerley JB, Lincoln DW (1973) The milk ejection reflex of the rat: a 20–40 fold acceleration in the firing of paraventricular neurones during oxytocin release. J Endocrinol 57:477–493

Wakerley JB, Noble R (1982) Electrophysiological behaviour of putative vasopressin neurones in intact brains and hypothalamic slices. In: Neuroendocrinology of vasopressin, corticolibenin and opiomelanocortins. Academic, London

Wakerley JB, Dyball REJ, Lincoln DW (1973) Milk ejection in the rat: the result of a selective release of oxytocin. J Endocrinol 57:557–558

Wakerley JB, Poulain DA, Dyball REJ, Cross BA (1975) Activity of phasic neurosecretory cells during haemorrhage. Nature 258:82–84

Wakerley JB, Poulain DA, Brown D (1978) Comparison of firing patterns in oxytocin- and vasopressin-releasing neurones during progressive dehydration. Brain Res 148:425–440

Watson SJ, Akil H, Fischli W, Goldstin A, Zimmerman E, Nilaver G, van Wimersma-Greidanus TB (1982) Dynorphin and vasopressin: common localization in magnocellular neurones. Science 216:85–87

Weber E, Evans DJ, Barchas JD (1982) Predominance of the animo-terminal octapeptide fragment of dynorphin in rat brain regions. Nature 299:77–79

Wittkowski W, Brinkmann H (1974) Changes of extent of neurovascular contacts and number of neuro-glial synaptoid contacts in the pituitary posterior lobe of dehydrated rats. Anat Embryol (Berl) 146:157–165

Yagi K, Iwasaki S (1977) Electrophysiology of the neurosecretory cell. Int Rev Cytol 48:141–186

Yagi K, Azuma T, Matsuda K (1966) Neurosecretory cell: capable of conducting impulse in rats. Science 154:778–779

Yamashita H, Inenaga K, Kawata M, Sano Y (1983) Phasically firing neurones in the supraoptic nucleus of the rat hypothalamus: immunocytochemical and electrophysiological studies. Neurosci Lett 37:87–92

Zarrow MX, Denenberg VH, Anderson CO (1965) Rabbit: frequency of suckling in the pup. Science 150:1835–1836

Zing HH, Baertschi AJ, Dreifuss JJ (1979) Action of γ-aminobutyric acid on hypothalamo-neurohypophysial axons. Brain Res 171:453–459

Coupling of Electrical Activity and Hormone Release in Mammalian Neurosecretory Neurons

D. A. POULAIN and D. T. THEODOSIS

Contents

1 Introduction

In the world of neurosecretion, the mammalian magnocellular neurons that secrete oxytocin and vasopressin provide excellent models for studying the relationship between electrical activity and hormone release. Their cell bodies are grouped in well-defined areas of the hypothalamus, the supraoptic and paraventricular nuclei; their axons leave the nuclei, course in the hypothalamo-neurohypophyseal tract and terminate in the neural lobe of the hypophysis. In the neurohypophysis, their secretory products are released directly into the bloodstream

Laboratoire de Neurobiologie des Comportements INSERM U176, University of Bordeaux II, 1 rue Camille Saint-Saens, Bordeaux, France

Current Topics in Neuroendocrinology, Vol. 9

and thus can be readily assayed by various methods. These magnocellular neurons constitute, then, a system whose anatomical organization, products of secretion, and patterns of hormone release are rather well established.

As neurons, magnocellular cells receive a very rich synaptic input, and represent the first site of integration of the afferent input of numerous neuroendocrine reflexes which control the release of hormone. In response to this afferent stimulation, the neurons generate action potentials. When one considers stimulus-secretion coupling in neurosecretory cells, the central question, in fact, is to understand how the electrical activity generated by their cell bodies actually governs the release of hormone from their terminals. This first question quickly gives rise to a second, namely, the effect on release of the temporal organization of action potentials generated during the various conditions that lead to secretion.

It should be noted from the start that neurosecretion in mammals does not easily lend itself to an intimate correlation of electrical events and secretion. Ideally, one would like to understand the mechanisms occurring at the level of a single cell with a time resolution close to the time-course of individual electrical events, which is of the order of milliseconds. However, at their best, most studies of this system have correlated an average rate of secretion from thousands of cells, during a period which is usually of the order of several minutes, with an electrical response to a stimulation regime during that period. Nevertheless, as we will see, the mammalian neurosecretory system has provided us with quite a unique repertoire of physiological patterns of electrical activity adapted to generate the temporal patterns of hormone release necessary to meet physiological demands.

This chapter will, in many respects, be quite limited in its scope. Only passing reference will be made to certain morphological and biochemical aspects of hormone secretion that have proved important for our understanding of the cellular mechanisms of release. Control mechanisms exerted on these neurons through their afferent pathways will also not be dealt with. Rather, what we hope to do is to show how the electrical activity of these neurosecretory cells is one of the essential means, and the fastest, by which their cell bodies control, moment after moment, the rate of release of their secretory products into the general circulation in reaction to afferent solicitation.

2 Characteristics of the Electrophysiological Activity of Magnocellular Neurons

Before attempting to understand how electrical activity is correlated to secretory events, it is necessary first to examine how electrical activity is organized within individual magnocellular neurons, along their different parts, and between different neurons located in different cell groups.

2.1 Action Potentials

Magnocellular neurons, like all other neurons, are capable of generating action potentials. An extensive discussion of the mechanisms controlling the electrical activity at the level of their cell bodies is beyond the scope of this article, but they can be briefly summarized into exogenous and endogenous mechanisms. Exogenous control mechanisms are represented by a rich afferent input which, electrophysiologically, results in excitatory and inhibitory postsynaptic potentials and eventually action potential discharge (Dudek et al. 1980; Mason 1983). Endogenous control mechanisms are represented by the ionic bases of somatic action potentials, and of more complex phenomena, such as the regenerative, calcium-dependent, slow potential, or "plateau" potential, underlying the phasic electrical activity of vasopressinergic neurons (Legendre et al. 1982; Andrew and Dudek 1984 a).

More important to our subject is that the neurosecretory axons are able to conduct action potentials. This was first inferred from experiments using electrical stimulation of the neurohypophysis, the magnocellular nuclei, or the afferent pathways to the neurons. Such stimulation evoked hormone release from the neurohypophysis, an effect which was abolished after lesion of the hypothalamo-neurohypophyseal tract (see Sect. 3.2). A direct demonstration of the ability of neurosecretory axons to conduct action potentials was first obtained by antidromic stimulation (Fig. 1 a): when the neurohypophysis is stimulated electrically, action potentials can be triggered in the cell bodies in the hypothalamus (Yagi, Azuma, and Matsuda 1966). Alternatively, electrical stimulation of the pituitary tract evokes orthodromically a compound action potential down to the neurohypophysis, both in vitro (Ishida 1970; Dreifuss et al. 1971; Nordmann and Stuenkel 1986) and in vivo (Fig. 1 b; Dyball and Leng 1987; Dyball et al. 1988). The axonal action potential appears to be of the classical sodium-potassium-dependent type since it is abolished by reducing the concentration of sodium or adding TTX to the medium (Dreifuss et al. 1971).

Action potentials are transmitted between cell bodies and endings in 10–15 ms, which corresponds to a conduction velocity of about 0.5 m/s. The refractory period of the antidromic potential being 3–5 ms, the axons can conduct at rates as fast as 200–300 Hz. Transmission down the axons is thus potentially very rapid, especially in comparison with the long time-course of the endocrine events following hormone release. For example, it takes about 15 s for a bolus of oxytocin released from the neurohypophysis to reach and act on the mammary gland to cause its contraction (Lincoln et al. 1973). However, transmission can be altered during long trains of high-frequency stimulation. In vitro, it was seen that with frequencies above 50 Hz, the evoked compound action potential decreases in amplitude (Dreifuss et al. 1971), while it may even fail from time to time at very slow rates (>1 Hz) of sustained stimulation (Nordmann and Stuenkel 1986). In vivo, transmission slows down and fails to evoke one-to-one antidromic action potentials within 1 min of steady stimulation at frequencies above 20 Hz. This phenomenon is certainly attributable to the small caliber of neurosecretory axons (0.2–0.5 μm in diameter), which would permit a significant rise in the concentration of extracellular potassium during sustained activation (Pittman 1983). Recent observations suggest, however, that such failures of transmission are due more to the in vitro experimental conditions, which do not allow a proper maintenance of the homeostasis of the extracellular space, than to any basic properties of the neurosecretory axons. As seen in Fig. 1 b, orthodromic action potentials re-

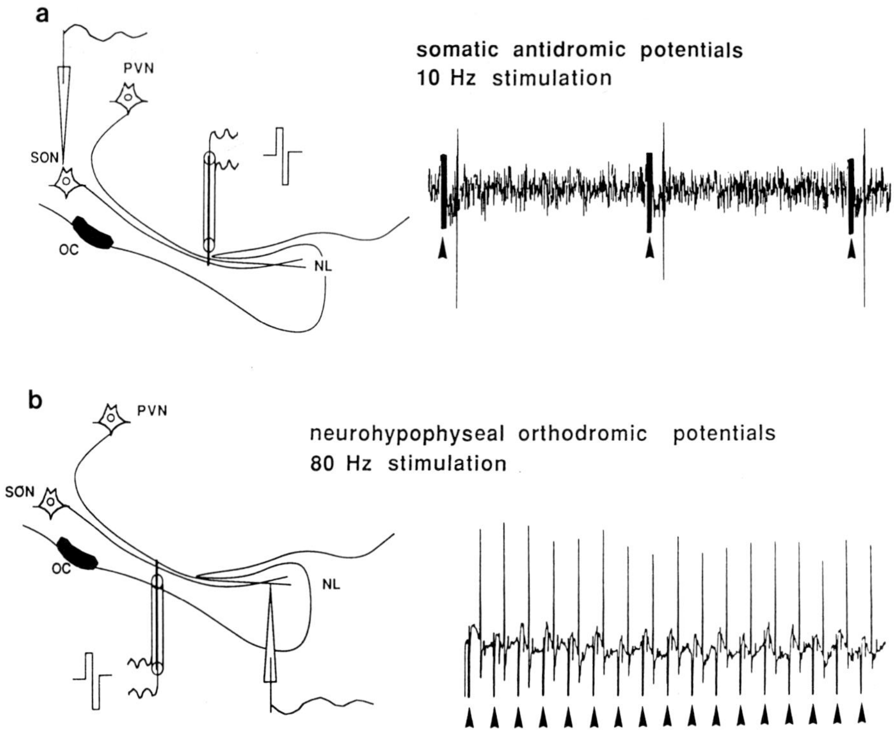

Fig. 1 a, b. Conduction of action potentials along the hypothalamo-neurohypophyseal tract. **a** Antidromic conduction. Using a dorsal approach to the hypothalamus, the neural stalk was electrically stimulated (biphasic pulse of 1 ms, 0.5 mA), and action potentials were recorded extracellularly within the supraoptic nucleus (*SON*) in a urethane-anesthetized rat. Each stimulus pulse (*arrows*; stimulus artifact masked in black) was followed, at the same latency (8 ms), by an action potential. In this experiment, 3-min stimulation at 10 Hz did not modify the latency or the shape of the action potential (personal data). **b** Orthodromic conduction. Using a ventral approach to the base of the brain, the neural stalk was electrically stimulated (biphasic pulses of 1 ms, 0.2 mA), and action potentials were recorded extracellularly from the neurohypophysis (*NL* neural lobe) in a urethane-anesthetized rat. During a 1-s train, note the ability of the axons to conduct orthodromic potentials at fast frequency after each pulse (*arrows*). *PVN*, paraventricular nucleus, *OC*, optic chiasma (from Dyball and Leng 1987)

corded from the neurohypophysis in vivo do follow very high rates of stimulation (80 Hz) for periods of time which are quite compatible with the physiological electrical behaviour of the cells (Dyball and Leng 1987; Dyball et al. 1988).

As for the terminals in the neurohypophysis, their precise electrical properties are still largely unknown. Electrophysiological and optical recordings from the neurohypophysis itself suggest that terminals display action potentials of brief duration (2–5 ms) in response to orthodromic stimulation of the hypothalamo-neurohypophyseal tract (Zeballos 1975; Rothballer and Zeballos 1980; Nordmann and Stuenkel 1986; Gainer et al. 1986; Dyball and Leng 1987; Dyball et al. 1988). However, because of the small size of the terminals (<2 μm in diameter), it is possible that the recorded potentials do not represent the activity of single terminals, but compound action potentials resulting from the activity of a small group of terminals. The issue is important and will be discussed at length in Sect. 3.4, since the electrochemical events set off by the incoming axonal action potentials are essential for stimulus-secretion coupling.

2.2 Physiological Patterns of Electrical Activity

Magnocellular neurons generate action potentials in succession, according to different temporal patterns, which can be described quantitatively by several parameters, although no single parameter will take into account all of their features. At the macroscopic level, so to speak, electrical activity may be considered in terms of frequency of discharge, or firing rate, which represents a number of action potentials per unit of time. In the hypothalamo-neurohypophyseal system, a convenient unit is the second, which provides sufficient resolution of firing patterns. For one given neuron, the record of successive firing rates (sequential record) may be analyzed to calculate the mean overall firing rate, that is, the average of all successive firing rates, a parameter which gives a good estimate of the "intensity" of activation of the neurons. Other analyses can be carried out to obtain histograms of the statistical distribution of firing rates, and, when required, specific parameters such as burst duration, intraburst firing rate, or periodicity in firing.

A further degree of resolution is provided by analyzing interspike intervals. This type of "microscopic" analysis, of the order of milliseconds, is of little help in studying the long-term parameters, of the order of several seconds or minutes, but provides some insight into the minute organization of the successive action potentials. As we will see, it does offer a valuable means of appreciating the efficacy of electrical activity in each type of neuron to the release of their respective hormones (see also Poulain and Wakerley 1982; Poulain et al. 1988).

2.2.1 Sequential Patterns of Firing Rates

Under basal conditions, vasopressinergic neurons generate a *slow irregular pattern* of discharge, characterized by a low mean overall firing rate (<1.5 spikes/s), and a skewed distribution of firing rates, with a peak at zero (Fig. 2). Upon steady activation, such as that observed under osmotic or cardiovascular stimulation, the neurons evolve a bursting or *phasic pattern* of electrical activity (Fig. 3). This consists of bursts of action potentials (range 5–100 s; mode 20–25 s) separated by periods with no action potentials (interburst intervals or "silences": range 5–100 s; mode 20–25 s), occurring more or less regularly. The intraburst firing rate varies between cells from 5 to 15 spikes/s, and the overall mean firing rate is above 2.5 spikes/s with a bimodal distribution of firing rates. Within a burst, there is often an initial peak firing rate, up to 20–30 spikes/s, followed by a stationary phase at a lower rate. In some cases, during a period of increasing stimulation, the neurons may evolve a *fast continuous pattern* of activity, but only temporarily (Fig. 4). In this case, the mean overall firing rate ranges from 3 to 15 spikes/s, but the distribution of firing rates is unimodal.

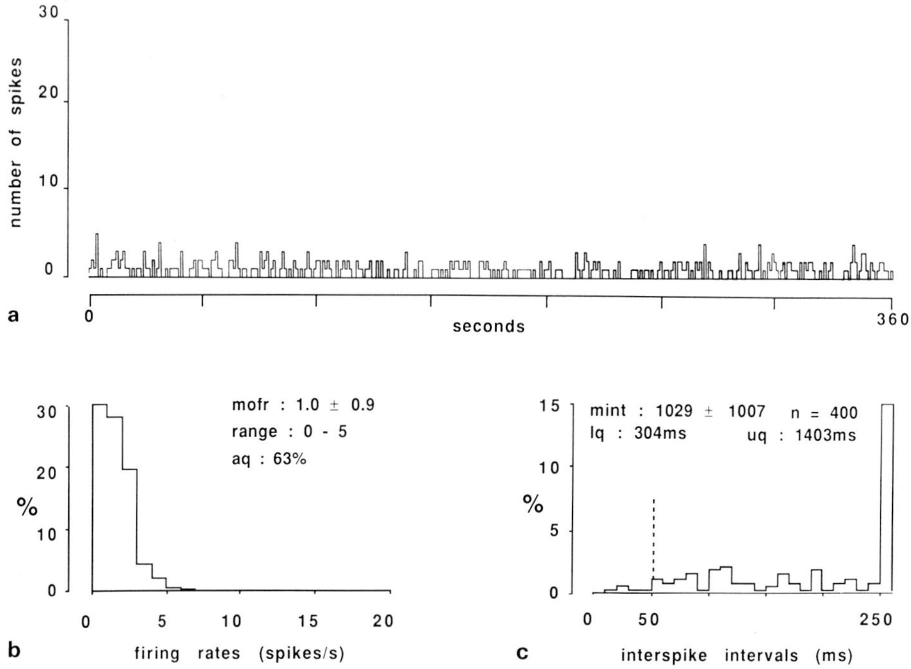

Fig. 2 a–c. *Slow irregular pattern* of electrical activity. **a** Sequential histogram of the successive rates of action potentials (in spikes/s) recorded extracellularly from a rat supraoptic magnocellular cell. **b** Histogram of the frequency distribution obtained from the sequential record above. Note the characteristic asymmetric distribution falling from zero. *mofr*, mean overall firing rate (± standard deviation); *aq*, activity quotient (i.e., proportion of firing rates greater than zero, an index of the amount of time the cell is active). **c** Histogram of the frequency distribution of interspike intervals. *mint*, mean interspike interval (± standard deviation); *n*, number of intervals analyzed; *lq*, lower quartile, i.e., 25% of the intervals are shorter than this value (that is, 25% of the action potentials occur at instantaneous firing rates $\geq 1/lq = 3.3$ spikes/s); *uq*, upper quartile, i.e., 25% of the intervals are greater than this value. The *dotted line* indicates the limit between intervals shorter and longer than 50 ms. The lower and upper quartiles provide an estimate of the dispersion of the intervals. Note that in this type of pattern, intervals have a very wide distribution, but that there is non-negligible proportion of short intervals below 50 ms (in this example 1.75%). The slow irregular pattern, often at a mofr close to 0 spikes/s, is the normal pattern of electrical activity under basal conditions, of both vasopressinergic and oxytocinergic neurons. Compare this with Figs. 3 and 4

During basal conditions, oxytocinergic neurons also display a *slow irregular pattern* of discharge (see Fig. 1) indistinguishable from that of vasopressinergic neurons. Under stimulation, however, the patterns shown by oxytocinergic cells vary according to the type of stimulation. During sustained stimulation (osmotic, cardiovascular), the neurons evolve a *fast continuous pattern* of activity which is similar to that displayed by vasopressinergic cells (see Fig. 4). On the other hand, during parturition and suckling in lactating animals, the neurons exhibit a highly specific activity superimposed on a background activity which is either slow irregular or fast continuous (Fig. 5). In the lactating rat, which nurses her young fre-

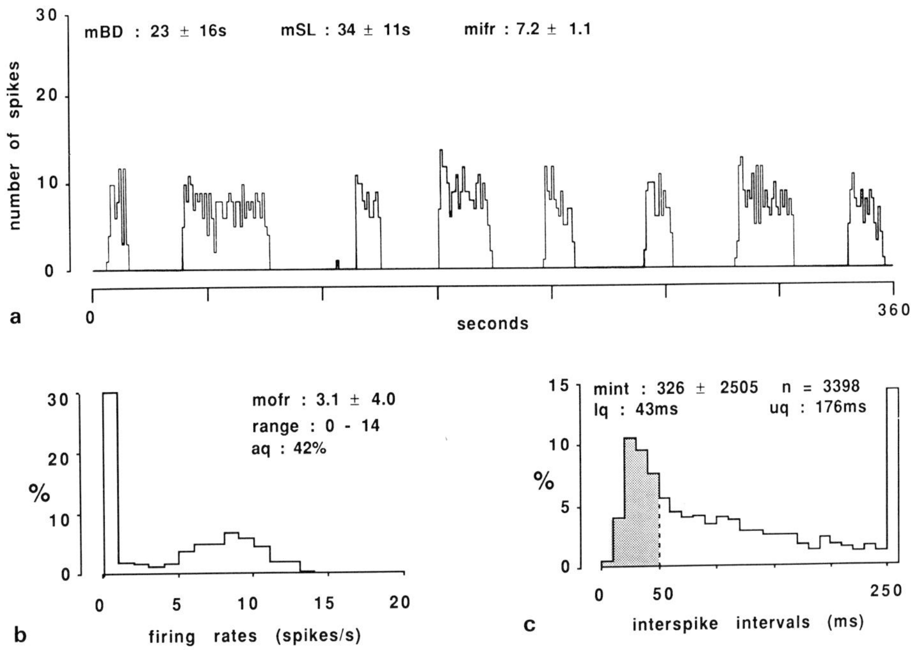

Fig. 3 a–c. *Phasic pattern* of electrical activity. As in Fig. 2, the sequential histogram (**a**) and the frequency distribution histogram (**b**) of firing rates are shown, as well as the frequency distribution histogram of interspike intervals (**c**) obtained from a rat supraoptic neuron. Note the periodicity of the activity (**a**), resulting in a characteristic bimodal distribution of firing rates (**b**), with one peak at 0 spikes/s (corresponding to the silent periods) and another peak at a higher rate (corresponding to the periods of activity). The organization of action potential discharge in periodic bursts results in a low *aq*, a low *mofr*, but a rather high *mifr*. The distribution of interspike intervals shows a large proportion of short intervals below 50 ms (*shaded area*), but yet 25% of the intervals are quite long, as a result of the clustering of action potential discharge in small groups separated by rather long intervals (see Fig. 14 for more details). The phasic pattern is typical of vasopressinergic neurons submitted to tonic stimulation. Abbreviation as in Fig. 2; *mBD*, mean burst duration (±SD); *mSL*, mean interburst interval (silence) duration; *mifr*, mean intraburst firing rate

quently, this consists of periodic *high-frequency discharges of action potentials*, every 3–5 min, that last 3–4 s and are characterized by an initial peak at about 30–100 spikes/s for 1 s, decreasing quite rapidly (Lincoln and Wakerley 1975). In the rabbit, which nurses her young only once a day, several high-frequency discharges occur prior to milk ejection, within a few minutes of each other (Paisley and Summerlee 1984). High-frequency discharges also occur just before the expulsion of each young at parturition (Summerlee 1981).

2.2.2 Organization of Interspike Intervals

There are several features of interest when we examine interspike intervals (see Figs. 2, 3, and 4). Even under strong activation, magnocellular cell bodies rarely exhibit high firing rates and never for a long time. Very short interspike intervals

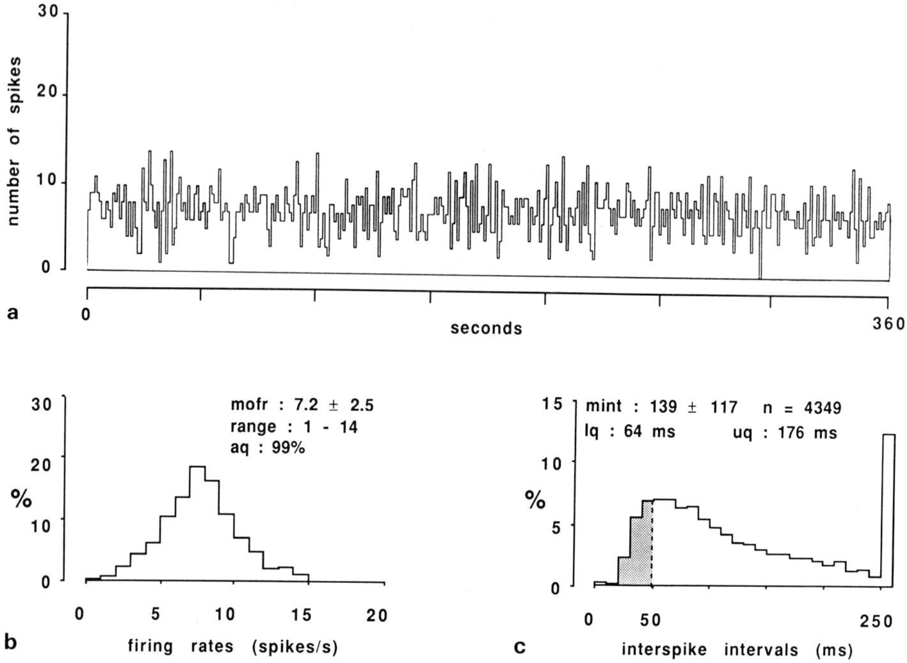

Fig. 4 a–c. *Fast continuous pattern* of electrical activity. As in Figs. 2 and 3, Fig. 4 shows the sequential histogram (**a**) and the frequency distribution histogram (**b**) of firing rates, as well as the frequency distribution histogram of interspike intervals (**c**) obtained from a rat supraoptic neuron. In this case, the activity is more regular, so that almost every second is occupied by the discharge of action potentials. The resulting activity quotient is near 100%. Note the rather symmetric, unimodal distribution of firing rates, in contrast to the bimodal distribution of the phasic pattern; the distribution of interspike intervals, on the other hand, has a similar shape for both types of pattern. As for the phasic pattern, note the high proportion of short interspike intervals below 50 ms (*shaded area*), the paucity of intervals below 20 ms, and the non-negligible proportion of large intervals (above 176 ms), as a result of the organization of action potential discharge in small clusters separated by rather long intervals. The fast continuous pattern is characteristic of oxytocinergic neurons under tonic stimulation. It is seen in vasopressinergic neurones only temporarily before they evolve, or return to, a phasic pattern. Abbreviations as for Fig. 3

below 20 ms (corresponding to an "instantaneous" firing rate above 50 Hz) are extremely rare (see Figs. 2–4), except briefly during a *high-frequency discharge* in oxytocinergic cells. However, the distribution histograms of interspike intervals in all patterns always exhibit a certain proportion of short interspike intervals under 50 ms (Fig. 6), which is always higher than would be expected given a random assortment of intervals. Moreover, a detailed analysis of the sequence of interspike intervals shows that action potentials, whatever the type of activity, tend to occur in little clusters (Poulain et al. 1988). This phenomenon, particularly conspicuous during phasic activity (see Figs. 3 and 14), is even apparent during a slow irregular pattern of discharge, and, as we will see, may be of great consequence to hormone release.

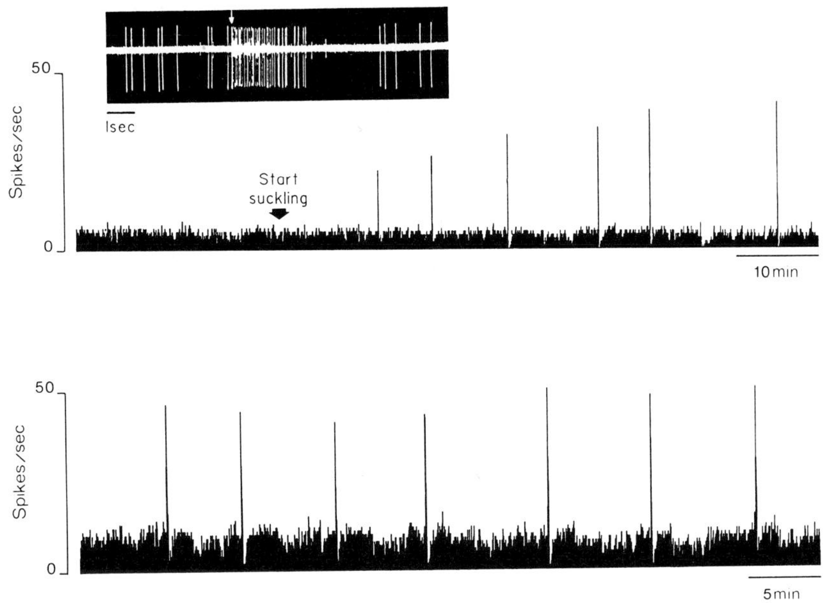

Fig. 5. Activity of oxytocinergic neurons during suckling. Examples of two supraoptic neurons recorded extracellularly from two different urethane-anesthetized lactating rats during suckling. The two sequential histograms of firing rates show the background electrical activity of the cells and the recurrent high-frequency discharges induced by suckling, each one leading to the release of a pulse of oxytocin and then to a milk ejection 12–15 s later. The *inset* shows the photograph of the oscilloscope trace of one such high-frequency discharge of action potentials. On the *upper histogram*, note that the background electrical activity was not influenced when the litter (10 pups) started suckling. High-frequency discharges increased progressively during the first four milk ejections, then reached their maximum firing rate. The *lower histogram* is an example of a fast continuous pattern. Note the regularity of high-frequency discharges from one milk ejection to the next and the short inhibition (about 20 s) following each discharge. Note also the relative irregularity of the pattern over a long time-period. Suckling-induced high-frequency discharges are specific to oxytocinergic neurons

2.2.3 Patterns of Population Activity

In addition to the electrical activity observed at the individual neuronal level, it is also necessary to consider electrical activity at the level of the whole neuronal population. Since vasopressinergic and oxytocinergic neurons occur in different structures in the hypothalamus (the paired supraoptic and paraventricular nuclei and in multiple accessory loci), two questions are particularly relevant in terms of the release of their hormones: first, that of synchronization of the electrical activity of the neurons, and second, that of recruitment, that is, the number of cells activated under stimulation.

Synchronization of neuronal firing has been studied both by occasional and systematic double recordings. In the former case, two different but adjacent neurons, recognizable by two spikes differing in size and shape, were recorded si-

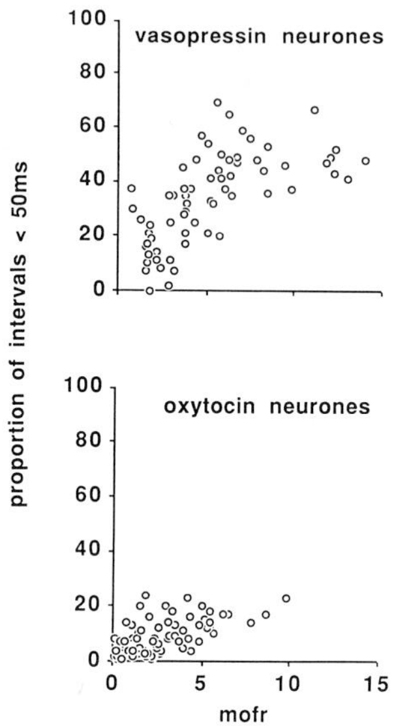

Fig. 6. Proportion of short interspike intervals in magnocellular neurons. Data from a population of 68 vasopressinergic and 77 oxytocinergic supraoptic neurons showing different levels of activity in various groups of dehydrated animals. The plots indicate that whatever the mean overall firing rate (*mofr*), there is a certain proportion of interspike intervals shorter than 50 ms, corresponding to action potentials occurring in small clusters at an instantaneous frequency of 20 Hz or more. In vasopressinergic neurons, the organization of the activity in a phasic pattern as soon as the mofr exceeds 2.5 spikes/s results in a significant increase in the proportion of short intervals, compared with that seen in oxytocinergic neurons at the same mofr. (Wakerley et al. 1978)

multaneously at the tip of the same extracellular electrode (Lincoln and Wakerley 1974). The more systematic approach consists in recording two neurons simultaneously with two different electrodes, a technique which also permits an appreciation of synchronization of neuronal activity between different nuclei (Belin et al. 1984; Belin and Moos 1985). Such recordings have revealed that adjacent vasopressinergic neurons display different levels of firing (in terms of mean overall firing rate) and often widely different patterns. For instance, in dehydrated animals with the same osmotic pressure, it was possible to record contiguous, phasically firing vasopressinergic neurons, and it was seen that burst duration varied from 1 to 10 between the two cells (Wakerley et al. 1978). Under sustained stimulation, therefore, there is no synchronization throughout the vasopressinergic population, although this does not preclude some correlation in the electrical activity between adjacent neurons (Fig. 7). As the intensity of stimulation for vasopressin

Fig. 8. Synchronization of high-frequency discharges of action potentials in oxytocinergic neurons. *Top*, sequential histograms of firing rates (spikes/s) from three different neurons recorded simultaneously during suckling in a lactating rat at the time of a reflex milk ejection. Two cells were recorded from the paraventricular nucleus with the same electrode (*PV1* and *PV2*) and further analyzed using a window discriminator (see Fig. 7), while the third neuron (*SO*) was recorded with a different electrode in the supraoptic nucleus. The three cells had a slow irregular pattern of activity. Note the simultaneous occurrence of the high-frequency discharges (numbers indicate the number of spikes in the burst). Nevertheless, on the expanded time-scales (*bottom*), the polygraph records of the three cells, where each vertical line corresponds to a spike, show that there was a time lag between the onset of the bursts from one cell to another, a time lag which was variable from one milk ejection to another. Moreover, there was no synchronization of action potentials between the cells during the bursts. (Adapted from Belin and Moos 1986)

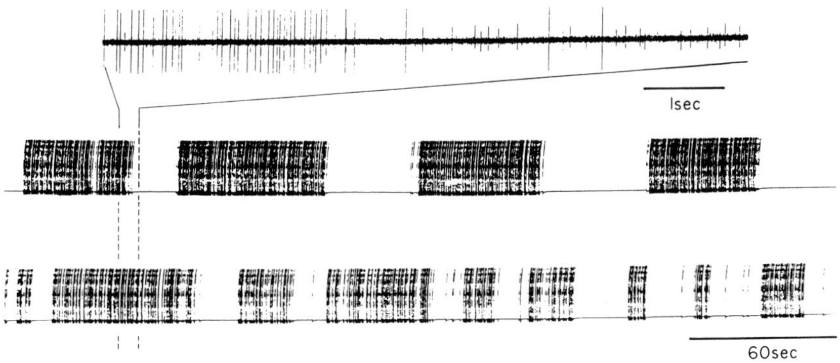

Fig. 7. Asynchrony of action potential discharge in vasopressinergic neurons. Examples of two supraoptic vasopressinergic neurons recorded from the same microelectrode in a urethane-anesthetized rat. The electrophysiological recording was stored on a PDP-11 computer after analog-to-digital conversion at 5 kHz. On the *expanded time-scale (top)*, the original trace replayed from the computer shows large and small action potentials which occur without synchrony (the variations in size of the potentials are due to round-up errors of the analog-to-digital conversion). By filtering out either the small potentials or the larger ones with a window discriminator, simultaneous records of the activity of the large spikes (*middle*) and of the small ones (*bottom*) were obtained on a polygraph, each vertical deflection of the pen corresponding to one spike. Note that the bursts are very different in duration and periodicity from one cell to the other

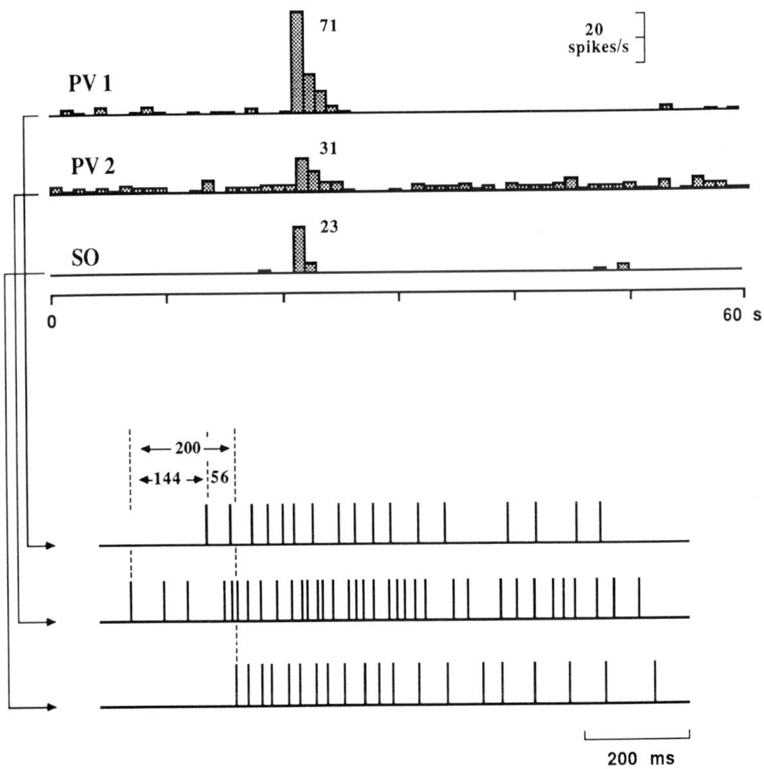

release progressively increases, more and more vasopressinergic cells evolve a phasic pattern of electrical activity. In other words, the vasopressinergic population is recruited into phasic activity with increasing stimulation. Synchronization in vasopressinergic neurons is extremely rare and is always very brief. For example, carotid occlusion, a powerful vasopressin-releasing stimulus (Dreifuss et al. 1976a), or vaginal distension, a stimulus for both vasopressin and oxytocin release during labor (Dreifuss et al. 1976b), can trigger a burst simultaneously in all phasically firing cells.

Oxytocinergic neurons also show no synchronization under normal circumstances. When stimulation is sustained, as during dehydration for example, there is a progressive recruitment of the cells into fast continuous activity, but they are still not synchronized (Wakerley et al. 1978). However, the oxytocinergic population displays a striking example of synchronization of neuronal activity during the milk ejection reflex induced by suckling. At that moment, all oxytocinergic neurons start a high frequency discharge simultaneously (Fig. 8): although there is no spike-to-spike synchronization between cells, the recruitment of the whole population throughout the hypothalamus is immediate and complete within less than 1 s (Belin et al. 1984; Belin and Moos 1985).Synchronization of high-frequency discharges in oxytocinergic cells is also noted at parturition, at the time of expulsion of each young (Summerlee 1981).

Magnocellular neurons thus offer different models of population activity, either asynchronous with progressive recruitment or synchronous with total recruitment. Are such complex organizations of electrical activity limited to their cell bodies or are they propagated down to their terminals? Although it was previously reported that transmission down the axons may fail at very high firing rates (see Sect. 2.1), recent in vivo observations have shown that neurosecretory axons are able to conduct action potentials at rates as fast as those seen in high-frequency discharges for the duration of these discharges (Dyball and Leng 1987); also, action potentials recorded in the neurohypophysis display phasic patterns indistinguishable from those observed at the cell bodies (Dyball et al. 1988).

3 Effect of Electrical Activity on Hormone Release

3.1 Methodological Aspects

Before assessing the role of electrical events in the control of hormone release from magnocellular neurons, we will first consider some methodological aspects of the most widely employed experimental approaches since, as we shall see, each has particular advantages and disadvantages that must be kept in mind for proper evaluation of the results obtained. As noted in the Introduction, the major handicap in these studies is that it is difficult to obtain a close correlation between the secretory and electrical events. Most studies have related an average rate of secretion from the entire gland that takes place in the space of several minutes with electrical responses which occur in a matter of milliseconds. The technological improvements of the past 20 years, both in recording the neurons and in assaying their secretory products, have aimed continuously at refining this correlation.

3.1.1 In Vivo Electrophysiological Methods

Most electrophysiological studies have consisted in electrical stimulation and/or recordings of the system under various experimental or physiological conditions that modify neurohormone release.

The anatomy of the hypothalamo- neurohypophyseal system makes it readily accessible to electrical stimulation, both at the level of the hypothalamus, where the neurosecretory cell bodies and dendrites are concentrated in well-delimited nuclei, and at the level of the pituitary tract and neurohypophysis, composed essentially of the neurosecretory axons and their terminals. This approach has permitted, inter alia, the study of the temporal relationship between electrical activity and hormone release from the neurohypophyseal terminals. Moreover, stimulation of the hypothalamo-neurohypophyseal tract synchronizes the electrical activity in all the fibers, hopefully transforming the entire gland into a "single" secretory terminal. Physiologically, however, the electrical activity of the magnocellular neurons is never synchronized, spike to spike, which may have important consequences in the maintenance of the homeostasis of the system.

Electrical stimulation must obey a certain number of criteria to be physiologically meaningful. Individual pulses must be short (usually in the range of 0.5–1 ms in vivo and up to 2 ms in vitro) and, if possible, biphasic, to avoid artifactual polarization of the stimulating electrode. Bipolar stimulation permits a more precise restriction of the area under stimulation. Stimulation is usually applied in trains of various frequencies, but sustained fast frequencies (>50 Hz) quickly lose their efficiency in terms of hormone release (see Sect. 3.3.2). Earlier experiments used very simple trains of stimulation, made of regularly spaced pulses. With the discovery that neurosecretory cells display complex patterns of electrical activity, a novel approach consists in using stimulation that mimics these patterns. One method is to stimulate through a generator with periodic trains of short duration (5–25 s) made of regularly spaced pulses. A much more accurate simulation consists in storing on a magnetic tape or a computer actual patterns of firing recorded from neurosecretory cells; the recording is then played back into a stimulator, which delivers one pulse to the preparation every time a recorded action potential is played back (Dutton and Dyball 1979; Shaw et al. 1984; Cazalis et al. 1985). We will see that this method has led to a considerable improvement of our understanding of the significance of electrophysiological patterns to hormone release.

To date, most recordings of the system have been conventional extracellular recordings of neurons in the hypothalamus, identified as magnocellular by antidromic stimulation from the neurohypophysis (see Poulain and Wakerley 1982). Recordings in the neurohypophysis are difficult because of the small size of the terminals (ca. 2 μm in diameter). Extracellular recordings may be facilitated by using suction electrodes (Nordmann and Stuenkel 1986). Intracellular recordings have not been made from the neurohypophyseal terminals, which leaves us with many questions related to stimulus-secretion coupling in this system. Recently, the indirect approach of optical recordings with potentiometric dyes (Salzberg et al. 1977; Grinvald et al. 1981) has allowed more precise recording of the time-course of action potentials in the neurohypophysis (Gainer et al. 1986). Another promising possibility is the use of patch clamp recordings of isolated neurohypophyseal terminals or neurosecretosomes (see Lemos et al. 1986).

A more indirect way of appreciating the effects of electrical activity on the release of hormone has been to correlate the electrophysiological activity and the amount of hormone released under conditions which induce a change in both parameters. For example, osmotic stimulation is accompanied by an enhanced release of hormone from the neurohypophysis and by a striking increase in the general activity of the neurons in the hypothalamus. A major inconvenience of these studies is that they do not permit a causal or even a temporal relationship to be made between spike activity and hormone release (for further discussion, see Sect. 3.2). Notwithstanding this disadvantage, such studies have permitted description and correlation of actual physiological patterns of electrical activity with hormone release during particular physiological conditions, a point which must be kept in mind if the aim is to understand the physiological significance of the various parameters of stimulus-secretion coupling.

3.1.2 In Vitro Methods

The fact that the neurohypophysis is fairly well circumscribed and easily accessible for dissection has given rise to many studies on the isolated neurohypophysis maintained under in vitro conditions. After decapitation, the gland can be quickly removed from the skull and maintained in a medium where it will remain viable for several hours. The advantages of such an approach are several: (a) the ionic composition of the medium bathing the gland can be readily modified, (b) different pharmacological agents can be applied, (c) the hormones can be assayed in the bathing medium, and (d) electrophysiological experiments can be performed by stimulating the stalk and recording from the terminals (for a more detailed discussion, see Douglas 1974). Nevertheless, the resolution afforded by such methods still suffers a number of disadvantages. For instance, the rate of sampling for hormone assay is considerably less than the time-course of the electrical and biochemical events actually related to hormone release. Moreover, for still unknown reasons, basal release of both neurohypophyseal hormones is very high in such preparations and such high levels of release may obscure small responses elicited by low-frequency stimulation. Also, until recently, most studies used preparations which in fact included not only the neurohypophysis, but also the adjacent pars intermedia. From recent observations, however, it appears that the presence of the intermediate lobe cannot be ignored since it can considerably affect the rate of at least vasopressin release (Knepel and Meyer 1983). All these factors may thus more or less blur the dynamics of hormone release and their fine relationship to the accompanying electrical phenomena. Recent technological refinements, such as cleaner dissection, the use of small perifusion chambers, which permit the collection of very small perifusates (about 50 μl) at relatively short intervals (1 min) (Bicknell et al. 1982), and the development of highly sensitive radioimmunoassays of the neuropeptides have all considerably improved such an experimental approach.

Another in vitro approach is to isolate the neurohypophyseal endings or neurosecretosomes (La Bella and Sanwal 1965) which, like synaptosomes, retain their electrophysiological properties after isolation. This method offers the possibility of separating the terminals from surrounding cellular elements, such as the pituicytes, and has permitted quite elegant pharmacological manipulations aimed at elucidating the ionic phenomena related to peptide release (see Cazalis et al. 1987a, b).

The entire hypothalamo-neurohypophyseal system can also be isolated and maintained in vitro (Sladek and Knigge 1977; Bourque and Renaud 1983; see also Armstrong et al. 1985). Such preparations offer the advantage of maintaining the axonal connections between the hypothalamic cell bodies and neurohypophyseal terminals relatively intact. A further advantage is the possibility of compartmentalizing each component, in which case each portion can be experimentally manipulated separately. Thus, electrical stimuli or various substances can be selectively applied to either the hypothalamic or pituitary portions and the medium bathing each portion subsequently assayed separately. However, the dissected hypothamic areas include structures other than the magnocellular nuclei, such as the perinuclear areas, which contain elements that may significantly affect the activation of the magnocellular neurons and therefore hormone release.

3.1.3 Evaluation of Hormone Release

Release of the neurohypophyseal hormones may be evaluated indirectly, by measuring other parameters known to be linked to hormone release, or directly, by various bio- or radioimmunological assays.

In vivo, the levels of circulating neurohypophyseal hormones can be assayed indirectly by monitoring the response of the target organ to the hormones as, for example, the vasopressor or antidiuretic response to vasopressin, or the contraction of the mammary gland or the uterus in response to oxytocin. Although this on-line approach can be very convenient in establishing the temporal relationship between an experimental manipulation and hormone release, the responses of the target organs have their own kinetics which may mask the kinetics of hormone release per se. For example, in lactating rats, 1 mU oxytocin injected intravenously causes a brisk milk ejection within 15 s; the same dose administered over 2 min will evoke no response, while a rate of 1 mU/min given over 10 min will evoke, after 2–4 min, recurrent intramammary pressure oscillations, whose periodicity has no counterpart in the plasma level of hormone, which remains constant (Poulain and Tasker 1985).

More direct bio- or radioimmunoassay procedures consist in assaying the levels of neurohypophyseal hormones in samples of plasma or media that have bathed the in vitro preparations. The bioassays are based on the physiological effects exerted by the hormones on their targets, such as the vasculature, kidney, mammary gland, and uterus. They are the oldest methods, and, although they are rather cumbersome to carry out, they have proven and continue to be highly sensitive. Moreover, they provide information about biologically active material.

The development of highly sensitive radioimmunoassays for vasopressin and oxytocin has several advantages, including the possibility of analyzing numerous samples. One disadvantage, however, is that both biologically active and inactive substances are assayed by such methods and this may lead to an incorrect appreciation of the actual dynamics of release of the biologically active principles (for further discussion, see Robinson 1985).

In vivo, both bio- and radioimmunoassays still necessitate relatively large amounts of blood for sampling. This is a major disadvantage in small animals where repetitive blood sampling results very quickly in "hemorrhage", a powerful stimulus for the release of both neurohypophyseal hormones, which then must be considered in addition to the original experimental situation. Finally, in vitro, to appreciate correctly the rate of secretion from the neurosecretory terminals, one has to take into account that the peptides diffuse slowly out of the gland to reach the medium in which they will be assayed (Ingram et al. 1982).

3.2 Action Potentials: A Prerequisite for Hormone Release

As we said earlier, the various stimuli received by the neurosecretory neurons through their synaptic connections set up impulses in their cell bodies which are propagated down to their terminals. Are action potentials per se then capable of and necessary for eliciting hormone release?

Electrophysiological observations obtained in vivo are of little help in giving a definite answer to this question. The electrical activity is recorded from one or at the most two neurons, within a time-span of seconds, but the amount of hormone released is that provided by the whole neuronal population, and over a time-course of minutes. Moreover, we now know that the electrical activity of the whole population of vasopressinergic cells during osmotic stimulation represents a wide spectrum of levels and patterns of firing (see Sect. 2.2.3). A direct causal relationship between hormone release and overall population electrical activity may be envisioned only for the oxytocinergic system when it is activated at milk ejection or parturition; under these stimuli, all oxytocinergic neurons show a similar pattern of electrical activity which is synchronized across the entire population and which systematically precedes the release of hormone (Lincoln and Wakerley 1975; Belin et al. 1984).

Nevertheless, it must be kept in mind that most of the afferent input to the hypothalamo-neurohypophyseal system is at the level of the cell bodies and dendrites in the hypothalamus, while hormone release takes place some millimeters away in the neurohypophysis. Very early experiments had shown that neurohypophyseal hormone release depends on the integrity of the hypothalamo-neurohypophyseal tract, the only connection between the magnocellular cell bodies and their terminals (Ranson et al. 1938), and that in terms of hormone release, this connection is electrical. Haterius and Ferguson (1938) had demonstrated that electrical stimulation of the tract enhanced uterine contractility in rabbits, an effect which was abolished by coagulating the tract. Later experiments revealed that such electrical stimulation also had appreciable effects on antidiuretic (Harris 1948) and milk-ejecting (Harris et al. 1969) activities. A step further in such reasoning consisted in studying the isolated neurohypophysis in vitro, and indeed, in such preparations, more hormone was released when the gland was stimulated electrically (Douglas and Poisner 1964; see also Douglas 1974).

Both in vivo and in vitro, the site of stimulation is distant from the site of release, so the effect on hormone output can be due only to action potentials that are triggered by the electrical stimuli and are propagated down the axons. This becomes particularly clear in in vitro preparations, where stimulation of the stalk evokes a compound action potential at the same time as it induces hormone release; blockade of axonal action potentials by TTX concomitantly arrests secretion (Dreifuss et al. 1971; see Douglas 1974).

3.3 Temporal Organization of Electrical Activity and Hormone Release

That action potentials are necessary for neurohypophyseal secretion does not mean that each action potential is equipotent, releasing a fixed amount of hormone, and that the amount of hormone released, therefore, depends solely on the number of action potentials arriving at the neurohypophyseal terminals. As in the secretion of transmitters at more classical synapses, current evidence has clearly shown that the effect of action potentials on neurohypophyseal hormone release depends on other parameters of the organization of spike discharge, such as its frequency and periodicity. Before we examine how the natural patterns of electrical activity govern hormone release, we should first consider certain basic principles obtained from experimental manipulations, namely, those of frequency facilitation and progressive "fatigue" of hormone release.

3.3.1 Frequency Facilitation

Frequency facilitation of hormone release consists in an increase in the amount of hormone released per pulse at relatively high frequencies of stimulation. In vivo, the response of the mammary gland to electrical stimulation of the neurohypophysis in lactating animals provides an excellent example of such frequency facilitation: the amplitude of milk ejections is maximal at stimulation frequencies of about 30–50 Hz (Harris et al. 1969), which corresponds to the greatest amount of oxytocin released in the blood (Ellendorff et al. 1982). A more accurate appraisal of the correlation between stimulus frequency and secretion can be obtained in vitro, where the amount of hormone released can be measured directly in the medium bathing the neurohypophysis, rather than from the response of a target organ (see Sect. 3.1.3). Thus, when the neurohypophysis is stimulated with a fixed number of electrical stimuli, there is more hormone released at frequencies around 30–50 Hz than at lower or higher frequencies (Fig. 9; Dreifuss et al. 1971). The upper limit of this phenomenon is reached at frequencies above 50 Hz, at which, as we noted previously (see Sect. 2.1), action potential propagation down the axons quickly fails after a few seconds, at least in vitro.

3.3.2 Influence of the Periodic Organization of Electrical Activity on Hormone Release

Given an optimal frequency of stimulation, the amount of hormone released depends on the number of stimuli, which is proportional to the duration of the train of stimulation (see Fig. 9). Thus, at 33 Hz, 2000 pulses given in 60 s release more hormone than 1000 pulses given in 30 s (Dreifuss et al. 1971). Yet there is also a concomitant process of "fatigue" as the duration of stimulation increases, such

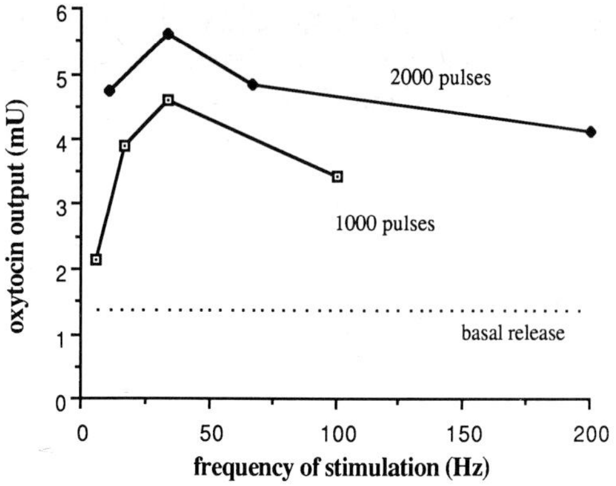

Fig. 9. Frequency facilitation of hormone release and influence of the number of stimuli on hormone release. Isolated neurohypophyses maintained in vitro were electrically stimulated with either 1000 or 2000 pulses applied at various frequencies (pulses of 6-ms duration, 0.5–1 mA amplitude). For each stimulation period (ranging from 30 to 180 s), the glands were incubated 10 min prior to hormone assay to allow for diffusion of hormone out of the gland. With 1000 pulses, note the sudden increase in hormone release when stimulation frequency rose from 5.6 to 16.7 Hz, reaching a maximum at 33.3 Hz. At the same frequencies of stimulation, there was more hormone released with the longer train of stimuli (i.e., when applying twice as many pulses). (Adapted from Dreifuss et al. 1971)

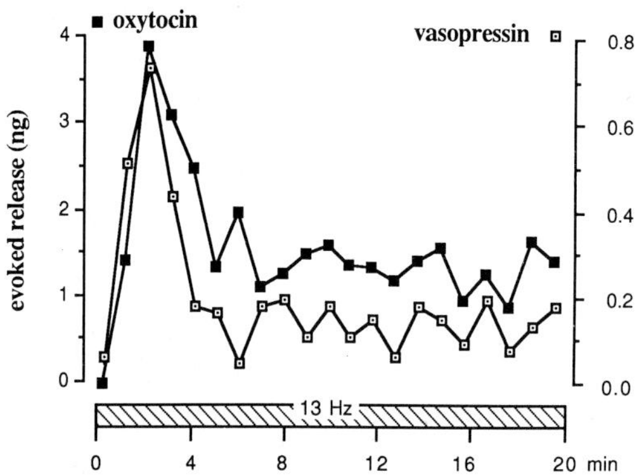

Fig. 10. Fatigue of hormone release during prolonged stimulation. Isolated neurohypophyses in vitro were electrically stimulated at 13 Hz for 20 min, and the perifusion medium was collected every 2 min for hormone assay (data corrected to take into account the low rate of diffusion out of the gland). After 2 min of stimulation, hormone output decreased markedly. Such fatigue was reversible, since after interrupting stimulation for 20 min, another stimulation train produced the same profiles of hormone output. Note that oxytocin output is much greater than vasopressin release. (Modified from Bicknell et al. 1984)

that the amount of hormone released per pulse progressively declines with time (Fig. 10). Thus, when neurohypophyses are submitted to prolonged periods of electrical stimulation at 13 Hz, there is a gradual decline in secretion so that the rate of release of vasopressin, for example, diminishes from an initial peak rate to a plateau level which corresponds to only 10%–20% of that released during the first 4 min of stimulation (Ingram et al. 1982; Bicknell et al. 1984). As we will see later (see Sect. 4), this does not result from a depletion of hormone in the neurosecretory terminals but rather from a progressive failure of the processes related to stimulus-secretion coupling. In any case, the process of fatigue is reversible: when stimulation is interrupted for 20 min, for example, a subsequent train of stimulation will again elicit a high rate of secretion.

3.3.3 Natural Patterns of Electrical Activity and Hormone Release

For a proper evaluation of the role played by electrical activity in the processes of neurohypophyseal hormone release, we should consider how facilitation and fatigue occur during the natural patterns of electrical activity displayed by oxytocin- and vasopressin-secreting neurons, under basal and stimulated conditions of hormone demand.

The high-frequency discharge of action potentials in oxytocinergic cells at milk ejection constitutes the most conspicuous example of a pattern of electrical activity organized to facilitate secretion. As pointed out by Lincoln (1974), the 9000 oxytocinergic cells of the rat hypothalamus produce simultaneously (within 3–4 s) a discharge of 60–100 spikes per cell, which leads to the release of a pulse of 0.5–1 mU oxytocin (i.e., $55–110 \times 10^{-8}$ mU/spike). Under basal conditions with a daily turnover of oxytocin of 25–30 mU (Jones and Pickering 1972), the same neurons have a mean firing rate of 1.0–2.5 spikes/s, thus releasing $1.5–4.0 \times 10^{-8}$ mU/spike. During a high-frequency discharge, therefore, there is about 25–100 times more hormone released per action potential than under basal conditions (see Lincoln 1974). This is certainly an underestimate since these calculations assume a constant firing rate during a high-frequency discharge while, in fact, firing rates reach a high peak rate during the first second, then decline exponentially very quickly during the next 2–3 s.

The phasic pattern of electrical activity of vasopressinergic cells also exemplifies the process of facilitation. In addition, it shows how such a pattern optimizes the efficiency of vasopressin release by overcoming the fatigue of stimulus-secretion coupling that accompanies continual stimulation. In the in vitro experiments of Dutton and Dyball (1979) (see Sect. 3.1.2), tape recordings of phasic patterns were used from various vasopressinergic cells to drive a stimulator and electrically stimulate isolated neurohypophyses (Fig. 11); the effects of these natural patterns were then compared with the effects obtained from regular trains of stimuli generated by the stimulator, taking care that the natural and regular trains produced the same number of stimuli. Such experiments clearly demonstrated that the natural trains of stimuli were considerably more efficient for hormone release, particularly at relatively low mean frequencies of action potential discharge.

The most obvious consequence of the patterning of electrical activity in bursts is that, for a given mean overall firing rate over a long period of time (that is, the total number of spikes during the period of analysis divided by the duration of that period), intraburst firing rates are much higher than the mean firing rate. For example, in the phasic pattern depicted in Fig. 3, the mean overall firing rate is 3.1 spikes/s, but the mean intraburst firing rate is 7.2 spikes/s. During the bursts, therefore, the neurohypophyses are stimulated at a higher rate, which would ex-

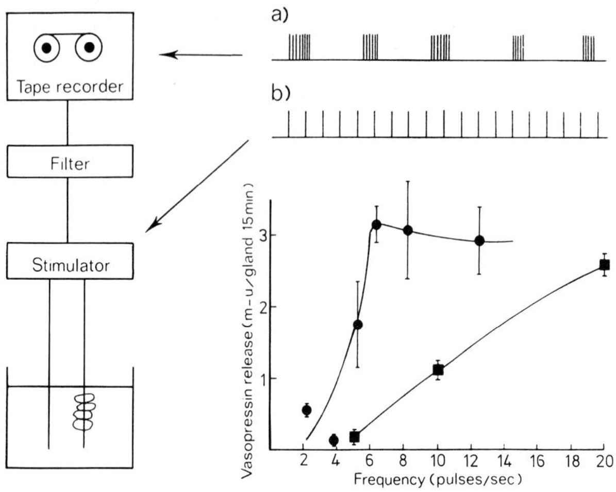

Fig. 11 a, b. Facilitatory effect of the phasic pattern on hormone release. Neurohypophyses incubated in vitro were stimulated electrically, and the amount of vasopressin released was assayed in the medium. The stimulator was triggered either (**a**) by phasic spike trains previously recorded on magnetic tape from vasopressinergic neurons at different levels of activity or (**b**) by trains of regularly spaced pulses derived from an electronic pulse generator. At a mean rate of stimulation above 4 Hz, pulses organized in a phasic pattern derived from the vasopressinergic neurons (*circles*) released more hormone than regular pulses (*squares*). (Adapted from Dutton and Dyball 1979)

plain the better effect on hormone release. However, in the phasic pattern, the intraburst firing rate is not the sole parameter to consider. Burst duration, interburst intervals, and the pattern of discharge within the bursts all contribute to maximize hormone output.

Subsequent in vitro experiments have studied the effects on hormone output by varying each one of these parameters. A first outcome of such studies is the paradoxical observation that the "silent" periods between bursts have a facilitatory effect on hormone release. Thus, stimulating a neurohypophysis with 4 bursts of 27 s, each separated by an interburst interval of 21 s, released more hormone than stimulating with the same 4 bursts with no interburst intervals (Fig. 12). By systematically varying bursts and/or interburst interval duration, it became obvious that hormone release is particularly enhanced for burst durations between 10–30 s and interval durations of about 15–25 s (Shaw et al. 1984; Cazalis et al. 1985). This range of values corresponds closely to those seen in most phasically firing neurons in vivo. In a systematic survey of vasopressinergic neurons in vivo during progressive dehydration, it was notable that, despite quite large variations from one cell to another, bursts and interburst intervals tended to stay at these values, whatever the degree of stimulation: at 6, 12, and 18 h of dehydration, the average burst durations were 20.4, 23.1, and 20.9 s, respectively, while the interburst intervals were 17.4, 12.9, and 13.5 s. In contrast, the intraburst firing rates were closely related to the degree of stimulation, reaching 6.3, 8.9, and 10.5 Hz, respectively (Wakerley et al. 1978).

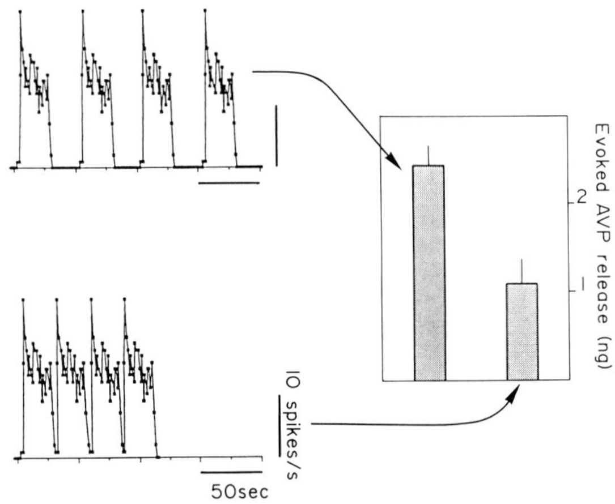

Fig. 12. Influence of the periodicity of stimulation on hormone release. A burst of action potentials previously recorded from a rat supraoptic vasopressinergic neuron was stored on a computer and played back into a stimulator to stimulate neurohypophyses in vitro. The burst was representative of the mean burst duration (27 s) and mean intraburst firing rate (13 Hz) for that cell, the mean interburst interval (silence) duration was 21 s. In this experiment the neurohypophyses were stimulated with four bursts separated by 21-s interval or by no interval. Note the facilitatory effect of intervals on vasopressin release. The evoked release corresponds to the quantity of hormone released during a 30-min incubation period following the onset of the first burst, minus the basal release during that period calculated on the basis of the release prior to stimulation. (Adapted from Cazalis et al. 1985)

Given optimal burst and interburst interval durations, the intraburst firing rate thus appears to be an essential factor for promoting hormone release. However, within a burst, action potentials do not occur regularly spaced. If we examine the burst profile for a cell, we see a clear initial peak of firing rates, lasting 2–3 s, followed by a stationary phase (see Figs. 3 and 12). This is particularly conspicuous for cells with a mean intraburst firing rate above 6.5 spikes/s. The peak of the averaged burst is usually twice this value. In addition, during the stationary phase in cells with a mean intraburst firing rate above 10 spikes/s, there is a significant positive serial correlation lasting up to 1 s between successive firing rates, calculated every 0.25 s. There is thus a certain amount of spike clustering during a burst, not only during its initial peak but also during its stationary phase (see Poulain et al. 1988).

In terms of hormone release, this particular organization of action potentials within a burst has a notable effect, and it is possible to see throughout the burst the processes of facilitation and fatigue coming into play. For example, frequency facilitation is apparent when a neurohypophysis is stimulated with a single burst of 27 s duration and a mean intraburst firing rate of 13 Hz: the natural burst has about twice as much effect on hormone release as a regular train of stimuli of the same duration and the same mean frequency of stimulation as the burst (Fig. 13).

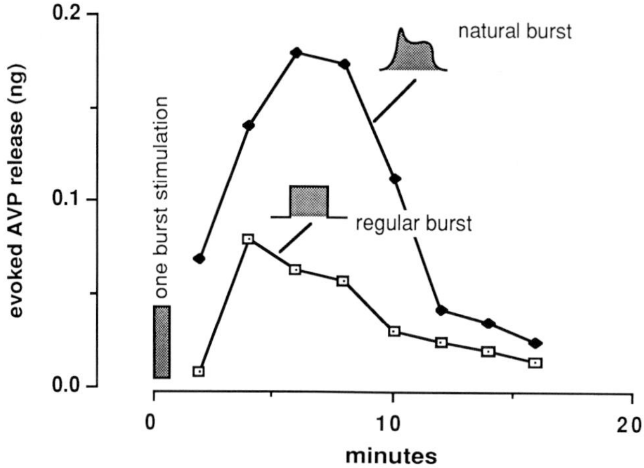

Fig. 13. Influence of the intraburst sequence of action potentials on hormone release. Neurohypophyses in vitro were stimulated electrically with a single train of stimuli (duration 27 s, mean frequency 13 Hz), and hormone release was assayed in the incubation medium, sampled every 2 min for 20 min. Note that the train triggered by the natural burst (the same as in Fig. 12) is about twice as efficient as the train made of regularly spaced stimuli. (Adapted from Cazalis et al. 1985)

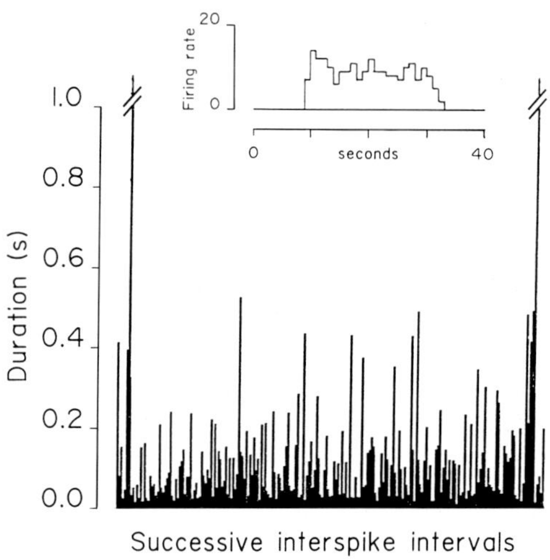

Fig. 14. Action potential discharge within a phasic burst. This burst of potentials derives from the same neuron as that depicted in Fig. 3 (4th burst from the left). The *inset* shows the successive firing rates within the burst. The plot of successive interspike interval durations during the burst clearly reveals how groups of very short intervals (< 50 ms) are separated by longer intervals (about 200 ms or more), a sequential arrangement which probably allows recovery from, or prevents, fatigue processes, even in the course of a burst (further explanation in the text, see Sect. 3.3.3). The very large initial and final intervals (truncated) correspond to the silent periods preceding and following the burst, respectively

Furthermore, the initial high rate of spike discharge within a burst is particularly efficient. By stimulating a neurohypophysis in vitro with the first third of a burst, then with the entire burst, it is possible to calculate that about 75% of the hormone released by the entire burst is in fact released during the first third; during that time, each pulse of a natural burst releases 1.5 times the amount of hormone released by a pulse in a regular train of stimuli. On the other hand, fatigue appears quite rapidly during a burst: in the experimental protocol just described, the amount of hormone released per pulse declined progressively during the last two-thirds (Cazalis et al. 1985).

High-frequency discharges in oxytocinergic cells and phasic patterns in vasopressinergic cells occur when the neurons are strongly activated and release a large amount of hormone. It must be kept in mind, however, that under basal conditions, most oxytocinergic and vasopressinergic cells display a slow irregular activity at a time when the levels of hormones are low (Wakerley et al. 1978). That such low levels of electrical activity contribute to basal hormone release has been difficult to demonstrate, mainly for technical reasons, such as the sensitivity of hormone assays and target organs, or the difficulties of sampling methods. Nevertheless, transections of the pituitary stalk have an immediate effect, inducing diabetus insipidus or stopping basal release of oxytocin, at a time when the gland is still replete with hormones. This suggests that release from the terminals, even under basal conditions, depends on the basal electrical activity of their cell bodies. More recently, in vivo and in vitro experiments have indicated more directly that, indeed, low frequency stimulation can elicit hormone release (Boer et al. 1980; Poulain and Tasker 1985) and, even more important, that natural slow irregular patterns of stimulation in vitro are more efficient for hormone release than regular patterns of the same mean frequencies (see Poulain and Theodosis 1988).

3.4 Stimulus-Secretion Coupling at Neurosecretory Terminals

When incoming action potentials arrive at neurosecretory terminals, they set off a whole series of events which will eventually lead to hormone release. We will not review here all the electrophysiological, biochemical, and morphological mechanisms involved but will limit our discussion to the immediate electrophysiological consequences. Extracellular recordings and optical recordings from the neurohypophysis (see Sect. 2.1) suggest that these terminals themselves display action potentials of brief duration (2–5 ms). We have often noted that the neurohypophyseal system is not amenable to an intimate analysis of electrical and secretory events and that the relationship between trains of action potentials recorded over several seconds or minutes and release from millions of terminals can only be grossly evaluated in comparison with the precise analysis obtained from single terminals, such as those in the giant synapse of the stellate ganglion of the squid or in invertebrate neurosecretory organs (see Cooke 1982). Until now, there have been no intracellular recordings from the mammalian neurohypophysis, and because of the very small size of the terminals, it is doubtful whether there ever will be. This is unfortunate because it prevents us from understanding the precise kinetics of the ionic exchanges essential to secretion and the basis of facilitation and fatigue.

3.4.1 Ionic Bases of Action Potentials in Neurohypophyseal Terminals

The seminal work of Douglas and his colleagues has been followed by numerous studies which now permit us to draw the general outlines of the concept of stimulus-secretion coupling (for detailed reviews, see Douglas 1974; Nordmann 1983). In brief, action potentials (i.e., the stimulus in Douglas' terminology) induce a depolarization in the terminal that permits the entry of calcium and ultimately the fusion of neurosecretory granules to the cellular membrane and exocytosis of their contents into the extracellular space.

The mechanisms leading to release are voltage-dependent, which explains why action potentials, which induce the necessary variations in transmembrane voltage in the terminals, are a prerequisite for hormone release. This was first demonstrated by the elegant series of in vitro experiments of Douglas and his colleagues (Douglas and Poisner 1964; review in Douglas 1974). In order to mimic the depolarizing effect of action potentials, isolated neurohypophyses were exposed to a medium containing a high concentration (56 m*M*) of potassium. Such a maneuver elicited a sustained depolarization. This has been recently confirmed by analyzing the fluorescence of a voltage-sensitive dye loaded into the neurohypophysis: the fluorescence intensity, which increases with depolarization, is also proportional to the concentration of external potassium (Nordmann et al. 1982). It was thus seen that in response to potassium-induced depolarization, hormone release increased in a manner comparable to that obtained by direct electrical stimulation of the gland.

Central to the concept of stimulus-secretion coupling is that the link between depolarization and hormone output is the influx of calcium into the terminal. Absence of calcium in the external medium or blockade of calcium channels prevents the release of hormone elicited either by electrical or potassium stimulation. In this respect, therefore, neurosecretion appears to be just another example of the essential role of calcium in all secretory processes, whether they take place at neuromuscular junctions, synapses, or endocrine and exocrine glands.

Other ions, however, also seem to play a part in the release process. Sodium is not indispensable since electrically or potassium-stimulated release can still take place in sodium-free medium or in the presence of sodium channel blockers. Nevertheless, comparison of in vitro observations after electrically stimulating neurohypophyses in the presence (Dreifuss et al. 1971) or absence (Nordmann and Dreifuss 1972) of sodium currents indicates that hormone release is greater after activation of sodium currents. Potassium also appears to intervene, apparently for two reasons. One is that potassium permits repolarization and thus ends the voltage-dependent calcium current; potassium channel blockers have a facilitatory effect on hormone release evoked by electrical stimulation of the gland (see further, Sect. 3.4.2). The other is that small fluctuations in the external potassium concentration take part in the maintenance of the level of polarization of the terminals. When the neurohypophysis is electrically stimulated in presence of differ-

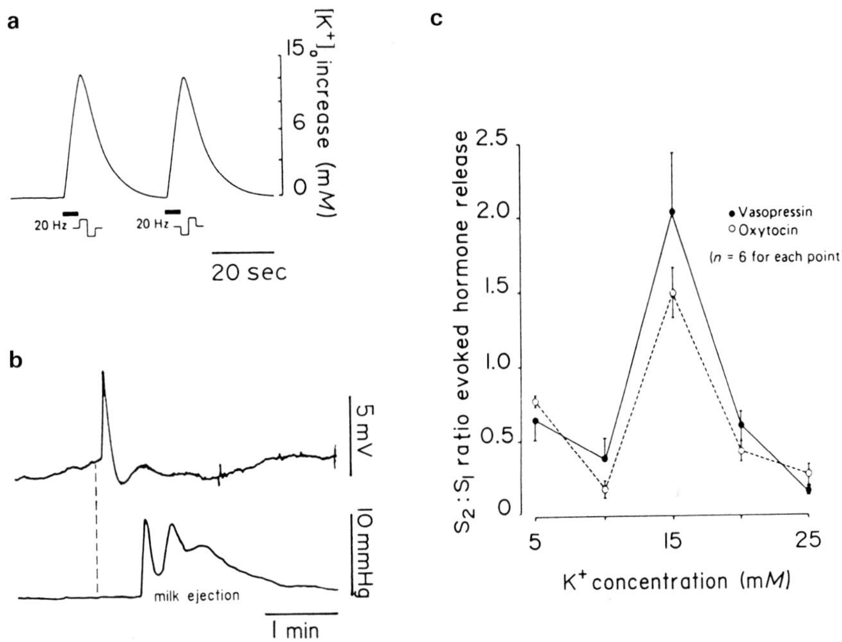

Fig. 15 a–c. Facilitation of hormone release by accumulation of extracellular potassium during electrical activity in the neurohypophysis. **a** Increase in potassium concentration within the neurohypophysis recorded with an extracellular potassium-sensitive electrode in vitro following a 5-s train of electrical stimulation of the stalk at 20 Hz. **b** Polygraph record showing the voltage change recorded from the neurohypophysis with a potassium-sensitive electrode (*upper trace*) along with the intramammary pressure (*lower trace*) in a suckled lactating rat. Note that the milk ejection was preceded by a transient rise in extracellular potassium concentration in the neural lobe, at a time corresponding to the occurrence of a high-frequency discharge of action potentials (see Fig. 5) in the oxytocinergic cell bodies. **c** Effect of external potassium concentration on hormone release. Isolated neurohypophyses were subjected to two identical series of stimulation during 5 min. Between the two trains (*S1, S2*), potassium concentration was raised, and the ratio of evoked release S2/S1 was calculated. Note the facilitatory effect of potassium on hormone output at a concentration of 15 m*M* (**a, b** Adapted from Leng and Shibuki 1987; **c** from Leng et al. 1987)

ent potassium concentrations in the external medium, hormone release is greatly enhanced at concentrations of 15 m*M* (Leng, Shibuki, and Way 1987; Fig. 15).

In electrophysiological terms, therefore, it appears that axonal action potentials in neurosecretory axons give rise to terminal action potentials which are sodium- and potassium-dependent, as are classic action potentials, and also calcium-dependent. It is interesting to note, therefore, that we find a number of membrane properties at the level of the terminals which are similar to those seen at the level of the cell bodies, where somatic action potentials are also sodium, potassium, and calcium dependent (see Andrew and Dudek 1985; Bourque and Renaud 1985).

3.4.2 Ionic Bases for Facilitation and Fatigue

As facilitation and fatigue are both related to the frequency and duration of action potential discharge, it is crucial to understand the time-course of the electrochemical events following the arrival of an impulse in the terminal. The terminal potential seems to have a rather short duration, so that calcium entry, which probably takes place through "late" calcium channels (see Nordmann 1983), must have a brief time-course. By analogy with findings at the neuromuscular junction, it is likely that, during a train of potentials, facilitation is due to an accumulation of calcium within the terminal. Studies of calcium uptake in the neurohypophysis show that hormone output indeed parallels calcium uptake, and that patterns of discharge which greatly facilitate hormone output (for example, the phasic pattern) also greatly increase calcium uptake (Cazalis et al. 1985). The question then is, how does calcium accumulate in the terminal?

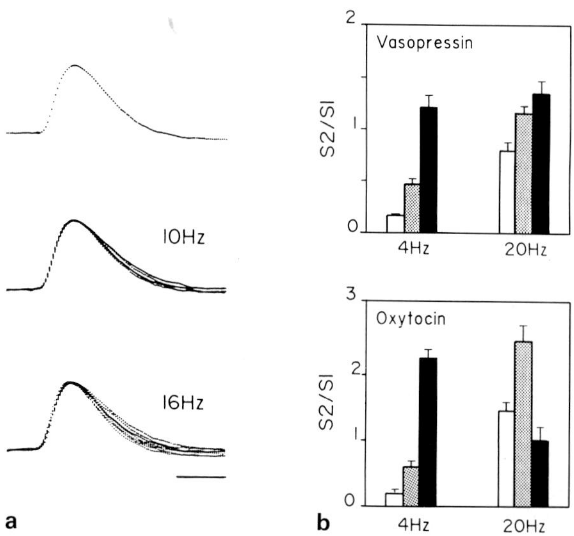

Fig. 16 a, b. Role of potassium currents in hormone release. **a** Optical recordings from a mouse neurohypophysis in vitro using the NK 2367 potentiometric probe. *Top*, single potential upon single pulse stimulation of the neural lobe. *Bottom*, the display shows that during a train stimulation, there was a progressive broadening of the spikes on their repolarizing slope, more evident at 16 Hz than at 10 Hz. Scale line: 5 ms. **b** Influence of potassium channel blockers on hormone release. Mouse neurohypophyses in vitro were stimulated at 4 Hz or 20 Hz in a normal medium (*open bars*) or in a medium containing either 4-aminopyridine (*hatched bars*) or the three blockers 4-aminopyridine, tetraethylammonium, and barium (*solid bars*). In normal medium, as expected, 20-Hz stimulation released more hormone than 4-Hz stimulation. For vasopressin, note that potassium channel blockers permitted an increased release so that, with all three blockers present, 4-Hz stimulation becomes as efficient as 20-Hz stimulation. For oxytocin, at 4 Hz, the blockers facilitated hormone release, but oxytocin release at 20 Hz was reduced with all three blockers. These data suggest that frequency facilitation of hormone release is based in part on the broadening of successive terminal action potentials due to inactivation of potassium channels, thereby permitting a larger calcium entry during the course of the enlarged potentials. (Adapted from Gainer et al. 1986; Bondy et al. 1987)

One possibility is that, during trains of action potentials, there is a gradual prolongation of the terminal potential (Fig. 16). This would result from inactivation of potassium conductances, so that repolarization would take place more slowly, and the voltage-dependent calcium currents would persist longer or increase. This mechanism has been demonstrated directly in various system, in particular in neurosecretory terminals of the crab sinus gland (see Cooke 1982). Evidence that such a phenomenon may also take place in the neurohypophysis has been provided by optical recordings from mouse neurohypophyseal terminals, which do show broadening of the compound action potential (Gainer et al. 1986). In addition, specific blockers of potassium ion channels, which prevent repolarization, enhance frequency-dependent hormone release (see Fig. 16), and this effect is particularly conspicuous at very low stimulation frequencies (ca. 4 Hz) when frequency facilitation is usually not apparent (Bondy et al. 1987). Under normal conditions, it is possible that potassium currents decrease because potassium has accumulated in the extracellular space during a burst of potentials (Leng and Shibuki 1987; see Fig. 15).

In addition to facilitation, we have seen that sustained stimulation leads to a progressive reduction in hormone output per pulse. That such fatigue results from a decrease in the store of hormone available for release can be excluded for various reasons (see Nordmann 1983). It seems, in fact, that there is a gradual uncoupling between the axonal action potential and hormone release. The question, then, is to determine whether such uncoupling is due to a progressive alteration of ionic currents set off in the terminals or to an alteration of other mechanisms taking place just before or during exocytosis. With respect to the terminal action potential, one possibility is that calcium channels are inactivated during maintained depolarization, as suggested by the decrease in calcium uptake noted during prolonged potassium-evoked depolarization (Nordmann 1976). Such inactivation would depend on several factors, all linked to the previous and on-going electrophysiological activity of the terminal itself, namely the level of depolarization of the terminal, previous calcium entry, and the level of external sodium (see Shaw et al. 1983). Alternatively or in addition to this inactivation, there may be a mechanism in the terminals analogous to that seen in magnocellular cell bodies, in which bursts of action potentials (which are also partially calcium-dependent) are followed by a prolonged period of hyperpolarization, possibly through calcium-activated potassium conductances (Andrew and Dudek 1984b).

Nevertheless, in permeabilized neurosecretosomes, hormone release is seen to decrease, despite an elevated concentration of calcium in the cytoplasm. This strongly suggests that the probability of secretory granules participating in exocytosis and thus releasing their contents depends not only on the participation of ionic currents (i.e., calcium entry), but also on the rate of "activation" and "inactivation" of other mechanisms which permit exocytosis (for further discussion see Cazalis et al. 1987b).

Whether such processes of fatigue actually occur physiologically is not certain. We have seen (in Sect. 2.2) that the natural patterns recorded from these neurosecretory cells are made up of short periods of activity, followed by periods with no action potential discharge. High-frequency discharges in oxytocinergic cells are rather brief (3–4 s), which makes it unlikely that fatigue has time to occur. A burst of phasic activity is longer (about 20 s on average) but shows within its time-course fluctuations of firing (see Fig. 12) corresponding to varying intervals between spikes (see Fig. 14). Fatigue can be produced experimentally in vitro during the course of a single burst (see Sect. 3.3.3), and there has been some suggestion that several minutes would be necessary for recovery (Nordmann and Stuenkel 1986). It must be kept in mind, however, that such fatigue may be due to the artifactual in vitro conditions. For example, conduction of action potentials down the stalk quickly fails in vitro, a phenomenon which is not apparent in the intact animal and which suggests that, in vitro, homeostasis of the extracellular space is far from normal. Moreover, in vitro, electrical stimulation is applied synchronously to all axons; such spike-to-spike synchronization throughout the entire gland does not occur in vivo (see Figs. 7 and 8), and may have a considerable influence on hormone release by modifying the external concentration of potassium.

In summary, then, when we consider the natural patterns of electrical activity in any individual neurosecretory cell, it is probable that the temporal organization of successive interspike intervals is such as first, to facilitate release during the small clusters of action potentials, and second, to prevent the establishment of, or to allow recovery from, fatigue during the long interspike intervals, which may reach several hundreds of milliseconds (see Fig. 14).

4 Relation of Electrophysiological Patterns to Pulsatile and Tonic Secretion of Hormone

In Sect. 2.2.3, we described the electrical activity of magnocellular neurons as it appears when considered at the population level. This aspect of neuronal activity is essential as it is in this way that the whole population of either oxytocinergic or vasopressinergic neurons can function as a single gland to meet the requirements of its target organs.

The different models of population activity that we have described correspond to different temporal patterns of hormone release. Thus, during suckling in lactating animals, the release of oxytocin occurs as a single large pulse of hormone that will then permit one milk ejection. The pulsatility of such release is due not so much to the significant activation of individual oxytocinergic neurons (i.e., the high frequency discharge) than to the strong synchronization of the neuronal reaction throughout the entire oxytocinergic population. This can be reproduced experimentally by electrically stimulating the pituitary stalk, or only one of the supraoptic nuclei. Stimulating the stalk with trains of various frequencies and durations shows that the amplitude of milk ejection is maximum for frequencies between 50–60 Hz and durations of 3–5 s, parameters which closely resemble those of the high-frequency discharge. However, if only part of the oxytocinergic population is stimulated with the same parameters, by stimulating a single magnocellular nucleus, the mammary gland response is always smaller.

Under other conditions, the release of either hormone from the gland is tonic. During basal conditions, the concentration of the hormones in plasma is low as a consequence of the slow, irregular, electrical activity displayed by the quasi-totality of the neurons. Under sustained stimulation, by a rise in osmotic pressure for example, there is a recruitment of many vasopressinergic cells into phasic activity, and of many oxytocinergic cells into fast continuous activity, but the activity from cell to cell is very variable and asynchronous. Although release may vary greatly from one moment to another for one neuron, and from neuron to neuron, the global effect for the whole neuronal population is that of a tonic release from the gland.

Thus, hormone output from the neurohypophysis under physiological conditions represents the integrated activity of the whole neuronal population, which tends to overcome the limitations of the activity of the individual neurons.

5 Conclusions

As described at length in this review, the electrical activity generated by the magnocellular cell bodies, in response to their afferent stimulation, is conveyed down to their terminals, where it induces a series of electrochemical events permitting release of hormone into the circulation. The temporal and spatial organization of this electrical activity within each neuron and within the population of neurons determines the amount of hormone released and the temporal sequence of this release in a manner closely adapted to physiological prerequisites.

Although electrical activity thus constitutes a major determinant of hormone release at the neuronal level, one should keep in mind that there are other factors which also play an essential role in the release process in neurosecretory cells. The afferent organization of the neuroendocrine reflexes in which neurosecretory cells represent the final common pathway is one such factor. Thus, the typically synchronized organization of the electrical activity of the oxytocinergic system during suckling-induced milk ejection is not seen during osmotic stimulation of the system. This shows that such population synchronization does not depend entirely on some intrinsic property of the oxytocinergic system, but, at least partly, on the functional organization of its afferences. Likewise, although vasopressinergic neurons have the endogenous property of developing a phasic activity, they show widely different levels of activation and patterns of firing when submitted to the same osmotic stimulus, and this may depend, in part, on afferent or intranuclear connections.

In addition, extrinsic regulation of hormone output can also be exerted on the efferent side of neurosecretory cells, that is, directly at the level of their terminals. For example, there is now quite convincing evidence that opioids inhibit oxytocin release from the neurohypophysis, even though the cell bodies display an intense electrical activity (see Bicknell 1985). Such an effect shows in fact that the control exerted by cell bodies on the secretory activity of their terminals can be uncoupled by a direct action on the terminals, in a form similar to presynaptic inhibition.

Finally, the close adaptation of the firing patterns generated by the magnocellular cell bodies to the secretory capabilities of their terminals – as, for example, the efficacy of phasic patterns to permit recovery from fatigue – raises the interesting question of a possible intraneuronal feedback system, whereby the cell body is informed of the secretory state of its terminal.

References

Andrew RD, Dudek FE (1984a) Analysis of intracellularly recorded phasic bursting by mammalian neuroendocrine cells. J Neurophysiol 51:552–566

Andrew RD, Dudek FE (1984b) Intrinsic inhibition in magnocellular neuroendocrine cells of rat hypothalamus. J Physiol (Lond) 353:171–185

Andrew RD, Dudek FE (1985) Spike broadening in magnocellular neuroendocrine cells of rat hypothalamic slices. Brain Res 334:176–179

Armstrong WE, Gallagher MJ, Sladek CD (1985) In vitro approaches to the electrophysiological analysis of magnocellular neurosecretory neurons. In: Schrier RW (ed) Vasopressin. Raven, New York, pp 395–405

Belin V, Moos F (1985) Paired recordings from supraoptic and paraventricular oxytocin cells in suckled rats: recruitment and synchronization. J Physiol (Lond) 377:369–390

Belin V, Moos F, Richard P (1984) Synchronization of oxytocin cells in the hypothalamic paraventricular and supraoptic nuclei in suckled rats: direct proof with paired extracellular recordings. Exp Brain Res 57:201–203

Bicknell RJ (1985) Endogenous opioid peptides and hypothalamic neuroendocrine neurones. J Endocrinol 107:437–446

Bicknell RJ, Chapman C, Leng G (1982) A perifusion system for studying neurosecretion from the isolated rat neurohypophysis in vitro. J Neurosci Methods 5:95–101

Bicknell RJ, Brown D, Chapman C, Hancock PD, Leng G (1984) Reversible fatigue of stimulus-secretion coupling in the rat neurohypophysis. J Physiol (Lond) 348:601–613

Boer K, Cransberg K, Dogterom J (1980) Effect of low-frequency stimulation of the pituitary stalk on neurohypophysial hormone release in vivo. Neuroendocrinology 30:313–318

Bondy CA, Gainer H, Russell JT (1987) Effects of stimulus frequency and potassium channel blockade on the secretion of vasopressin and oxytocin from the neurohypophysis. Neuroendocrinology 46:258–267

Bourque CW, Renaud LP (1983) A perfused in vitro preparation of hypothalamus for electrophysiological studies on neurosecretory neurons. J Neurosci Methods 7:203–214

Bourque CW, Renaud LP (1985) Activity dependence of action potential duration in rat supraoptic neurosecretory neurones recorded in vitro. J Physiol (Lond) 363:429–439

Cazalis M, Dayanithi G, Nordmann JJ (1985) The role of patterned burst and interburst interval on the excitation-coupling mechanism in the isolated rat neural lobe. J Physiol (Lond) 369:45–60

Cazalis M, Dayanithi G, Nordmann JJ (1987a) Hormone release from isolated nerve endings of the rat neurohypophysis. J Physiol (Lond) 390:55–70

Cazalis M, Dayanithi G, Nordmann JJ (1987b) Requirements for hormone release from permeabilized nerve endings isolated from the rat neurohypophysis. J Physiol (Lond) 390:71–92

Cooke IM (1982) Electrical activity in relation to hormone secretion in the X-organ-sinus gland system of the crab. In: Farner DS, Lederis K (eds) Neurosecretion: molecules, cells, systems. Plenum, New York, pp 235–247

Douglas WW (1974) Mechanism of release of neurohypophyseal hormones: stimulus-secretion coupling. In: Knobil E, Sawyer WH (eds) Endocrinology. American Physiological Society, Washington, pp 191–224 (Handbook of physiology, vol 4, part 1)

Douglas WW, Poisner AM (1964) Stimulus-secretion coupling in a neurosecretory organ: the role of calcium in the release of vasopressin from the neurohypophysis. J Physiol (Lond) 172:1–18

Dreifuss JJ, Kalnins I, Kelly JS, Ruf KB (1971) Action potentials and release of neurohypophyseal hormones in vitro. J Physiol (Lond) 215:805–817

Dreifuss JJ, Harris MC, Tribollet E (1976a) Excitation of phasically firing hypothalamic supraoptic neurones by carotid occlusion in rats. J Physiol (Lond) 257:337–354

Dreifuss JJ, Tribollet E, Baertschi AJ (1976b) Excitation of supraoptic neurones by vaginal distension in lactating rats; correlation with neurohypophyseal hormone release. Brain Res 113:600–605

Dudek FE, Hatton GI, MacVicar BA (1980) Intracellular recordings from the paraventricular nucleus in slices of rat hypothalamus. J Physiol (Lond) 301:101–114

Dutton A, Dyball REJ (1979) Phasic firing enhances vasopressin release from the rat neurohypophysis. J Physiol (Lond) 290:433–440

Dyball REJ, Leng G (1987) Action potential recordings from the rat neural lobe in vivo. J Physiol (Lond) 394:122P

Dyball REJ, Grossmann R, Leng G, Shibuki K (1988) Spike propagation and conduction failure in the rat neural lobe. J Physiol (Lond) (to be published)

Ellendorff F, Forsling ML, Poulain DA (1982) The milk ejection reflex in the pig. J Physiol (Lond) 333:577–594

Gainer H, Wolfe SA, Obaid AL, Salzberg BM (1986) Action potentials and frequency-dependent secretion in the mouse neurohypophysis. Neuroendocrinol 43:557

Grinvald A, Cohen LB, Lesher S, Boyle MB (1981) Simultaneous optical monitoring of activity of many neurons in invertebrate ganglia using a 124-element photodiode assay. J Neurophysiol 45:829–840

Harris GW (1948) The excretion of an antidiuretic substance by the kidney after electrical stimulation of the neurohypophysis in the unanaesthetised rabbit. J Physiol (Lond) 107:430–435

Harris GW, Manabe Y, Ruf KB (1969) A study of the parameters of electrical stimulation of unmyelinated fibers in the pituitary stalk. J Physiol (Lond) 203:67–81

Haterius HO, Ferguson JKW (1938) Evidence for the hormonal nature of the oxytocin principle of the hypophysis. Am J Physiol 124:314–321

Ingram CD, Bicknell RJ, Brown D, Leng G (1982) Rapid fatigue of neuropeptide secretion during continual electrical stimulation. Neuroendocrinology 35:424–428

Ishida A (1970) The oxytocin release and the compound action potential evoked by electrical stimulation on the isolated neurohypophysis of the rat. Jpn J Physiol 20:84–96

Jones CW, Pickering BT (1972) Intra-axonal transport and turnover of neurohypophyseal hormones in the rat. J Physiol (Lond) 227:553–564

Knepel N, Meyer DK (1983) The effect of naloxone on vasopressin release from rat neurohypophysis incubated in vitro. J Physiol (Lond) 341:507–515

La Bella FS, Sanwal M (1965) Isolation of nerve endings from the posterior pituitary gland. J Cell Biol 25:179–191

Legendre P, Cooke IM, Vincent JD (1982) Regenerative responses of long duration recorded intracellulary from dispersed cell cultures of fetal mouse hypothalamus. J Neurohypophysiol 48:1121–1141

Lemos JR, Nordmann JJ, Cooke IM, Stuenkel EL (1986) Single channels and ionic currents in peptidergic nerve terminals. Nature 319:410–412

Leng G, Shibuki K (1987) Extracellular potassium changes in the rat neurohypophysis during activation of the magnocellular neurosecretory system. J Physiol (Lond) 392:97–111

Leng G, Shibuki K, Way S (1987) Facilitation of stimulus-evoked hormone release from the rat neurohypophysis by elevated extracellular potassium concentrations. J Physiol (Lond) 388:14P

Lincoln DW (1974) Dynamics of oxytocin secretion. In: Knowles FGW, Vollrath L (eds) Neurosecretion: the final neuroendocrine pathway. Springer, Berlin Heiderlberg New York, pp 129–133

Lincoln DW, Wakerley JB (1974) Electrophysiological evidence for the activation of supraoptic neurones during the release of oxytocin. J Physiol (Lond) 242:533–554

Lincoln DW, Wakerley JB (1975) Factors governing the periodic activation of supraoptic and paraventricular neurosecretory cells during suckling in the rat. J Physiol (Lond) 250:443–461

Lincoln DW, Hill A, Wakerley JB (1973) The milk ejection reflex of the rat: an intermittent function not abolished by surgical levels of anaesthesia. J Endocrinol 57:459–476

Mason WT (1983) Electrical properties of neurons recorded from the rat supraoptic nucleus in vitro. Proc R Soc (Lond) B 217:141–161

Nordmann JJ (1976) Evidence for calcium inactivation during hormone release in the rat neurohypophysis. J Exp Biol 65:669–683

Nordmann JJ (1983) Stimulus-secretion coupling. Prog Brain Res 60:281–304
Nordmann JJ, Dreifuss JJ (1972) Hormone release evoked by electrical stimulation of rat neurohypophyses in the absence of action potentials. Brain Res 45:604–607
Nordmann JJ, Stuenkel EL (1986) Electrical properties of axons and neurohypophysial nerve terminals and their relationship to secretion in the rat. J Physiol (Lond) 380:521–539
Nordmann JJ, Desmazes JP, Georgescauld D (1982) The relationship between the membrane potential of neurosecretory nerve endings, as measured by a voltage-sensitive dye, and the release of neurohypophysial hormones. Neuroscience 7:731–737
Paisley AC, Summerlee AJS (1984) Activity of putative oxytocin neurones during reflex milk ejection in conscious rabbits. J Physiol (Lond) 347:465–478
Pittman Q (1983) Increases in antidromic latency of neurohypophyseal neurons during sustained activation. Neurosci Lett 37:239–243
Poulain DA, Tasker JG (1985) Recurrent mammary gland contractions induced by a low tonic release of oxytocin in rats. J Endocrinol 107:89–96
Poulain DA, Theodosis DT (1988) Electrical activity of peptidergic neurones and its relation to hormone release. In: Pickering BT, Wakerley JB, Summerlee AJS (eds) Neurosecretion: Cellular aspects of the production and release of neuropeptides. Plenum Press, New York (to be published)
Poulain DA, Wakerley JB (1982) Electrophysiology of hypothalamic magnocellular neurones secreting oxytocin and vasopressin. Neuroscience 7:773–808
Poulain DA, Brown D, Wakerley JB (1988) Statistical analysis of patterns of electrical activity in vasopressin- and oxytocin-secreting neurones. In: Leng G (ed) Pulsatility in neuroendocrine systems. CRC, New York (to be published)
Ranson SW, Fischer C, Ingram WR (1938) The hypothalamo-hypophysial mechanism in diabetus insipidus. Res Publ Assoc Res Nerv Ment Dis 17:410–432
Robinson ICAF (1985) Radioimmunoassay of oxytocin: the standard. In: Amico JA, Robinson AG (eds) Oxytocin, clinical and laboratory studies. Excerpta Medica, Amsterdam, pp 24–30
Rothballer AB, Zeballos GA (1980) Multiple unit activity in rat neurohypophysis. Neuroendocrinology 30:268–274
Salzberg BM, Grinvald A, Cohen LB, Davila HW, Ross WN (1977) Optical recording of neuronal activity in an invertebrate central nervous system: simultaneous monitoring of several neurons. J Neurophysiol 40:1281–1291
Shaw FD, Dyball REJ, Nordmann JJ (1983) Mechanisms of inactivation of neurohypophyseal hormone release. Prog Brain Res 60:305–317
Shaw FD, Bicknell RJ, Dyball REJ (1984) Facilitation of vasopressin release from the neurohypophysis by application of electrical stimuli in bursts. Relevant stimulation parameters. Neuroendocrinology 39:371–376
Sladek CD, Knigge KM (1977) Cholinergic stimulation of vasopressin release from the rat hypothalamo-neurohypophyseal system in organ culture. Endocrinology 101:411–420
Summerlee AJS (1981) Extracellular recordings from oxytocin neurons during the expulsive phase of birth in unanaesthetised rats. J Physiol (Lond) 321:1–9
Wakerley JB, Poulain DA, Brown D (1978) Comparison of firing patterns in oxytocin- and vasopressin- releasing neurones during progressive dehydration. Brain Res 148:425–440
Yagi K, Azuma T, Matsuda K (1966) Neurosecretory cell: capable of conducting impulse in rats. Science 154:778–779
Zeballos GA, Thornborough JR, Rothballer AB (1975) Neurohypophyseal electrical activity in the anesthetized cat. Neuroendocrinology 18:104–114

The Bag Cell Neuroendocrine System of *Aplysia**

F. STRUMWASSER

Contents

1 Introduction

In the opisthobranch mollusc *Aplysia* one aspect of reproduction, egg-laying, is controlled by a neuropeptide hormone named egg-laying hormone (ELH). The primary structure of ELH from *A. californica* has been determined; it has 36 amino acid residues and the C-terminal lysine is amidated (Chiu et al. 1979). ELH is synthesized by the bag cell neurons, which are located in two clusters of about 400 neurons each at the anterior pole of the abdominal ganglion. There are at least three genes coding for ELH or ELH- like peptides in *Aplysia* (Scheller et al. 1983 b). Two of these genes are expressed in the atrial gland, an exocrine gland (Beard et al. 1982) at the end of the reproductive tract (large hermaphroditic duct) which leads to the external genital aperture. The function of these ELH-like peptides, called califins, in the atrial gland are not known, but it has been speculated that they may be pheromones to induce egg-laying in nearby *Aplysia* (Rothman et al. 1986). The third gene is expressed in the bag cells and codes for ELH. This

* Original research presented in this article has been supported by an NIH grant (NS 21046) to the author
Marine Biological Laboratory, Woods Hole, MA 02543, USA

Current Topics in Neuroendocrinology, Vol. 9

chapter deals primarily with the bag cell system in *Aplysia* but some comparative information is included. In the freshwater snail *Lymnaea stagnalis* the caudodorsal neurons synthesize an ELH and are located in the cerebral ganglion (Joosse and Geraerts 1983).

2 Primary Structure of ELH

Figure 1 illustrates the primary structure of three ELHs in two species of *Aplysia* and in the freshwater snail *L. stagnalis*. In spite of about 300 million year divergence between marine and freshwater snails, ELH is 36 residues long in both groups. Furthermore, there is a 40% homology in amino acid residues of ELH of the two *Aplysia* species with *Lymnaea*. It is particularly impressive that there is identical charge conversation in the first 18 amino acid residues of all three species. This implies that the charge distribution in this portion of the molecule may be important in some general property of the polypeptide such as its general conformation, whereas the charge distribution in the remaining half of the molecule may determine species specificity of the interaction with the ELH receptor.

3 The ELH Prohormone

Early studies by Arch (1972), using radiolabeled amino acids to examine the biosynthesis of ELH, indicated that it was processed from a precursor with an apparent molecular weight of 25000 daltons, as estimated from SDS-polyacrylamide (5%) gels. Later studies by Berry (1981) estimated the precursor as 27000–32000 daltons from electrophoresis on SDS-polyacrylamide gels (8%). The intermediate polypeptides, generated during processing, were found to have apparent molecular weights of 16000–20000, 13000–14500, 6000–7000 (pI 7.2), 4500 (pI 4.1) and 2000 (pI 7.5) daltons. These studies were limited by the absence of amino acid composition or sequence data on the intermediates.

Considerable insight into the preprohormone structure was obtained when the gene for ELH was cloned (Scheller et al. 1983b). Poly A mRNA was obtained from bag cells, cDNA was synthesized from it using reverse transcriptase, and a genomic library, constructed from *A. californica* sperm, was screened by ^{32}P-labeled cDNA. It was determined that the gene for bag cell ELH coded for a preprohormone of 271 amino acid residues with eight putative cleavage sites. ELH consists of residues 206–241 within the precursor. After cleavage of the signal peptide, the calculated molecular weight of the ELH precursor is 33000 daltons (Scheller et al. 1983a), which agrees well with the estimate made by Berry (1981) discussed above.

In a recent study, 11 peptides, excluding ELH, have been isolated from bag cell homogenates whose amino acid compositions indicate that they are various fragments of the precursor (Newcomb and Scheller 1987). Table 1 lists the known peptides generated from the precursor in terms of amino acid residue numbers

```
A. c.: H-Ile-Ser-Ile-Asn-Gln-Asp-Leu-Lys-Ala-Ile-Thr-Asp-Met-Leu-Leu-Thr-Glu-Gln-Ile-Arg-Glu-Arg-Gln-Arg-Tyr-Leu-Ala-Asp-Leu-Arg-Gln-Arg-Leu-Leu-Glu-Lys-NH2
                              -       +               -                   -           +   -   +       +               -       +       +           -   +

A. p.: H-Ile-Ser-Ile-Asn-Gln-Asp-Leu-Lys-Ala-Ile-Ala-Asp-Met-Leu-Ile-Val-Glu-Gln-Lys-Gln-Glu-Arg-Glu-Lys-Tyr-Leu-Ala-Asp-Leu-Arg-Gln-Arg-Leu-Leu-Asn-Lys-NH2
                              -       +               -                   -       +       -   +   -   +               -       +       +               +

L. s.: H-Leu-Ser-Ile-Thr-Asn-Asp-Leu-Arg-Ala-Ile-Ala-Asp-Ser-Tyr-Leu-Tyr-Asp-Gln-His-Trp-Leu-Arg-Glu-Arg-Gln-Glu-Glu-Asn-Leu-Arg-Arg-Arg-Phe-Leu-Glu-Leu-NH2
                              -       +               -                   -                   +   -   +       -   -           +   +   +           -
```

Fig. 1. Primary structure of ELH from two *Aplysia* species and a freshwater snail. A.c., *Aplysia californica*; A.p., *Aplysia parvula*; L.s., *Lymnaea stagnalis*. The primary structure of ELH of A.c. is taken from Chiu et al. (1979); ELH of A.p. is taken from Nambu and Scheller (1986); ELH of L.s. is from Ebberink et al. (1985)

Table 1. Peptides isolatable from bag cells that correspond to various parts of the ELH precursor

Peptide	Function
ELH 33– 93	?
ELH 96–100 (β-BCP)	?
ELH 103–107 (γ-BCP)	?
ELH 103–148	?
ELH 110–148	?
ELH 110–144	?
ELH 150–158 (α-BCP 1–9)	Excitatory/inhibitory transmitter?
ELH 150–157 (α-BCP 1–8)	Excitatory/inhibitory transmitter?
ELH 185–203	?
ELH 188–203	?
ELH 245–271 (acidic peptide)	Presumed counter ion in granule

and known or putative functions. As can be seen, functions are known for only two of the peptides, ELH and α-bag cell peptide (α-BCP). The acidic peptide (AP; pI 4.8) which occurs at the end of the precursor is thought to be used as a counter-ion for ELH when stored in the neurosecretory granule. Its function would be similar to that of neurophysin for vertebrate posterior pituitary hormones.

4 Release of ELH

A spontaneous discharge of action potentials always occurs in the bag cells of intact *Aplysia* about 30 min prior to egg-laying (Dudek et al. 1979). These important observations have been made on intact *Aplysia* with cuff electrodes around the posterior pleuroabdominal connectives, the nerves connecting the abdominal ganglion to the pleural ganglia in the head of the animal. The findings clearly indicate that in the intact animal every bout of egg-laying is preceded by a bag cell discharge. The signal inducing this bag cell discharge presumably emanates from one of the head ganglia (cerebral, pleural, pedal ganglia) but neither its exact origin nor what triggers it is known. Gonadectomy does not interfere with the expression or frequency of spontaneous bag cell discharge in otherwise intact *Aplysia*, at least up to 9 days after gonadectomy (Ferguson et al. 1986). This result implies that there is no feedback from the ripening of eggs, in the gonad, to the mechanism in the head ganglia generating the spontaneous bag cell discharge.

In vitro experiments on bag cell clusters have helped to identify the products released during bag cell discharge. When an isolated bag cell cluster is synaptically stimulated for a few seconds, through the pleuroabdominal connectives, an afterdischarge is induced which outlasts the stimulus by about 30 min (Kupfermann and Kandel 1970; Kaczmarek et al. 1978). During the afterdischarge, ELH and AP are released, as well as the nonapeptide α-bag cell factor (α-BCP) and α-BCP 1–8 (Fig. 2). These products have been identified either by using appropriate radiolabeled amino acids in the extracellular medium and allowing adequate time

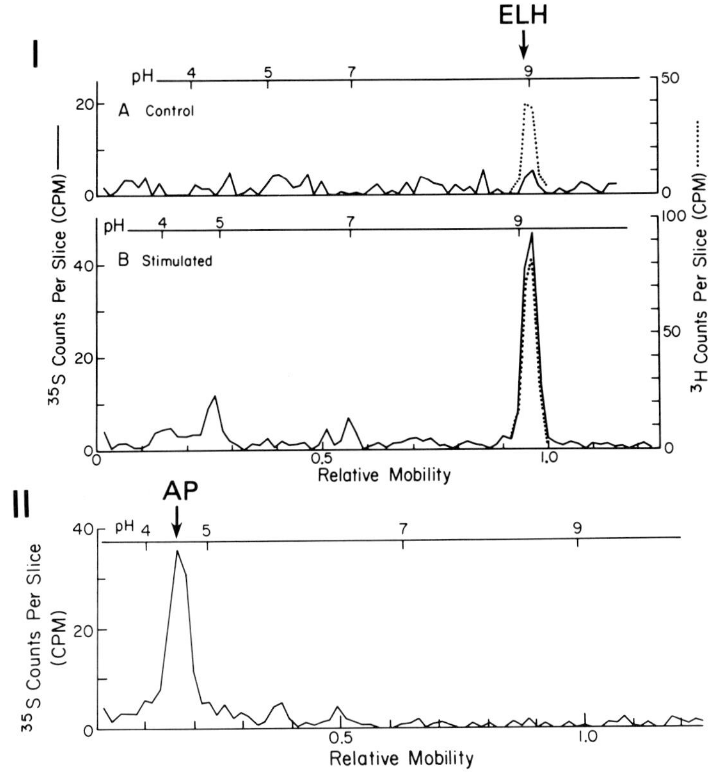

Fig. 2 I, II

Fig. 2 I–IV. Release of ELH, acidic peptide (AP), α-bag cell peptide (α-BCP) and α-BCP 1–8 from isolated bag cell clusters (**I, II, III**) and abdominal ganglion (**IV**) during afterdischarge. In **III**, an isolated bag cell cluster was labeled in ^{3}H-arginine and ^{14}C-leucine simultaneously for 24 h followed by 6 h of rinse medium prior to beginning the experiment. It was then placed in 1.0 ml medium. During the 1-h control period (**III**A) the bag cell cluster was not stimulated but electrical recordings were made. All the medium was removed at the end of the control period and processed as described below. At the beginning of the next hour (**III**B) the bag cell was stimulated to produce an afterdischarge. The afterdischarge persisted for 25 min. The medium was removed and 0.5 ml was applied to a Bio-Gel P-6, 400-mesh gel filtration column kept at 4 °C. Fractions were counted for ^{3}H (———) and ^{14}C (----) with crossover correction. Markers, not run concurrently, are blue dextran 2000 MW 2 000 000 and bovine pancreatic trypsin inhibitor, MW 6500 (●); cytochrome c, MW 12 384 (▲); glucagon, MW 3485 (*); α-bungarotoxin, MW 7904 (▼); bacitracin, MW 1411 (■); leucine (△); and $^{3}H_2O$ (○). Neither cytochrome c or α-bungarotoxin eluted appropriately according to molecular weight. *V*, void peak; peaks 1, 2, 3 are unidentified In **I**A, **I**B and **II** the isolated cluster was first labeled in ^{35}S-methionine as described in **III** above, and after P-6 gel filtration the ELH peak was run on an isoelectric focusing gel to verify that it was ELH (**I**B). The *dotted line* in **I** is ^{3}H-labeled purified ELH which was used as a marker. In **II**, the peak eluting just prior to ELH after P-6 gel filtration (**III**B) was identified from its pI as the acidic peptide (AP). In **IV**, the perfusates of six abdominal ganglia during a 30-min control period (*A*) and during 30 min of an afterdischarge period (*B*) were injected onto a reverse-phase HPLC column (Supelco, LC_{18} DB) and eluted with a gradient of *n*-propanol in pyridine acetate, pH 4.0. *1–7* and *1–8* are fragments of α-BCP (*1–9*) (*D*). Peptides were detected by the fluorescamine reaction. **I, II** and **III** are from Stuart et al. (1980); **IV** is from Sigvardt et al. (1986)

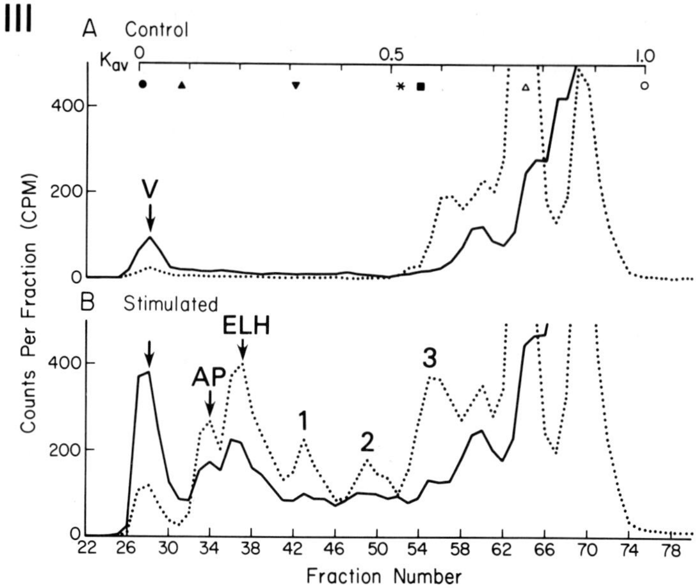

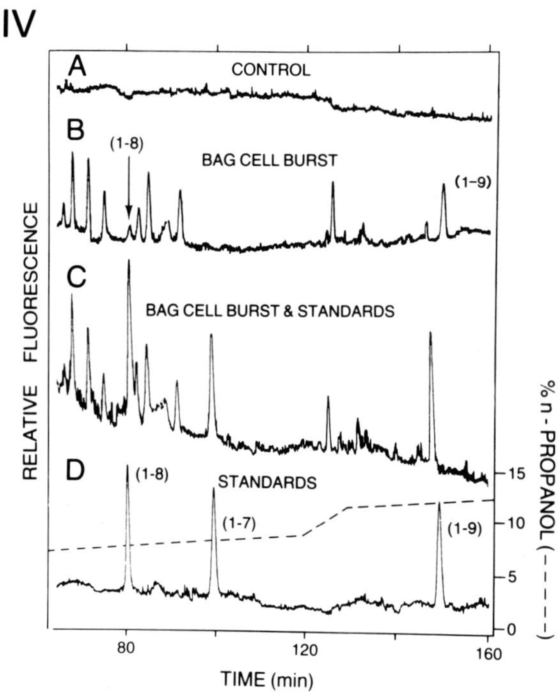

Fig. 2 III, IV (Legend see page 109)

for their incorporation into newly synthesized prohormone and their processing and packaging, or by sensitive detection of non-radioactive peptides by fluorescamine (Stuart et al. 1980; Sigvardt et al. 1986). ELH and AP can be identified by gel permeation chromatography and isoelectric focusing. The molecular weights and isoelectric points of ELH and AP are 4385 daltons and 9.1 (pI) and 4000 daltons and 4.8 (pI) respectively. α-BCP has been identified by its elution time on a C_{18} reversed-phase HPLC column. As Fig. 2 IVD indicates, only two of 13 peaks in the HPLC elution profile have been positively identified (α-BCP 1–9 and 1–8), while in Fig. 2 III only ELH and AP have been identified by isoelectric focusing (Fig. 2 I and II). Assuming that ELH and AP are among the remaining 11 peaks in the HPLC profile, there would still be nine peaks that remain to be identified at the moment.

In the recent study of proteolytic processing of ELH, referred to above, 11 peptides were isolated from bag cell homogenates; these were characterized by amino acid composition and by elution time using HPLC (Newcomb and Scheller 1987). It is difficult without further information to relate these peptides, except for ELH, AP and α-BCP, to the nine other peaks in the bag cell release experiments, because different protocols were used during the HPLC runs.

5 Targets of ELH Action

There is considerable evidence that ELH has direct actions on the gonad as well as the nervous system. The microscopic structure of the gonad has been described by Coggeshall (1970) and Dudek et al. (1980). The unit repeating element in the gonad is the follicle. The follicle contains three types of cells: oocytes and sperm in various stages of maturation, and follicle cells which are purportedly support or nurturing cells. Around each follicle are muscle cells with long processes which are thought to contract and squeeze the eggs out of the follicle. Coggeshall (1970, 1972) argued, on morphological grounds, that ELH caused contraction of the muscle cells around the follicle. Dudek and Tobe (1978) first demonstrated that bag cell extracts have a direct effect on the isolated gonad, inducing egg release. Later, Rothman et al. (1983 a) provided evidence that purified ELH was able to cause egg release in isolated cubes of gonad. Egg release occurred in a dose-dependent manner with applied ELH in the range 1–100 n*M*. The slope of egg release with dose of purified ELH was rather shallow though, with only a two-fold increase in eggs released over a 100-fold to 1000-fold range of ELH.

It is not clear that the muscle cells around the follicle are the target of ELH. Dudek et al. (1980) found that 110 m*M* external K^+ applied to the isolated cubes of gonad did not cause egg release. Based on this finding, they argue that if muscle was involved, the high potassium treatment should have produced contraction and subsequent egg release. This argument, however, can be countered. While a transient or sustained contraction may be expected from the muscle fibers surrounding the follicles in response to high potassium, ELH may induce periodic pacemaker-like contractions in these muscle cells. The periodic contractions may be important in actually getting eggs out of the follicle. There is evidence (see below) that ELH actually induces pacemaker activity in certain neurons.

ELH also has direct actions on neurons in the abdominal, buccal and pedal ganglia. It is interesting that all actions of ELH described to date are excitatory. The neurons activated in the abdominal ganglion include the LB and LC clusters in the left lower quadrant (Mayeri et al. 1985) and R15 in the right lower quadrant (Branton et al. 1978). None of the abdominal ganglion neurons can play an important role in the overt behavior of egg-laying, because in *Aplysia* with the abdominal ganglion surgically removed, normal egg-laying with associated behaviors can be induced by injecting a bag cell extract containing ELH (Strumwasser et al. 1972). Some of the neurons activated in the abdominal ganglion may play

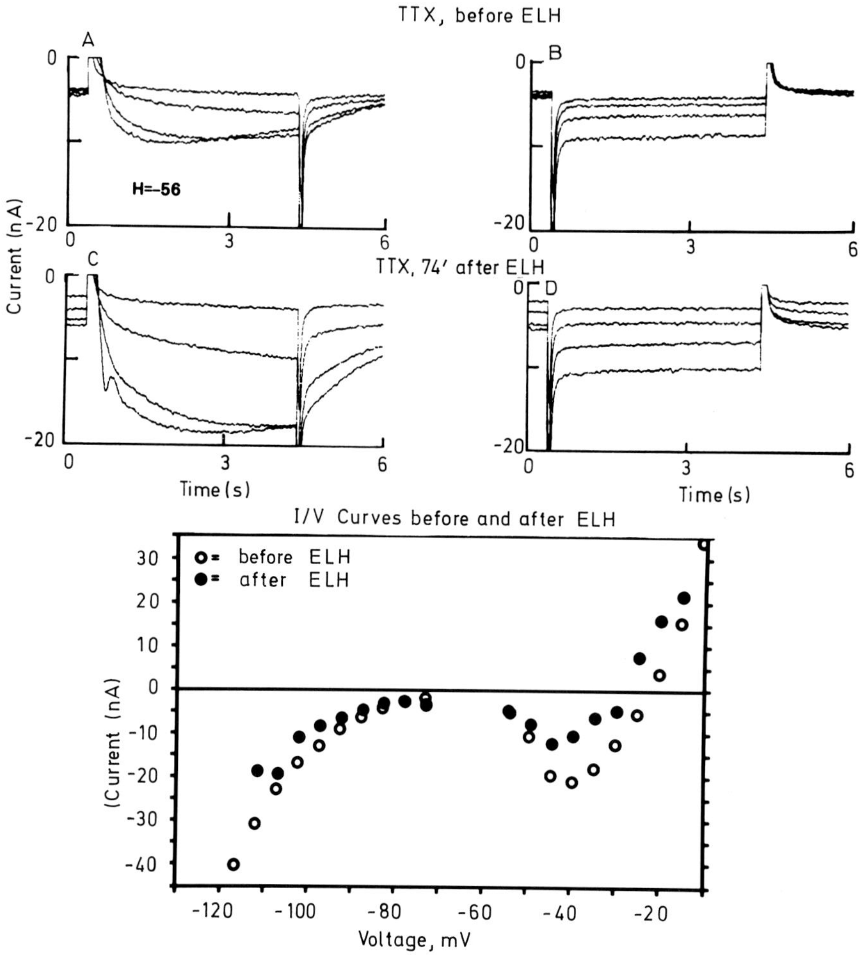

Fig.3. Ionic currents (*top* frames) and I/V relationship (*bottom* frame) obtained in R15, by voltage clamp, before and after application of 18 μM ELH to the bath. The holding potential was -56 mV throughout the records and curves illustrated here. The *left upper* frames are responses to depolarizing commands while the *right upper* frames are responses to hyperpolarizing commands. A sustained inward current (*left* frames) is enhanced after ELH, as well as the anomalous rectifier conductance (*right* frames). (From F. Strumwasser, unpublished, 1986)

a role in respiratory adjustments that may take place during egg-laying. During a bag cell discharge, the frequency of interneuron II bursts, a premotor interneuron for the gill and siphon, is enhanced, resulting in more frequent and larger amplitude contractions of these organs (Schaefer and Brownell 1986).

Targets for ELH in the buccal ganglion may play an important role in the inhibition of feeding that occurs after ELH release (Stuart and Strumwasser 1980). If *Aplysia* starved for 24 h are exposed to 1 g algal food 20 min after an injection of ELH there is no feeding, while control animals injected with head ganglion extracts feed at about 4 min after food is offered. In another behavioral test, food was presented at 10 min after injection of ELH or head ganglia homogenate. Experimental animals started eating at 2 min after food was offered but stopped at 7 min, having only consumed 40% of their food, whereas six of seven control animals continued eating for 12 min until the 1 g food was consumed. These behavioral tests suggest that in the intact animal a signal for inhibition of feeding occurs approximately 17 min after ELH injection. Since eggs are released at 32 min, the inhibition of feeding is independent of the external appearance of eggs.

At least two neurons in each buccal hemiganglion respond to ELH (Stuart and Strumwasser 1980). One neuron has its axon in buccal nerve 3 (see Fig. 1 in Stuart and Strumwasser) and the other has its axon in the cerebrobuccal connective nerve. The former neuron has been identified by intracellular recording as the B16 motoneuron (Ram 1983) which innervates the accessory radula closer (ARC) muscle (Cohen et al. 1978). This muscle keeps the radula of the buccal mass pulled in and could be one of the mechanisms inhibiting feeding. There is some other information about the B16 motoneuron. It is a cholinergic cell which is excited also by serotonin (Ram et al. 1986; Sossin et al. 1987) and inhibited by FRMFamide (Sossin et al. 1987), a cardioactive tetrapeptide discovered by Price and Greenberg (1977). Modulation of the neuronal circuits mediating feeding is said to occur at all levels of the hierarchical organization (central pattern generators, premotor neurons, motoneurons and muscles).

The nature of the ion channels in the membrane that are modulated by ELH are currently under investigation. Kirk and Scheller (1986) find that ELH induces an inward shift in the holding current of a voltage-clamped B16 neuron as well as enhancing a voltage-dependent slow inward current. The nature of this ion channel is not known. In R15, a slow inward current is also enhanced by ELH, as is the inward current due to a sustained hyperpolarizing pulse, the anomalous rectifier channel (Levitan et al. 1987; F. Strumwasser, unpublished 1986; see Fig. 3).

6 Structure-Function Relationship in ELH

Egg-laying hormone has been synthesized by manual or automatic stepwise solid-phase peptide synthesis on a benzhydrylamine resin (Kent and Clark-Lewis 1985). After hydrogen fluoride (HF) cleavage of the product from the resin, purification was performed by reverse-phase HPLC on a Vydac C4 column. Synthetic

ELH 1–36 amide induced normal egg-laying with associated behaviors in *A. californica* in all seven animals tested with doses ranging from 70 to 200 μg (Strumwasser 1984; Strumwasser et al. 1987). More recent studies indicate that about 50% of warm-adapted *A. californica* will respond to 1.5 μg of ELH. Egg-laying is associated with a specific set of behaviors which include inhibition of locomotion, extrusion of the egg string, adherence of the egg string to the substrate and winding of the egg string onto the substrate. All of these components of egg- laying behavior were normal with synthetic ELH. In addition, synthetic ELH induced egg-laying with normal latency and the quantity of egg string produced was normal. We can conclude, therefore, that ELH is sufficient to induce all the behavioral components of egg-laying and that a role for the other peptides released from the precursor during bag cell discharge remains to be established.

In order to investigate structure-activity relationships in ELH, various fragments of ELH have been tested in their ability to cause egg-laying (Strumwasser et al. 1987). Any removal of amino acid residues at the N- terminal end of the polypeptide results in inactivity. Thus ELH 2–36 amide, 3–36 amide, 4–36 amide, 8–36 amide and 14–36 amide are unable to induce egg-laying, even when used at quantities 500–1000 times the threshold for intact ELH (s. above). Subtle changes at the N-terminus such as substituting leucine for isoleucine, do not interfere with egg-laying activity. Large changes at the C-terminus, such as ELH 1–29 amide, result in an inactive molecule, but minor changes, such as ELH 1–35 amide, and even ELH 1–34 amide, still allow-egg-laying.

There is no information, to date, on the tertiary structure of ELH. Another polypeptide in the same size class as ELH is pancreatic polypeptide, which has 36 amino acid residues. The crystal structure of avian pancreatic polypeptide (APP) has been worked out with 0.98-A resolution (Glover et al. 1983). It is interesting that APP is a U-shaped molecule with a reverse turn at Pro 13. In addition, Arg 33 is hydrogen-bonded to residues near the N-terminus (Gln 4, Pro 5). These findings indicate that there are intramolecular interactions between residues near the C- and N-termini in APP. Presumably the U shape of APP plays an important role in how this hormone binds its specific receptor. Whether APP will turn out to be a model of how polypeptide hormones in this size class are shaped and interact with their receptor remains to be determined.

7 Afterdischarge

7.1 General Features

The mechanism by which ELH and related peptides are released from the bag cells is through the afterdischarge property of these cells. The bag cells are ordinarily quiescent cells when studied in the isolated abdominal ganglion or isolated bag cell cluster. When a brief train of synaptic stimuli is induced in the bag cells, one-to-one following responses are generated during the train. After the train of synaptic stimuli, the bag cells start to discharge at a relatively high frequency (4–5 Hz); this discharge peaks within 1 min (Fig. 4). Subsequently, the discharge be-

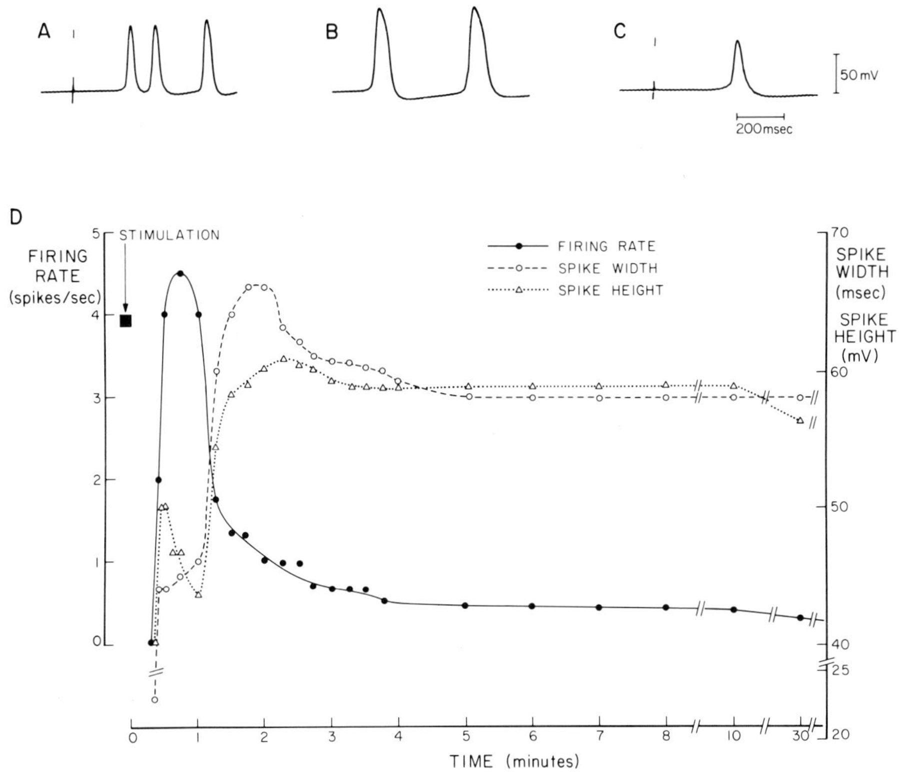

Fig. 4 A–D. Intracellularly recorded bag cell action potential traces. **A** Spikes evoked by extracellular stimulation (20 V, 2.5 ms) of a pleuroabdominal connective nerve at the onset of a bag cell afterdischarge. **B** Shape of the enhanced spontaneous action potentials 10 min after the onset of afterdischarge. **C** An action potential evoked after the end of afterdischarge. **D** Plot of the firing rate, spike width and spike height in the early part of a bag cell afterdischarge triggered by extracellular stimulation (20 V, 2.5 ms, 1 Hz, 10 s) of a pleuroabdominal connective nerve in a normal seawater medium. (From Kaczmarek et al. 1982)

comes more burst-like and is of lower frequency (0.5 Hz). The average duration of afterdischarge at 15 °C is 30 min (Kaczmarek et al. 1978). During afterdischarge, intracellularly recorded spike height and spike width increase with a time course slightly later than that of firing rate (Fig. 4).

7.2 cAMP Mediates Afterdischarge

The mechanisms of this long-lasting afterdischarge have been investigated with good success. Within 1 min of the start of afterdischarge, the earliest practical time point for measurement, there is a rise in cAMP, which subsides within 5 min (Kaczmarek et al. 1978). This rise in cAMP plays an important role in the genesis of the afterdischarge. When membrane-permeable, phosphodiesterase-resistant analogs of cAMP (Miller et al. 1980) are applied to the intact bag cell cluster, afterdischarge is initiated without providing any electrical stimulation to the preparation (Kaczmarek et al. 1978). This finding indicates that the measured increase in cAMP is not a correlative metabolic change with afterdischarge but plays some important role in its genesis.

7.3 Isolated Bag Cells Have Afterdischarge Properties

Bag cells can be maintained in cell culture as isolated cells (Strumwasser et al. 1978), and under these conditions regenerate their neurites and couple electrically with other bag cell neurons (Kaczmarek et al. 1979). Such isolated bag cells, in cell culture, are normally quiescent, that is produce no spontaneous action potentials as is also the case in the intact cluster. When cAMP analogs are added to the medium, these cells begin to produce spontaneous action potentials (Kaczmarek and Strumwasser 1981). Of particular interest is the fact that when a brief depolarizing pulse is used to induce repetitive action potentials, after spontaneous activity due to cAMP has started, the rate of spontaneous activity transiently increases after the depolarizing pulse.

The action potentials of bag cells are primarily calcium spikes, since they are partially or totally resistant to tetrodotoxin but blockable by Co^{2+} (Strumwasser et al. 1981). As Fig. 5 shows, there is a significant rise in intracellular concentration of calcium, as measured by Arsenazo III, when a train of bag cell action potentials is produced in normal external Ca^{2+} (Woolum and Strumwasser 1983). When Ca^{2+} is increased by a factor of 9, intracellular Ca^{2+} increases by about a factor of 3 after the same train of action potentials (Fig. 5). The finding that there is a significant Ca^{2+} influx when action potentials occur in bag cells suggests that after cAMP priming, Ca^{2+} entry provides an additional enhancement of the spontaneous discharge in bag cells.

7.4 The Role of Protein Phosphorylation

The current view is that cAMP mediates cellular actions in eukaryotic cells through protein phosphorylation (Nestler and Greengard 1984; Krebs 1983). Phosphorylation of two specific proteins is enhanced during bag cell afterdischarge (Jennings et al. 1982). These two proteins, BC-2 and BC-1, have apparent molecular weights of 21000 and 33000 daltons respectively. When measured at 2 min and 20 min into afterdischarge, the phosphorylation of BC-1 is increased by $82\% \pm 14\%$ (SEM) and $69\% \pm 43\%$ respectively, compared with quiescent bag cell clusters. These changes are statistically significant at $p=0.005$ and $p=0.05$ (one-tailed paired t test) respectively. Phosphorylation of the BC-2 protein is unchanged at 2 min ($-19\% \pm 28\%$) into afterdischarge, but significantly increased at 20 min ($92\% \pm 23\%$; $p=0.02$).

There is more information on the "late" phosphorprotein (BC-2) during afterdischarge because it is a more abundant protein than BC-1, as based on Coomassie blue staining after separation on a 10% SDS-polyacrylamide gel. BC-2 has

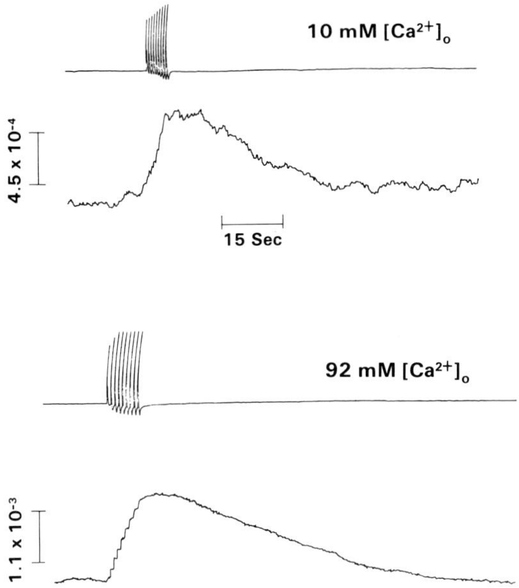

Fig. 5. Increasing external Ca^{2+} enhances calcium influx due to evoked action potentials in a bag cell. Membrane potential (*upper* trace) and differential absorbance (A_{700}–A_{660}) (*lower* trace). *Top pair* of traces in 10 m*M* Ca^{2+}; *bottom pair* of traces in 92 m*M* Ca^{2+}. Note the greater sensitivity of the absorbance trace in the normal Ca^{2+} solution. (From Woolum and Strumwasser 1988)

been partially sequenced after electroelution of the band, excised from the gel. Fourteen of the first 23 amino acid residues are positively identified and three are tentatively identified by a sensitive gas phase sequenator. An amino acid composition was also obtained on the electroeluted BC-2 band. Serine and threonine residues were detected, as would be expected if BC-2 is a phosphoprotein.

It is unlikely that BC-2 plays an important role in the genesis of afterdischarge, because it is phosphorylated between 2 min and 20 min into afterdischarge. There is information suggesting that BC-2 is part of the ELH precursor. According to Rothman et al. (1985), the 14 positively identified residues of BC-2 are in perfect agreement with a segment of the ELH precursor that begins 30 residues after the initiation methionine residue and extends six residues into the 80-residue insertion coding for α-BCP, β-BCP, and γ-BCP. They find that the correlation coefficient for the comparison of the computed amino acid composition of a 21 000-dalton fragment, obtained from the nucleotide sequence, with the actual amino acid composition of the electroeluted band has an r value of 0.575 and a p value of 0.05. These findings certainly suggest that BC-2 may be part of the N-terminal end of the ELH precursor.

This possibility was tested for, in part, by Jennings et al. (1982), who compared the position of the radiolabeled (^{3}H-leucine) 29 000-dalton ELH precursor and ^{32}P-labeled BC-2 on the same gel, after phosphorylation of a bag cell cell-free extract. BC-2 migrated faster than the 29 000-dalton ELH precursor. It is still possible, however, that the two proteins are related but that the 29 000-dalton ELH precursor is not phosphorylatable until it is further processed. In summary, BC-2 is possibly a 21 000-dalton N-terminal fragment of the ELH precursor which is phosphorylated during afterdischarge, but not all of the available evidence fits this hypothesis. When Newcomb and Scheller (1987) recovered fragments of the ELH precursor in their study of prohormone processing, their largest fragment was a 61 amino acid-containing fragment (residues 33–93, labeled "Kl"). This fragment could include the N-terminal part of BC-2 but is substantially shorter than would be needed to include a 21 000-dalton protein.

BC-1 remains a reasonable candidate for playing some role in the genesis of afterdischarge. The fact that it is a minor component in bag cells, based on Coomassie blue staining, is compatible with the low concentration in the cell of most membrane proteins. However, further work with BC-1 is difficult until probes, possibly monoclonal antibodies, are developed which in particular are function-interfering. A start has been made in this direction (Strumwasser et al. 1985).

7.5 Voltage Clamp Studies of Bag Cells

Two outward currents are reduced in isolated bag cells in the presence of cAMP. One of the outward currents is relatively sustained with 1-s command steps (Strumwasser et al. 1982; Kaczmarek and Strumwasser 1984; Strong 1984) and is insensitive to 40 m*M* tetraethylammonium ions extracellularly or EDTA intracellularly. On this basis it is unlikely that this current is a calcium-activated potassium current, but it could be the delayed rectifier potassium current. The second outward current that is suppressed by cAMP is the A current, a transient potassium current (Kaczmarek and Strumwasser 1984; Strong and Kaczmarek 1986). This current is sensitive to 4-aminopyridine. The reduction of these two potassium currents with applied cAMP plays an important role in the genesis of the pacemaker activity and the broadening of the action potential duration during afterdischarge.

Recently another messenger system has been implicated in the afterdischarge process, namely diacylglycerol (DAG), which activates protein kinase C. Extracellular application of phorbol ester, which mimics DAG, enhances the calcium action potential amplitude in isolated bag cells, as does the injection of protein kinase C (DeRiemer et al. 1985). Treatment of isolated bag cells with phorbol esters or synthetic DAGs causes the appearance of a new class of calcium channels (Strong et al. 1987). It is presumed that these processes occur in the intact bag cell cluster during afterdischarge, but evidence has not been provided for this to date. The unmasking of these covert calcium channels in bag cells may play an additional role, independent of the cAMP-dependent decrease in potassium channels, in the enhancement of the action potential amplitude during afterdischarge (see Fig. 4). Such enhancements in the amplitude and duration of the action potentials, so far only reported in somata, will enhance stimulus-secretion coupling, if similar changes take place in the secretory terminals.

8 Does α-Bag Cell Peptide Act to Perpetuate or Initiate Afterdischarge?

Since α-BCP has been shown to be capable of initiating a bag cell discharge in vitro (Rothman et al. 1983 b), it is natural to wonder what role it might play in the afterdischarge mechanism. Perhaps the release of α-BCP at the start of an electrically initiated afterdischarge plays some role in maintaining the afterdischarge by acting as an autoexcitatory agent. Recently, Kauer and Kaczmarek (1987) found that α-BCP is inhibitory to bag cells in their experiments. After electrically initiating an afterdischarge, local application of 1 μ*M* of any of the three forms of α-BCP causes a premature termination of the afterdischarge. This inhibition of afterdischarge is correlated with a reduction of cAMP when measured at 7 min into afterdischarge, α-BCP being applied at 2 min into the afterdischarge.

While the exact nature of the differences in the protocols of the two laboratories remains to be determined, these discrepant findings were produced with in vitro experiments. In an attempt to determine what might be occurring in vivo, three sexually mature *Aplysia* were injected with α-BCP 1–8, the most active form according to Rothman et al. (1983 b). If α-BCP does induce bag cell discharge, the expectation would be that egg-laying would be produced. Three doses were used (420, 630 and 1050 μg). None of the animals laid eggs to α-BCP 1–8 during the 2.5-h postinjection observation period. Following this observation period all three animals were injected with synthetic ELH (150 μg) and responded with normal latency and behavior by egg-laying (F. Strumwasser, unpublished, 1987). Thus we must conclude that α-BCP is unlikely to be an autoexcitatory agent to bag cells in vivo.

9 Integration by the Gene for ELH

These latter findings go to the heart of a deeper issue. It was stated by Scheller et al. (1983 b) that "the entire repertory of behaviors associated with egg laying cannot simply be elicited by ELH alone." This conclusion was based in part on the fact that bag cell peptides other than ELH have electrophysiological effects on the abdominal ganglion. Another factor leading to this conclusion was the unravelling of the structure of the prohormone for ELH by gene cloning. The large size of the prohormone compared with ELH forced investigators to attempt to account for the functions of the other peptides that would be post-translationally produced. These factors led to the following interesting speculation: "The ELH gene expresses a polyprotein precursor which contains ELH along with several additional neuropeptides. It is therefore tempting to assume that the behavioral repertory is mediated by a small set of neuropeptides, all encoded by a single gene, expressed in a single polyprotein, cleaved and stored together, facilitating their coordinate release" (Scheller et al. 1983 b).

Since synthetic ELH can elicit normal egg-laying with the associated behaviors of attachment and winding of the egg-string on a substrate, and since α-BCP does not induce egg-laying, we must conclude in this instance that the actual behavior of egg-laying is strictly due to ELH itself. Furthermore, not every peptide fragment in a behavioral prohormone need have a "behavioral" function. The present evidence indicates that the AP has no electrophysiological functions but may act as the counter- ion in the granule for basic ELH. The other peptide fragments released with ELH may have metabolic or trophic functions for which there are no easy assays at the moment. Thus the gene coding for a behavioral prohormone may use one peptide for behavior (ELH), another as a counter-ion in the granule (AP) and yet other peptides for trophic or metabolic signals. In this way the ELH gene still accomplishes integration of a coordinated response, but over a broader spectrum than just behavior.

Acknowledgments. The structure-activity studies reported herein are part of a collaborative project with Drs. D. Schiller and S. B. H. Kent of the Division of Biology at California Institute of Technology.

References

Arch S (1972) Biosynthesis of the egg-laying hormone (ELH) in the bag cell neurons of *Aplysia californica*. J Gen Physiol 60:102–119

Beard M, Millecchia L, Masuoka C, Arch S (1982) Ultrastructure of secretion in the atrial gland of a mollusc (*Aplysia*). Tissue Cell 14:297–308

Berry RW (1981) Proteolytic processing in the biogenesis of the neurosecretory egg-laying hormone in *Aplysia*: I. Precursors, intermediates and products. Biochemistry 21:6200–6205

Branton WD, Arch S, Smock T, Mayeri E (1978) Evidence for mediation of a neuronal interaction by a behaviorally active peptide. Proc Natl Acad Sci USA 75:5732– 5736

Chiu AY, Hunkapiller MW, Heller E, Stuart DK, Hood LE, Strumwasser F (1979) Purification and primary structure of the neuropeptide egg-laying hormone of *Aplysia californica*. Proc Natl Acad Sci USA 76:6656– 6660

Coggeshall RE (1970) A cytolytic analysis of the bag cell control of egg laying in *Aplysia*. J Morphol 132:461–486

Coggeshall RE (1972) The muscle of the follicle of the ovotestis in *Aplysia* as the probable target organ for bag cell extract. Am Zool 12:521–523

Cohen JL, Weiss KR, Kupfermann I (1978) Motor control of buccal muscles in *Aplysia*. J Neurophysiol 41:157–180

DeRiemer SA, Strong JA, Albert KA, Greengard P, Kaczmarek LK (1985) Enhancement of calcium current in *Aplysia* neurones by phorbol ester and protein kinase C. Nature 313:313–316

Dudek FE, Tobe SS (1978) Bag cell peptide acts directly on ovotestis of *Aplysia californica*: basis for an in vitro bioassay. Gen Comp Endocrinol 36:618–627

Dudek FE, Cobbs JS, Pinsker HM (1979) Bag cell electrical activity underlying spontaneous egg laying in freely behaving *Aplysia*. J Neurophysiol 42:804–817

Dudek FE, Soutar B, Tobe SS (1980) Reproduction in *Aplysia californica*: correlations between egg laying in vivo and egg release in vitro. Can J Zool 58:2163–2166

Ebberink RHM, van Loenhout H, Geraerts WPM, Joosse J (1985) Purification and amino acid sequence of the ovulation neurohormone of *Lymnaea stagnalis*. Proc Natl Acad Sci USA 82:7767–7771

Ferguson GP, Parsons DW, ter Maat A, Pinsker HM (1986) Spontaneous and elicited bag cell discharges in gonadectomized *Aplysia*. J Exp Biol 123:159–173

Glover I, Haneef I, Pitts J, Wood S, Moss D, Tickle I, Blundell T (1983) Conformational flexibility in a small globular hormone: x-ray analysis of avian pancreatic polypeptide at 0.98-A resolution. Biopolymers 22:293–304

Jennings KR, Kaczmarek LK, Hewick RM, Dreyer WJ, Strumwasser F (1982) Protein phosphorylation during afterdischarge in peptidergic neuros of *Aplysia*. J Neurosci 2:158–168

Joosse J, Geraerts WPM (1983) In: Saleuddin ASM, Wilbur KM (eds) The mollusca, vol 4. Academic, New York, pp 317–406

Kaczmarek LK, Strumwasser F (1981) The expression of long lasting afterdischarge by isolated *Aplysia* neurons. J Neurosci 1:626–634

Kaczmarek LK, Strumwasser F (1984) A voltage-clamp analysis of currents underlying cyclic AMP-induced membrane modulation in isolated peptidergic neurons of *Aplysia*. J Neurophysiol 52:340–349

Kaczmarek LK, Jennings KR, Strumwasser F (1978) Neurotransmitter modulation, phosphodiesterase inhibitor effects, and cyclic AMP correlates of afterdischarge in peptidergic neurites. Proc Natl Acad Sci USA 75:5200–5204

Kaczmarek LK, Finbow M, Revel JP, Strumwasser F (1979) The morphology and coupling of *Aplysia* bag cells within the abdominal ganglion and in cell culture. J Neurobiol 10:535–550

Kaczmarek LK, Jennings KR, Strumwasser F (1982) An early sodium and a late calcium phase in the afterdischarge of peptide-secreting neurons of *Aplysia*. Brain Res 238:105–115

Kauer JA, Kaczmarek LK (1987) α-Bag cell peptide directly modulates the excitability of the neurons that release it. J Neurosci 7:3623–3632

Kent S, Clark-Lewis I (1985) Modern methods for the chemical synthesis of biologically active peptides. In: Alitalo K, Partanen P, Vaheri A (eds) Synthetic peptides in biology and medicine. Elsevier, Amsterdam, pp 29–57

Kirk MD, Scheller RH (1986) Egg-laying hormone of *Aplysia* induces a voltage-dependent slow inward current carried by Na^+ in an identified motoneuron. Proc Natl Acad Sci USA 83:3017–3021

Krebs EG (1983) Historical perspectives on protein phosphorylation and a classification system for protein kinases. Phil Trans Roy Soc Lond (B) 302:3–11

Kupfermann I, Kandel ER (1970) Electrophysiological properties and functional interconnections of two symmetrical neurosecretory clusters (bag cells) in abdominal ganglion of *Aplysia*. J Neurophysiol 33:865–876

Levitan ES, Kramer RH, Levitan IB (1987) Augmentation of bursting pacemaker activity by egg-laying hormone in *Aplysia* neuron R15 is mediated by a cyclic AMP-dependent increase in Ca^{2+} and K^+ currents. Proc Natl Acad Sci 84:6307–6311

Mayeri E, Rothman BS, Brownell PH, Branton WD, Padgett L (1985) Nonsynaptic characteristics of neurotransmission mediated by egg-laying hormone in the abdominal ganglion of *Aplysia*. J Neurosci 5:2060–2077

Miller JP, Boswell KH, Meyer RB Jr, Christensen LF, Robins RK (1980) Synthesis and enzymatic and inotropic activity of some new 8-substituted and 6,8-disubstituted derivatives of adenosine cyclic 3′,5′-monophosphate. J Med Chem 23:242–251

Nambu JR, Scheller RH (1986) Egg-laying hormone genes of *Aplysia*: Evolution of the ELH gene family. J Neurosci 6:2026–2036

Nestler EJ, Greengard P (1984) Protein phosphorylation in the nervous system. Wiley, New York

Newcomb R, Scheller RH (1987) Proteolytic processing of the *Aplysia* egg-laying hormone and R3–14 neuropeptide precursors. J Neurosci 7:854–863

Price DA, Greenberg MJ (1977) Structure of a molluscan cardioexcitatory neuropeptide. Science 197:670–671

Ram JL (1983) Neuropeptide activation of an identifiable buccal ganglion motoneuron in *Aplysia*. Brain Res 288:177–186

Ram JL, Heller KA, Levran Z (1986) Sensitivity of a peptide activated neuron in *Aplysia* to serotonin and cyclic AMP relevant agents. Comp Biochem Physiol [C] 83:279–283

Rothman BS, Weir G, Dudek FE (1983a) Egg-laying hormone: direct action on the ovotestis of *Aplysia*. Gen Comp Endocrinol 52:134–141

Rothman BS, Mayeri E, Brown RO, Yuan P-M, Shively JE (1983b) Primary structure and neuronal effects of α-bag cell peptide, a second candidate neurotransmitter encoded by a single gene in bag cell neurons of *Aplysia*. Proc Natl Acad Sci USA 80:5753–5757

Rothman BS, Mayeri E, Scheller RH (1985) The bag cell neurons of *Aplysia* as a possible peptidergic multitransmitter system: from genes to behavior. In: Zomzely-Neurath C, Walker WA (eds) Gene expression in brain. Wiley, New York, pp 235–274

Rothman BS, Hawke DH, Brown RO, Lee TD, Dehghan AA, Shively JE, Mayeri E (1986) Isolation and primary structure of the califins, three biologically active egg-laying hormone-like peptides from the atrial gland of *Aplysia californica*. J Biol Chem 261:1616–1623

Schaefer M, Brownell PH (1986) Modulation of a respiratory motor program by peptide-secreting neurons in *Aplysia*. J Neurobiol 17:121–126

Scheller RH, Rothman BS, Mayeri E (1983a) A single gene encodes multiple peptide-transmitter candidates involved in a stereotyped behavior. TINS 6:340–345

Scheller RH, Jackson JF, McAllister LB, Rothman BS, Mayeri E, Axel R (1983b) A single gene encodes multiple neuropeptides mediating a stereotyped behavior. Cell 32:7–22

Sigvardt KA, Rothman BS, Brown RO, Mayeri E (1986) The bag cells of *Aplysia* as a multitransmitter system: identification of alpha bag cell peptide as a second neurotransmitter. J Neurosci 6:803–813

Sossin WS, Kirk MD, Scheller RH (1987) Peptidergic modulation of neuronal circuitry controlling feeding in *Aplysia*. J Neurosci 7:671–681

Strong JA (1984) Modulation of potassium current kinetics in bag cell neurons of *Aplysia* by an activator adenylate cyclase. J Neurosci 4:2772–2783

Strong JA, Kaczmarek LK (1986) Multiple components of delayed potassium current in peptidergic neurons of *Aplysia*: modulation by an activator of adenylate cyclase. J Neurosci 6:814–822

Strong JA, Fox AP, Tsien RW, Kaczmarek LK (1987) Stimulation of protein kinase C recruits covert calcium channels in *Aplysia* bag cell neurons. Nature 325:714–717

Strumwasser F (1984) The structure of the commands for a neuropeptide-mediated behavior, egg-laying, in an opisthobranch mollusc. In: Hoffmann J, Porchet M (eds) Biosynthesis, metabolism and mode of action of invertebrate hormones. Springer, Berlin Heidelberg New York, pp 36–43

Strumwasser F, Schlechte FR, Bower S (1972) Distributed circadian oscillators in the nervous system of *Aplysia*. Fed Proc 31:405

Strumwasser F, Kaczmarek LK, Viele D (1978) The peptidergic bag cell neurons of *Aplysia*: morphological and electrophysiological studies of dissociated cells in tissue culture. Soc Neurosci Abstr. 4:207

Strumwasser F, Kaczmarek LK, Jennings KR, Chiu AY (1981) Studies of a model peptidergic neuronal system, the bag cells of *Aplysia*. In: Farner DS, Lederis K (eds) Neurosecretion: molecules, cells, systems. Plenum, New York, pp 251–270

Strumwasser LK, Kaczmarek LK, Jennings KR (1982) Intracellular modulation of membrane channels by cyclic AMP-mediated protein phosphorylation in peptidergic neurons of *Aplysia*. Fed Proc 41:2933–2939

Strumwasser F, Viele DP, Lovely KD (1985) Monoclonal antibody blocks the postburst hyperpolarization in R15 and bag cell neurons. Biophys J 47:52a

Strumwasser F, Schiller DL, Kent SBH (1987) Synthetic neuropeptide egg-laying hormone (ELH) of *Aplysia californica* induces normal egg-laying: structure-activity studies. Soc Neurosci Abstr 13:38

Stuart DK, Strumwasser F (1980) Neuronal sites of action of neurosecretory peptide, egg-laying hormone, in *Aplysia californica*. J Neurophysiol 43:499–519

Stuart DK, Chiu AY, Strumwasser F (1980) Neurosecretion of egg-laying hormone and other peptides from electrically active bag cell neurons of *Aplysia*. J Neurophysiol 43:488–498

Woolum JC, Strumwasser F (1983) Dynamic Ca^{2+} measurements in isolated *Aplysia* bag cells. Biophys J 41:59a

Woolum JC, Strumwasser F (1988) Calcium changes in isolated peptidergic neurons during activation by a cAMP analog. Brain Res 444:1–9

Electrophysiological Characteristics of Peptidergic Nerve Terminals Correlated with Secretion *

E. L. STUENKEL [1] and I. M. COOKE [2]

Contents

1 Introduction

1.1 History

This article reviews studies correlating electrical with secretory activity of a peptidergic neurosecretory system of crabs known as the X-organ – sinus gland system (XOSG). Justification for giving such attention to an invertebrate model derives from the unique observations obtainable by reason of the relatively huge size of axon terminals (in certain species) and the discrete anatomical segregation of the system. These permit (1) experimentation on an intact, purely peptidergic neurosecretory system removed to a chamber, (2) simultaneous intracellular recording from electrodes placed under visual control into somata and terminals, and (3) monitoring of secretion separately from both somata and terminal regions while recording. The XOSG is analogous to the vertebrate hypothalamic-neuro-

* Work on the crab XOSG has been supported by a series of NSF and NIH grants to I.M.C., including currently NSF grant BNS84-04459 and NIH grant NS15453, as well as by funds from the University of Hawaii Foundation
[1] Department of Physiology, University of Michigan, Ann Arbor, MI, 48109, USA
[2] Békésy Laboratory of Neurobiology University of Hawaii, Honolulu, HI 96822, USA

Current Topics in Neuroendocrinology, Vol. 9

hypophysial system in function as well as in those details of physiological mechanisms for which comparable information is available. Generalizability of the information obtainable only from the XOSG to other neurosecretory systems thus seems likely.

The mystery implied in the naming of the X-organ and sinus gland (Hanström 1931) from histological studies of crustacean eyestalks dissipated with the discovery of a tract of axons connecting the two structures (Bliss 1951; Passano 1951): it became clear that these were components of a single major neurosecretory system. "X-organ" has now come to refer to a clump of about 200 biosynthetically active neuronal somata whose terminals constitute the bulk of the sinus gland and form a now classical example of a neurohemal organ (Bliss and Welsh 1952; Potter 1956; reviews: Gabe 1966; Chaigneau 1983; Andrew 1983; referencing of work in this review attempts to provide entry to the literature, but must be considered indicative only).

Ablation and extract reinjection studies early implicated the XOSG in the control of a number of hormonally mediated responses. These included mediation of retinal and hypodermal pigment movements (Kleinholz 1936; Brown and Cunningham 1939; Welsh 1941), inhibition of molt (Brown and Cunningham 1939; Scudamore 1947), elevation of hemolymph glucose levels (Abramowitz et al. 1944) and others. Four decades of further work has now implicated the XOSG in the control of nearly all physiological and homeostatic responses as well as in growth and maturation processes involving endocrinological mediation (reviews: Cooke and Sullivan 1982; Keller 1983; Adiyodi 1985; Skinner 1985; Mattson 1986).

1.2 Anatomy

In fresh material, removal of carapace, muscles and superficial connective tissue from the eyestalk reveals the sinus gland as an iridescent white sphere or disk of about 1 mm diameter at the periphery of the eyestalk optic ganglia (Fig. 1 A). The iridescence is attributable to refraction from secretory granules packed into the densely aggregated nerve terminals that constitute the bulk of the sinus gland. In some preparations, the tract of axons from which the terminals arise can be seen to emerge from the medulla terminalis (the most proximal of the eyestalk ganglia). The approximately 200 somata form a group or groups, often recognizable in fresh material by their iridescence, at the periphery of the ganglion diametrically opposite the sinus gland. A number of generalizations can be made from an extensive literature pertaining to the anatomy of the XOSG of a number of

Fig. 1 A–D. Anatomy of the crab X-organ – sinus gland (XOSG) neurosecretory system. **A** Freshly dissected neural tissue of the eyestalk: the clump of neurosecretory somata (*X-organ*), part of the axon tract and the densely aggregated secretory terminals forming a neurohemal organ (*sinus gland*) are iridescent white (*OP*, optic peduncle; *MT*, medulla terminalis, the most proximal of the eyestalk ganglia) (courtesy T. Weatherby). **B** Light micrograph of a section through the sinus gland of a biosynthetically radiolabeled XOSG (5-h pulse of ^{3}H-leucine on somata only, 19-h chase, glutaraldehyde-fixed, plastic-embedded,

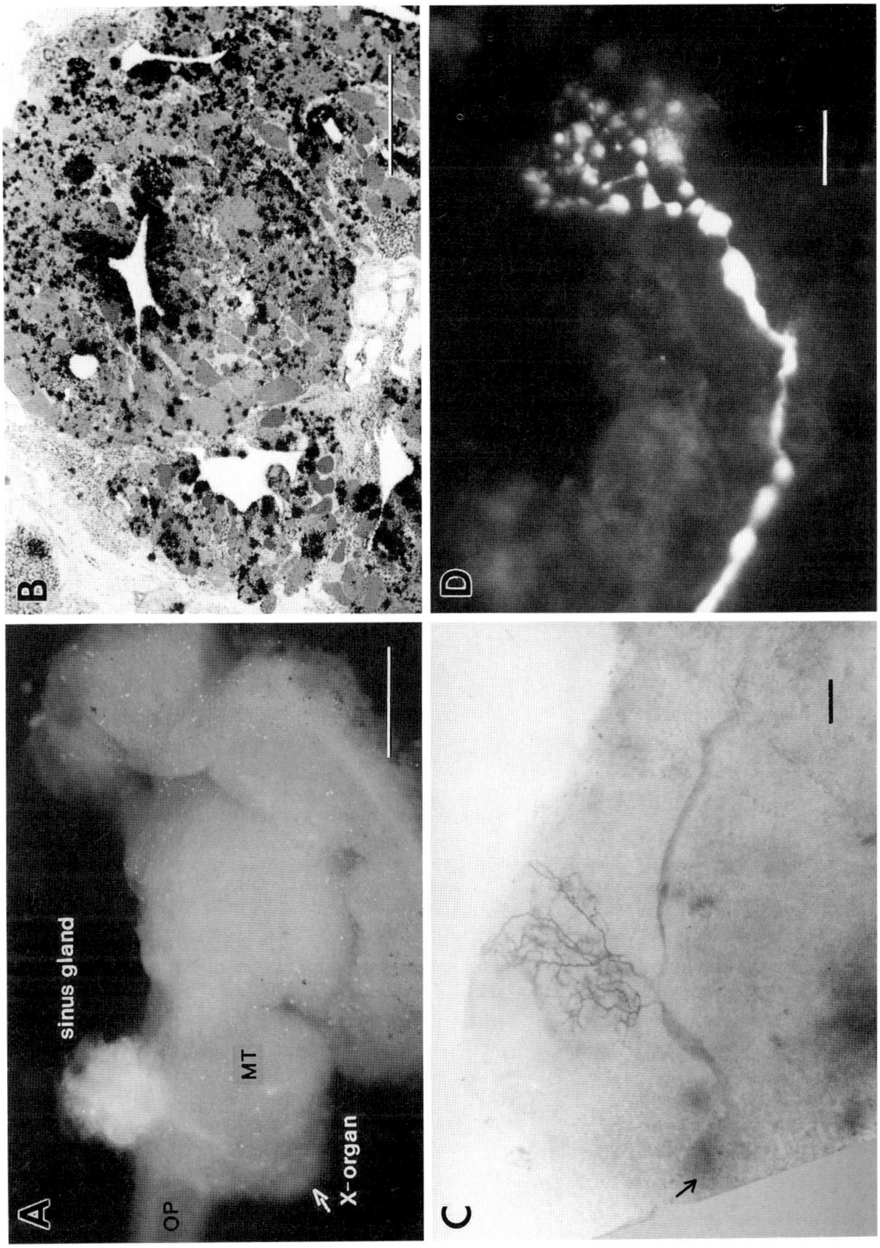

autoradiographic exposure, 7 days, stained with methylene blue). Note concentration of radiolabel in terminals abutting the hemolymph sinuses (E. Stuenkel and E. Gillary, unpublished). **C** Intracellular injection of an X-organ neuron (out of plane of focus, *arrow*) with $CoCl_2$ permits visualization in a cleared whole mount of the arborization of neurite collaterals in the neuropil of the medulla terminalis. **D** Terminal dilatations of a single peptidergic axon visualized in a cleared whole mount of the sinus gland by intracellular injection of lucifer yellow into one terminal (courtesy M. Nagano). *Scale bars*: **A** 1 mm, **B, C, D** 50 µm. **A, B, C** *Cardisoma carnifex*; **D** *Podophthalmus vigil*

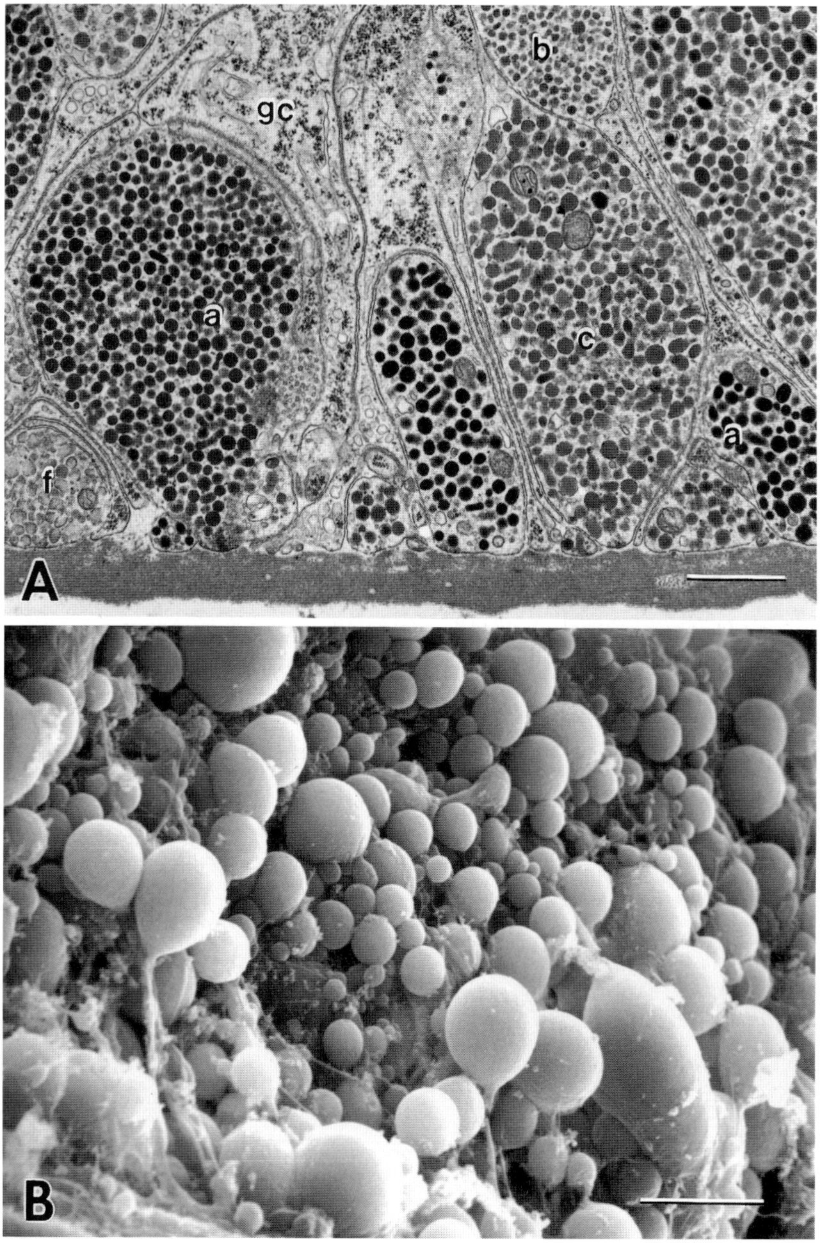

Fig. 2 A, B. Morphology of the crab sinus gland (*Cardisoma carnifex*). **A** Transmission electron micrograph of a section showing axon terminals against the neurolemma lining a hemolymph sinus (lower edge of photo). Four of the six types are indicated (*a, b, c, f*); types *a* and *c* predominate. Each terminal profile is surrounded by glial cell (*gc*) processes except at the point of contact with the neurolemma. **B** Scanning electron micrograph of the external surface of the sinus gland showing terminals protruding into the hemolymph sinus. *Scale bars*: **A** 1 μm; **B** 10 μm. (Courtesy T. Weatherby)

crustacean groups at the levels of both light microscopy (Potter 1956, 1958; Rehm 1959) and electron microscopy (e.g., Bunt and Ashby 1967, 1968; Silverthorn 1975; Shivers 1976; Weatherby 1981):

1. At least 90% of the cell somata giving rise to terminals of the sinus gland lie in a single cluster (e.g., crabs) or in two distinct clusters (in certain crustacean groups, e.g., crayfish) in the medulla terminalis (the X-organ).
2. The cell bodies contain large amounts of rough endoplasmic reticulum, Golgi and developing secretory granules typical of cells involved in sustained production of secretory proteins.
3. Morphological assessment of cell size and histochemical staining of cytoplasm and granules have suggested the system to be heterogeneous with respect to cell type, with as many as six types of cells and corresponding terminals (Fig. 2 B) distinguishable (Potter 1956; Weatherby 1981). It remains, however, unsettled whether this typing process reliably recognizes distinct cell types rather than variation in the amount of peptide packaged in the granules or maturation state of the cell or its secretory contents, or whether it may be a reproducible artifact of fixation and staining (see Sect. 1.3).
4. Consistent with invertebrate neural architecture, a collateral arbor arises from the proximal axon segment of each cell (Fig. 1 C) and enters into the ganglion neuropil (Andrew et al. 1978; Jaros 1978; Glantz et al. 1983; Cooke and Stuenkel 1985; Nagano 1986 a). This may be assumed to be the site of regulatory or modulatory synaptic interaction (Nagano 1983, 1986 b; Glantz et al. 1983; Iwasaki and Satow 1971; see Sect. 2.3).
5. The sinus gland is a true neurohemal structure in that it is composed entirely of axon terminal dilatations, glial cells and supportive cells juxtaposed with hemolymph sinuses (Figs. 1 B, 2 A). As revealed by intracellular injection of lucifer yellow dye (Nagano 1986 a), each axon divides within the sinus gland to form an extensive arborization of varicosities and terminals (Fig. 1 D). Terminals are exposed to hemolymph both at the surface (Fig. 2 B) and where they are palisaded against a neurolemma lining internal sinuses (Fig. 2 A). Portions of the outer boundary of the sinus gland have a neurolemmal sheath. The largest dilatations are found at the periphery. Smaller axon dilatations abut the neurolemma lining the internal hemolymph sinuses. It is here that omega figures suggestive of exocytotic events have been observed in electron-microscopic studies (Weatherby 1981; Weatherby and Haylett 1985), pointing to these as sites of hormone release.

1.3 Neurohormones

We cannot here review the extensive literature describing factors obtained from the XOSG having biological activity, and the efforts to isolate and characterize them (reviews: Cooke and Sullivan 1982; Keller 1985). Such studies were hampered by the difficulty of obtaining sufficient material, difficulties in devising specific, sensitive bioassays, and confusion arising from species differences. Thus far, all of the active factors appear to be peptides. Examination of the peptide and

Table 1. Peptides of the crustacean X-organ – sinus gland

Peptide	Species	Reference
Peptides for which primary structures have been determined:		
1. Red pigment-concentrating hormone (RPCH) ⟨ELNFSPGW-NH_2⟩	*Pandalus borealis*	Fernlund and Josefsson (1972)
	Cardisoma carnifex[a]	Newcomb (1987)
	Carcinus maenas[a]	Keller and Kegel (1984)
	Orconectes limosus[a]	Keller and Kegel (1984)
	Eriocheir sinenses[a]	Keller and Kegel (1984)
2. Light-adapting hormone (LAH, DRPH) NSGMINSILGIPRVMTEA-NH_2	*Pandalus borealis*	Fernlund (1976)
Pigment-dispersing hormone (PDH) NSELINSILGLPKVMNDA-NH_2	*Uca pugilator*	Rao et al. (1985)
3. H and related peptides RSADGFGRME[S]LLTSL [R]GSAESPAALGEASAAHPLE ├── I ──┤ ├── D ──┤ ├── C ──┤ ├── F ──┤ ├ E ┤	*Cardisoma carnifex*	Newcomb (1987)
Peptides for which amino acid composition has been determined:		
1. Crustacean hyperglycemic hormone (CHH)	*Orconected limosus*	Keller (1981)
	Carcinus maenas	Keller (1981)
	Cardisoma carnifex[b]	Newcomb (1983)
	Porcellio dilatatus	Martin et al. (1984)
	Eriocheir sinenses	Keller and Kegel (1984)
	Procambarus bouvieri	Huberman and Aguilar (1986)
2. Melanophore-dispersing hormone (MDH)[c]	*Eriocheir sinenses*	Keller and Kegel (1984)
3. Molt-inhibiting hormone (MIH)	*Homarus americanus*	Chang et al. (1987)
	Carcinus maenus	Webster and Keller (1986)
	Cardisoma carnifex[d]	Newcomb (1983, 1987)

[a] Preliminary amino acid compositions only
[b] Peptides J and L; melanophore dispersing activity inseparable from Peptide J
[c] Structural homology with LAH
[d] By similarity of amino acid composition, peptide K is likely to be MIH

protein composition of the XOSG from a number of crustacean species by gel electrophoresis (review: Keller 1983), immunocytochemistry (e.g., Jaros 1979; Van Herp and Van Buggenum 1979; Mangerich et al. 1986), and high-performance liquid chromatography (HPLC) (Newcomb 1983; Keller and Kegel 1984; Keller et al. 1985) shows that there is variation in peptide content between crustacean species. All groups are, however, characterized by having the bulk of stored sinus gland peptides represented by relatively few peptide groups. Table 1 summarizes the peptides for which primary structures or amino acid compositions have been determined. Red pigment-concentrating hormone (RPCH) of several diverse species is identical. Distal retinal pigment-dispersing hormone (DRPH, also referred to as light-adapting hormone) and crustacean hyperglycemic hormone (CHH) differ in different crustacean groups (Keller et al. 1985), as probably molt-inhibiting hormone (MIH) does also (Chang et al. 1987; Webster and Keller 1986; Newcomb 1987).

In evaluating studies correlating electrical and secretory activity, it becomes important to know how heterogeneous is the population of neurosecretory cells. For the tropical land crab, *Cardisoma carnifex*, on which most of the studies to be discussed were made, Newcomb (1983, 1987) has provided analyses, by quantitative HPLC, of all the peptides of less than 10000 M_r stored in the sinus gland. A total of 11 peptides are present in an individual sinus gland. Included are RPCH (Fernlund and Josefsson 1972), seven novel peptides sequenced by Newcomb (1987) and three peptides of closely related composition which have been tested for an exhibit the activities and amino acid compositions of CHH (Keller and Kegel 1984) and DRPH (Fernlund 1976) (it has not been possible to separate these activities). This information together with data on biosynthesis (Stuenkel 1983, 1986; Andrew and Saleuddin 1979), make it possible to propose a processing scheme that suggests that the bulk (>90%) of the peptides stored in the sinus gland of this crab are derived from a single prohormone of 14000 M_r (Stuenkel 1986). The peptides cleaved from this precursor can be grouped into two categories: (1) the peptides having CHH-like composition, including activities corresponding to CHH, DRPH, and MIH (Chang et al. 1987; Webster and Keller 1986; Newcomb 1987), and (2) the seven novel peptides represented by peptide "H" and smaller peptides derived by cleavage from it, whose function(s) have yet to be determined (Newcomb 1983, 1987). RPCH represents about 3% of the stored peptides in the *Cardisoma* sinus gland. Recent immunohistochemical studies with antibodies directed against CHH and against the N-terminal tetrapeptide portion of RPCH (Mangerich et al. 1986) are consonant with this scheme. The large cells constituting the bulk of the X-organ were positive to the CHH antibody, and a group of about 20 smaller cells (in *Carcinus maenas*) reacted to anti-RPCH. Thus there appears to be much less biochemical heterogeneity in the population of X-organ neurons than the diversity of morphological terminal types first suggested.

2 Electrophysiological Characterization

2.1 Intracellular Recording: Comparison of Terminals with Axons and Somata

The large size of axon terminal dilatations (up to 30 μm) present in certain species of crabs (e.g., *Cardisoma* ssp., *Podopthalmus vigil*) has permitted intracellular recording and comparison of the electrical responses of terminals with those recorded from axons and somata (Stuenkel 1985; Cooke 1985; Nagano and Cooke 1987). These studies add to earlier observations from crayfish X-organ somata (Iwasaki and Satow 1971). Several features of the responses recorded from terminals differ from those of other regions of the neurons and imply specialization of the terminal membrane (Fig. 3). Because intracellular recordings average the contributions from large areas of membrane, they are not ideally suited to distinguishing regional differences in membrane responses and underestimate the extent of such differences.

In view of the essential role of Ca in secretion by this system (as in neurosecretory systems generally), the ability of the terminal region (but not axons) to produce regenerative impulses in tetrodotoxin (TTX)-containing saline or nearly Na-free saline is significant, as it indicates a rich endowment of terminal membrane with voltage-dependent Ca channels. Enrichment of terminal membrane with Ca channels has been observed in the vertebrate neurohypophysis (Obaid et al. 1985) as well as at synapses, for example, in the squid stellate ganglion (Katz and Miledi 1969a), frog neuromuscular junction (Katz and Miledi 1969b), lobster neuromuscular junction (Niwa and Kawai 1982) and barnacle photoreceptor (Edgington and Stuart 1979). In all of these, observation of regenerative Ca-mediated responses required the addition of tetraethylammonium ion (TEA) to suppress competing K currents. By contrast, such responses can be obtained from the crab neurosecretory terminals without the addition of TEA.

Recordings from axons of the crab XOSG (Fig. 3B) show them to have purely Na-mediated impulses, a conclusion reached on less direct evidence for the crayfish XOSG (Iwasaki and Satow 1971). Recordings from somata showed variability in the extent of impulse invasion of the soma. This was seen also in the crayfish (*Pacifastacus* spp., Glantz et al. 1983), but impulses were reported to be consistently overshooting in *Procambarus clarkii* by Iwasaki and Satow (1971). In crab X-organ somata having overshooting impulses, regenerative responses show mixed Na- and Ca-dependence (as in crayfish; Iwasaki and Satow 1971). A study of crayfish X-organ somata using whole-cell patch clamp techniques (Garcia et al. 1985) reports that the major inward currents are blocked by Cd (a Ca-channel blocker) in axotomized cells, although TTX-sensitive currents are seen if the axon is present. This suggests that the mixed ionic dependence seen in microelectrode recordings results from contamination of somal Ca currents by axonal Na currents.

Action potentials of somata show less increase in duration in TEA than those of terminals, suggesting that fewer slowly inactivated inward current (presumably Ca) channels or fewer TEA-sensitive K channels are present in the soma than in terminals. Axonal spikes are relatively unaffected by TEA (Fig. 3C).

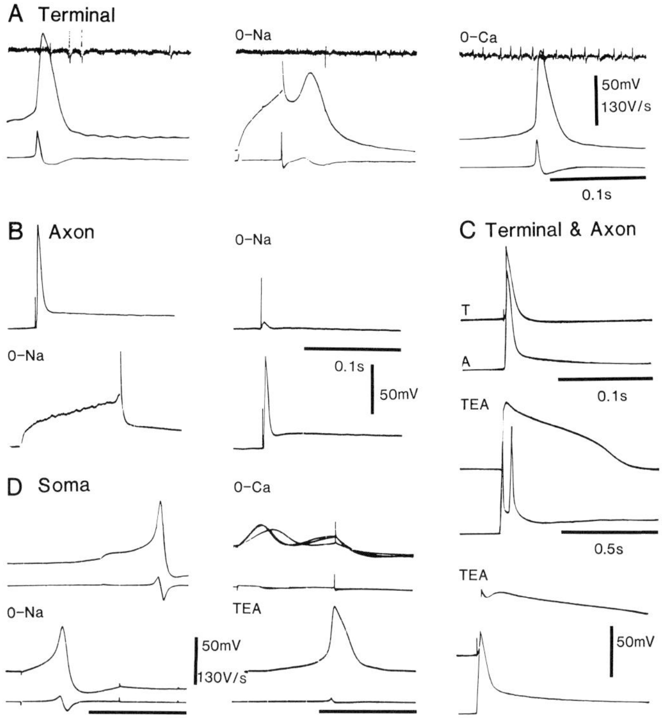

Fig. 3 A–D. Intracellular recordings from neurosecretory terminals, axons and a soma of the isolated crab X-organ – sinus gland system: effect of altered salines. **A** Terminal of *Podophthalamus vigil*: sinus gland nerve ligatured ca. 0.6 mm proximal to the terminal. *Top traces*: at ca. +15 mV relative to intracellular trace, extracellular recording from vaseline barrier proximal to ligature across sinus gland nerve (uncalibrated: impulses, left frame, ca. 50 μV). *Middle traces*: intracellular potential (at beginning of left frame, −60 mV). *Lower traces*: dV/dt. All records from the same terminal. *Left*: spontaneous impulse in normal saline. *Middle*: after 11 min perfusion with Na-free (choline-substituted) saline, resting potential (r.p.) is −76 mV, no spontaneous impulses; response to depolarizing current through the electrode (note current-off artifact). The peak of the regenerative response is ca. −5 mV. *Right*: after a period in normal saline and 12 min after commencing Ca-free saline perfusion; spontaneous impulse; r.p. −64 mV. **B** An axon (*P. vigil*) penetrated near entry to sinus gland. *Top left*: extracellularly stimulated impulse in normal saline (r.p. −84 mV). *Top right*: same, 8 min after introducing Na-free saline (r.p. −74 mV). *Bottom left*: 9 min in Na-free saline; no response to depolarizing current (1.5 nA); upward deflection is current-off transient. *Bottom right*: response 3 min after restoring normal saline (r.p. −74 mV). **C** Simultaneous intracellular recording from an axon (*A*) and a terminal (*T*) of different neurons (*Cardisoma carnifex*). *Top*: normal saline (time scale applies also to bottom frame). *Middle and bottom*: in 50 m*M* tetraethylammonium (*TEA*). Note greatly lengthened impulse in the terminal but not in the axon. **D** Intracellular recording (*upper trace*) and dV/dt (*lower trace*) from the same soma of *C. carnifex*. *Top left*: spontaneous impulse in normal saline (r.p. −56 mV). *Top right*: 7 min after commencing perfusion with Ca^{2+}-free (Mg-substituted) saline. Three sweeps superimposed, one with a spontaneous potential, two during depolarizing current (r.p. −36 mV); membrane potential is in process of depolarizing toward −30 mV. *Bottom left*: 9 min in Na-free saline; impulse evoked by depolarizing current. *Bottom right*: after restoring normal perfusion, then 7 min after introducing 50 m*M* TEA. Spontaneous impulse; membrane is held near −36 mV. Note relatively small duration increase in TEA relative to increase shown by terminal in **C**. (Recordings by M. Nagano, from Cooke and Stuenkel 1985)

A particularly interesting feature of the responses of many terminals, not seen in somata recordings, is a progressive increase in the duration of impulses during repetitive activity (Fig. 4C). The effects on impulse broadening of imposed changes in the terminal resting potential are consistent with a mechanism involving voltage-dependent inactivation of voltage-dependent K conductance, as delineated for spike broadening in a molluscan neuron (Ruben and Thompson 1984). Thus, the recordings show regional differences in the nature and number of K conductance channels as well as in the distribution of Na and Ca channels in the XOSG neurons.

Spontaneous activity is recorded from XOSGs not only when in situ in the eyestalk but also after isolation, and includes irregular firing, pacemaker-like ac-

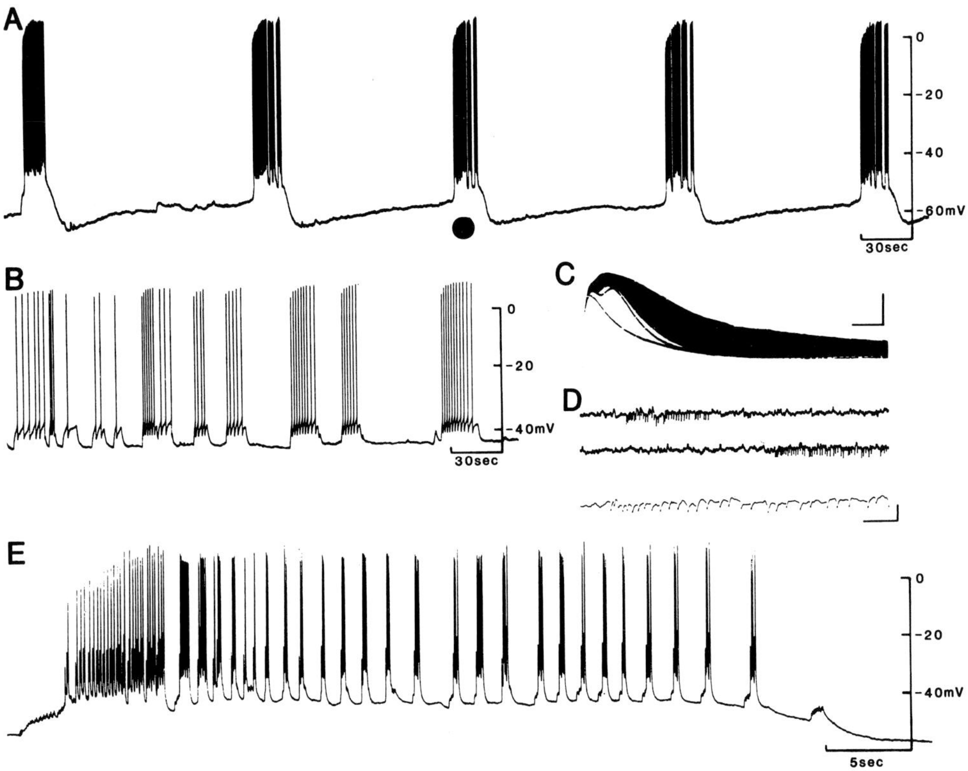

Fig. 4 A–E. Spontaneous impulse bursting recorded from in vitro crab (*Cardisoma carnifex*) X-organ – sinus gland systems. **A, B** Intracellularly recorded grouped discharge of impulses from a sinus gland terminal dilatation and an X-organ somata respectively. Note the depolarizing plateau underlying each burst. **C** Spike broadening of successive impulses within a burst, recorded simultaneously with the early portion of third terminal burst (●) shown in **A. D** Bursts of axonal impulses recorded extracellularly from the sinus gland nerve (note the bursts of impulses in a single unit). Two traces continuous, *bottom trace* shows a subsequent burst on an expanded scale. Polarity indicates propagation toward the terminals. **E** Bursting impulse pattern of sinus gland terminal dilatation demonstrating grouped impulse discharge within a single burst (Recordings by E. Stuenkel, from Cooke and Stuenkel 1985)

tivity and bursting in a variety of patterns (Fig. 4). Demonstration of burst pattern phase shifts in reponse to intracellular current passing provided evidence for endogenous generation of bursting recorded in crayfish X-organ somata (Iwasaki and Satow 1969). Both spike broadening and bursting are features frequently associated with neurosecretory or presumptive neurosecretory cells (review: Cooke and Stuenkel 1985). It is inviting to suggest that these are mechanisms for enhancing the entry of Ca and facilitating secretion. For somata of bursting neurons in molluscs there is evidence for progressively increased entry of Ca with successive impulses of a burst, and a marked increase in the amount of Ca entering with increased impulse duration (Gorman and Thomas 1978). For the neurohypophysis of rats there is evidence for facilitated release of hormone per impulse during bursting (Dutton and Dyball 1979). For the XOSG, efforts to obtain similar data on release of RPCH proved inconclusive (B. Haylett and I. Cooke, unpublished).

2.2 Patch Clamp Analysis of Ionic Channels of Terminals

The axon terminal dilatations of the *Cardisoma* sinus gland make gigaohm seals with fire-polished micropipets without enzymatic treatment, and hence permit application of the several configurations of the "patch clamp" technique (Hamill et al. 1981). Initial observations were obtained on preparations of dissociated terminal dilatations isolated by gentle mechanical teasing of the sinus gland (Lemos et al. 1986). Such treatment results in hundreds of spherical structures having diameters up to 30 μm. Electron-microscopic examination of such preparations shows membrane-bound profiles filled with neurosecretory granules. These profiles show the same variety of morphology as seen in sections of sinus gland (Nordmann et al. 1986). Depletion of the granules is observed following treatments known to stimulate secretion.

Observations of macroscopic currents under the "whole-terminal" voltage clamp configuration revealed responses to depolarizing voltage steps consisting of initial inward followed by later outward current. Tests with TTX and Cd confirmed the presence of both Ca- and Na-mediated components of inward current. Block of outward current after substitution of CsCl for KCl in the internal solution confirms that outward current is K-mediated. Outward current was strongly inhibited by TEA.

Inside-out patches of terminal membrane showed conspicuous unitary current fluctuations which were not voltage-gated. They have been characterized by their kinetics and conductance as fast (f-) and slow, or second (s-) channels. The f-channels can be found in nearly every patch tested, although s-channels are rare. The s-channels characteristically have long openings with flickerings to the closed state. The f-channels, by contrast, have "bursty" openings with many brief transitions. Both types are cation-selective, showing equal conductance to Na and K and failure to pass divalents or anions. They differ in that only the s-channel will pass Cs. Conductances in symmetrical 310 m*M* KCl solutions are 213 pS and 69 pS for s- and f-channels respectively. The s-channels are activated by increases in $[Ca]_i$ to μ*M* levels; at higher concentrations activation is transient. The f-channels are activated by $[Na]_i$ exceeding 40 m*M*. Like the s-channels, they are inhibited by high $[Ca]_i$ (Lemos et al. 1986).

Recently, it has proven feasible to obtain gigaohm seals on dilatations at the exposed surface of the isolated, but otherwise intact, sinus gland (Fig. 2A). It has been possible to routinely isolate patches including f-channels and to show that their characteristics are indistinguishable from those observed in membrane of dissociated terminals (Ruben and Cooke 1987). A Ca-activated cationic current has been reported in whole-cell patch clamp studies of axotomised crayfish X-organ cells (Valdiosera et al. 1986). The role served by f- and s-channels is not clear. It is interesting that channels exhibiting similar characteristics have also been observed in patches from dissociated terminals of rat neurohypophysis prepared in a manner similar to the crab terminal dilatations (Lemos and Nordmann 1986). Their conductance characteristics would permit them to play a role in broadening spikes or maintaining the plateau seen to underlie bursting in crab terminals.

Exploration and categorization of the repertoire of channels present in membrane of the peptidergic terminal regions is just beginning. The opportunity to utilize patch clamp methods on acutely dissected, non-cultured material is relatively rare. A report of patch clamp recording from undissociated rat neurohypophysis has appeared (Mason and Dyball 1986). An interesting question to be addressed in our material is whether Ca channels are highly localized at potential release sites or distributed more generally. Exocytotic profiles have thus far been observed only where small processes extending from the larger dilatations make contact with the neurolemmal lining of hemolymph sinuses (Weatherby 1981). However, the most external dilatations are apparently exposed to a hemolymph space without an intervening neurolemmal sheath (Fig. 2A; T. Weatherby, unpublished). These are the surfaces to which the patch electrodes have ready access. Are they sites of secretion?

2.3 Electrophysiological Evidence Concerning the Control of Secretion

Direct evidence (to be reviewed below) is available that action potentials propagated to sinus gland terminals cause release of peptide hormones (Cooke et al. 1977). The presence of axon collaterals extending into regions of central neuropil provides an anatomical basis for suggesting synaptic control of the peptidergic neurons. In view of the consistent presence of "spontaneous" activity in the XOSG recordings, inhibitory as well as excitatory modulation can be considered. Since different physiological situations will demand release of different peptides, specific central control over neurons releasing different peptides would be anticipated, and different transmitters might be involved at the synapses. Because they are neurosecretory the XOSG neurons are very well supplied with hemolymph and might be modulated by neurohormones or endocrine hormones. Fragmentary but suggestive evidence bearing on these possibilities is available.

The color changes mediated by factors released from the sinus gland have been utilized to test responses to injections of putative transmitters or neuromodulators. More recently, release rates of chromatophorotropins from isolated eyestalk neural tissue of fiddler crabs (*Uca pugilator*) have been determined by bioassay in the presence and absence of substances, with and without general electrical stimulation (Quackenbush and Fingerman 1984; review: Fingerman 1985). Thus, for example, dopamine and met-enkephalin stimulated release of red and black pigment-concentrating factors; gamma-aminobutyric acid (GABA) inhibited release of these; 5-hydroxytryptamine (5-HT) released a red pigment-dispersing hormone. There is evidence for the presence of these substances in crustacean neural tissue. Moreover, dopamine and 5-HT are released as neurohormones from another neurohemal organ, the pericardial organs (review: Cooke and Sullivan 1982), thus raising the question of a possible hormonal influence of these substances on the release of material from XOSG.

Direct evidence for synaptic modulation of the XOSG comes from observation of synaptic potentials in intracellular recordings from crayfish X-organ somata following stimulation of the optic peduncle (Iwasaki and Satow 1971; Garcia and Aréchiga 1986). Glantz et al. (1983), utilizing relatively intact crayfish, observed excitatory postsynaptic potentials recorded from the neurite near the collateral arbor following illumination of the ipsilateral eye.

Nagano (1986b) simultaneously recorded intracellularly from both somata and terminals and extracellularly from the axon tract of crab XOSGs during bath application of putative transmitters. A Vaseline barrier through which the axon tract passed separated compartments, permitting independent applications of substances to the somata and collaterals or to the terminals of isolated XOSGs. Consistent inhibitory responses were obtained to 5-HT in *Cardisoma* preparations and to GABA in *Podopthalmus* recordings. The substances were effective only if the collaterals were exposed to them. There was a decrease in the spontaneous impulse traffic in the sinus gland tract, and recordings from somata showed an increase of resting potential, with an accompanying decrease of impulse firing rate. Although recordings from terminals reflected the decreased impulse firing rates, changes in resting potential were not observed. Application of substances to the terminals generally produced little change. These observations are consistent with the suggestion that receptors are localized to collaterals. A similar conclusion was reached in a study of the localization of GABA responses in the crayfish XOSG (Garcia and Aréchiga 1986). The concentrations of the substances required to obtain the inhibitory effects (5-HT: 10^{-6}–10^{-4} *M*; GABA: 10^{-4}–10^{-3} *M*) are consistent with a role as synaptic transmitters but not as neurohormones. A possible problem in evaluating the sensitivity of preparations to substances by introducing them into the perfusate, as in Nagano's study, is that desensitization can occur if the concentration of the substance in the bath increases gradually.

Responses were observed to a number of other putative neurotransmitter substances (M. Nagano, unpublished), but none produced effects on overall spontaneous activity recorded extracellularly, and the number of examples of intracellularly recorded responses obtained were insufficient to permit their characterization. Application of extracts of the XOSG did not have an effect. Dopamine at 10^{-6}–10^{-4} *M* brought on or increased spontaneous firing rate in eight preparations of the crab, *Podopthalmus*, tested in a rapidly perfused but not divided chamber. Resting potentials were not changed, but input resistance was increased in some cases.

In summary, available evidence supports the suggestion that secretion from the XOSG system is controlled, or at least modulated, by input from the CNS by way of synapses on collaterals of the neurosecretory cells. The evidence is inadequate to establish which transmitters are involved. Inconsistency of responsiveness may reflect heterogeneity of the neurosecretory cells and specificity in their synaptic relations with the CNS. The possibility of modulation of the XOSG by neurohormones secreted from the pericardial organs or other sites, or by other hormones, remains to be adequately tested. Modulation of XOSG activity by the system's own peptides appears not to occur. However, the time frame of observation afforded by intracellular recording from isolated neurosecretory systems may be too short to observe such modulation, if it occurs.

3 Studies of Neurohormone Secretion

3.1 Responses to Axonal Stimulation

Initial studies of secretion from the sinus gland evoked by electrical stimulation of the sinus gland nerve (Cooke et al. 1977) correlated the appearance of RPCH in the perfusate with action potentials recorded extracellularly from the sinus gland. The remarkable sensitivity of the bioassay (detection of an absolute amount of 1 fmol in a volume of 0.2 ml is routine) made it possible to study secretion by single sinus glands. The results supported the Ca hypothesis (Douglas and Poisner 1964 b): an increase in release of RPCH over unstimulated levels was detectable when the stimulus intensity was sufficient to evoke a compound action potential (CAP), was greatest when the largest CAP was observed and did not further increase (and in some cases decreased) at higher stimulus intensities. Release rates were of the order of 3 fmol/min. Release, but not propagated electrical activity, was blocked in the absence of Ca.

Patterned stimulation (trains of five stimuli at 5/s every 10 s) was effective in obtaining release and gave a well-sustained CAP. However, the bioassay, with an uncertainty of half a log unit, was not sufficiently quantitative to determine whether patterning results in greater release than steady stimulation at an equivalent average rate, or whether different stimulus rates (given an equal number of stimuli) affect the release per impulse.

3.2 Responses to Elevated Saline [K]

Elevation of $[K]_o$ has been widely used as a secretory stimulus. It is believed that the evoked membrane depolarization causes calcium entry through specific ionic channels in a manner similar to the depolarizing effect of action potentials in vivo (Douglas and Poisner 1964 a, b; Katz and Miledi 1967). Clearly elevation of $[K]_o$ causes unphysiological changes in the ionic composition of nerve terminals. Yet the relevance of using it as a secretory stimulus is well established and lies in analysis of secretory mechanisms and not in physiological reproduction of in vivo secretion. Unlike most preparations, in the XOSG we can directly record the membrane depolarization produced by high K in the somata and terminals and can simultaneously monitor secretion.

Peptide secretion by the XOSG has been quantitatively monitored using two separate assay techniques. The first utilizes a bioassay for RPCH (Cooke et al. 1977). The second utilizes systems receiving a biosynthetic pulse-chase regime with radiolabeled amino acid(s) (^{3}H-leucine or ^{35}S-cysteine) and subsequent assay for secretion through monitoring radiolabel efflux (Stuenkel 1985; Newcomb et al. 1985). The relevance of monitoring label efflux as a measure of neuropeptide secretion has been substantiated by a number of tests, most directly through identification of released label using HPLC.

Knowledge of the amino acid composition of the neurosecretory peptides for *Cardisoma carnifex* (Table 1; Newcomb 1983, 1987) has allowed differential labeling of particular peptides. Nearly equal amounts of the incorporated ^{3}H (ca. 45% each) are found in the CHH and the peptide H groups when ^{3}H-leucine is the label (Stuenkel 1983, 1986). RPCH accounts for considerably less (<5%). Substituting ^{35}S-cysteine results in incorporation of the radiolabel into the CHH peptides, but the peptide H group, which lacks cysteine or cystine (Stuenkel 1986), remains unlabeled. The biosynthetic pulse-chase studies utilized a split-chamber

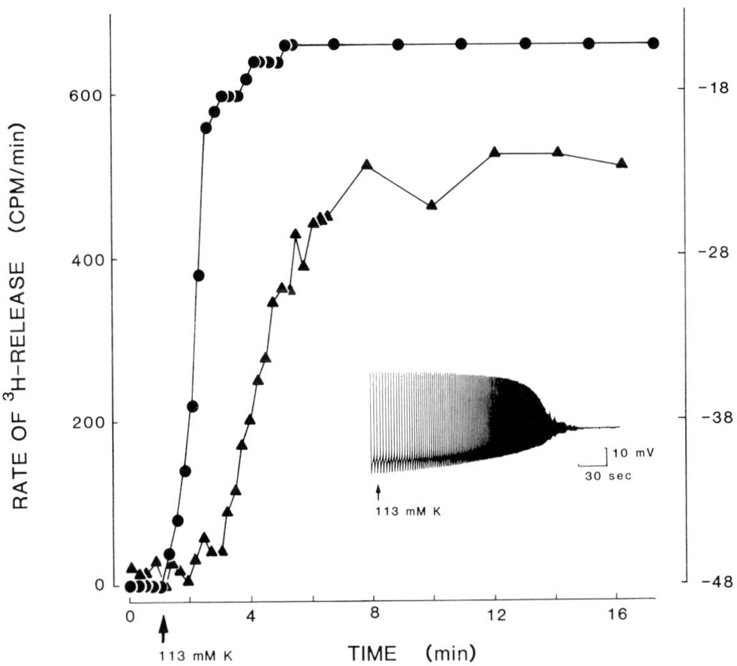

Fig. 5. Comparison of the onset of axon terminal depolarization (●) with the rate of ^{3}H release (▲) when perfusion of the terminals region is switched from normal to high-K saline (*arrow*); time resolution is 14 s. *Inset*: intracellularly recorded response of an axon terminal. An isolated X-organ – sinus gland of *Cardisoma carnifex* was radiolabeled by a 5-h pulse of ^{3}H-leucine on the X-organ side of a divided chamber (see inset, Fig. 7), followed by a 19-h chase. (From Stuenkel 1985)

configuration (Fig. 7 A, inset) allowing application of the label to be restricted to the somata, thus ensuring that radiolabel present in the sinus gland represented transported material (Fig. 1 B). The two parts of the chamber were independently perfused, which permitted secretion to be monitored simultaneously and independently from the portion including the somata, proximal axons and collaterals, and from that having the sinus gland, i.e., the axons terminals.

Application of depolarizing concentrations of $[K]_o$ (113 m*M*) to the axon terminal region of radiolabeled XOSGs resulted in a rapid and several-fold increase of terminal ^3H label efflux (Fig. 5). A time resolution of 14 s was possible for observations on a single XOSG. Maximum ^3H efflux rates (400 cpm/min) were observed within 2 min and were maintained during continued high K perfusion (Stuenkel 1985). With prolonged elevated K application the rate ultimately declined, exhibiting a $t_{1/2}$ of 47 min. The secretory time course was identical for both ^3H and ^{35}S efflux in response to prolonged elevation of saline [K] (Stuenkel, unpublished). Thus, this secretory time course is characteristic for CHH secretion and perhaps also for the H peptide and its cleavage products.

Significant differences in secretory responses turned up when the time course of RPCH secretion was compared with that of biosynthetically radiolabeled peptides (Fig. 6). The time resolution for following RPCH secretion from an individ-

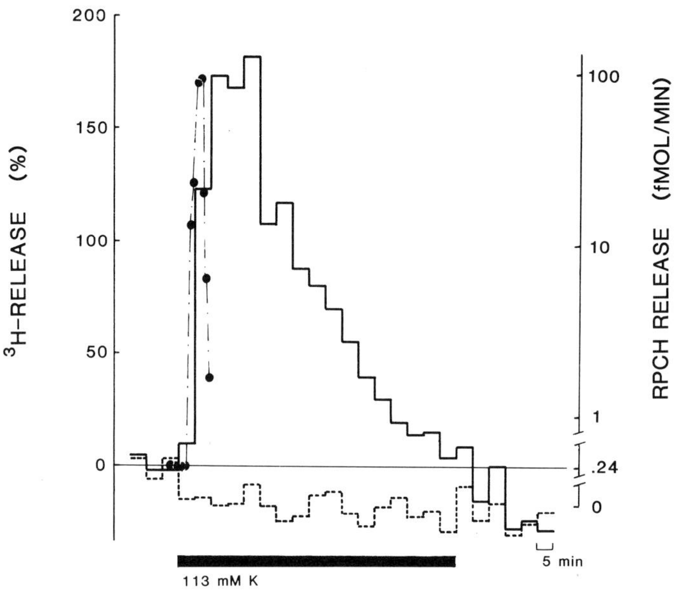

Fig. 6. Comparison of the time course of secretion of ^3H and of red pigment-concentrating hormone (*RPCH*) during perfusion of the terminals region with high-K saline (*bar*). *Solid line*, ^3H release from terminals region; *broken line*, simultaneously monitored release from compartment including somata and collaterals (see inset, Fig. 7). Release is expressed as percent of mean prestimulation basal release; *filled circles*, rate of RPCH release (note log scale) as determined by bioassay of 1-min fractions of the perfusate from the terminals region. Secretion of RPCH falls off rapidly ($t_{1/2} = 6$ min) compared to radiolabeled peptide release ($t_{1/2} = 47$ min). Isolated X-organ – sinus gland of *C. carnifex* radiolabeled as in Fig. 5. (E. Stuenkel, unpublished)

ual XOSG was 0.5 min. The secretion of RPCH rapidly (within 5 min) reached a peak rate (average of 30 fmol/min) and immediately fell off reaching levels only slightly above unstimulated rates within another 2 min (Cooke and Haylett 1984; Stuenkel 1985). The rapid return to near basal levels for RPCH is in sharp contrast to the prolonged secretory response for ^{3}H label (see further below).

The ionic dependency of ^{3}H label and RPCH secretion appear to be identical. Both the increased efflux of ^{3}H label and of RPCH in response to elevation of $[K]_o$ show susceptibility to removal of saline Ca or to ionic blockers of Ca current (e.g., Cd, Mn; Fig. 7 A, B), indicating that Ca entry is necessary for these secretory responses. Both addition of Cd (1 m*M*) or substitution of Mn (26.3 m*M*) for Mg while maintaining normal saline [Ca] are able to suppress elevated K-induced secretion. Replacement of Na with choline had no effect on the duration of the elevated K-induced secretory response for RPCH or ^{3}H label. It also had no effect on the amount of radiolabel released, and slightly enhanced the release of RPCH in response to elevated K perfusion. An enhancement of secretory response following reduction of saline [Na] has been reported in other preparations, for example, the rat neurohypophysis (Nordmann 1976).

3.3 Inactivation

Depolarization is important in initiating entry of extracellular Ca, and it has also been suggested in a number of cases to exert a governing influence on the time course of secretion via voltage-dependent inactivation of inward Ca current. The marked differences between the secretory time course for RPCH ($t_{1/2}$ = 6 min) and for ^{3}H efflux ($t_{1/2}$ = 47 min) upon exposure to elevated K suggests that the secretory processes governing release differ among neurosecretory terminals. Our evidence suggests that the rapid decline of RPCH release, as contrasted with sustained release of ^{3}H-labeled hormones, reflects a voltage-dependent inactivation of the RPCH release, perhaps attributable to inactivation of Ca channels and lack of such inactivation in the majority of terminals responsible for ^{3}H-labeled peptide secretion. If a sinus gland is first perfused with a Ca-free, high-K saline, no release of RPCH or ^{3}H peptides occurs. If Ca is restored to the perfusate while continuing to hold the sinus gland in high K, release of ^{3}H-labeled peptides occurs on the same time course and in the same amounts as from a first exposure of the preparation to high-K saline. By contrast, there is very little or no release of RPCH. If, however, the preparation is returned to normal saline for 20–30 min and then challenged with high-K (normal-Ca) saline, RPCH release occurs as if this were a first exposure to high K. Hence, the K-induced depolarization in the absence of hormone release inactivates RPCH secretory responsiveness, but not ^{3}H-labeled secretion. Other observations supporting this conclusion are that application of saline containing Cd or Mn, before (Fig. 7 A) or following onset of K-induced secretion of ^{3}H-labeled peptides, resulted in a block or a sharp reduction of efflux of radiolabel. Removal of Cd or Mn during continued high-K perfusion led to a resurgence of label efflux. Hence, we expect to find electrophysiological evidence that terminals differ in the characteristics of their Ca channels: a minority showing marked voltage-dependent inactivation of Ca currents, the majority showing a lack of voltage-dependent inactivation.

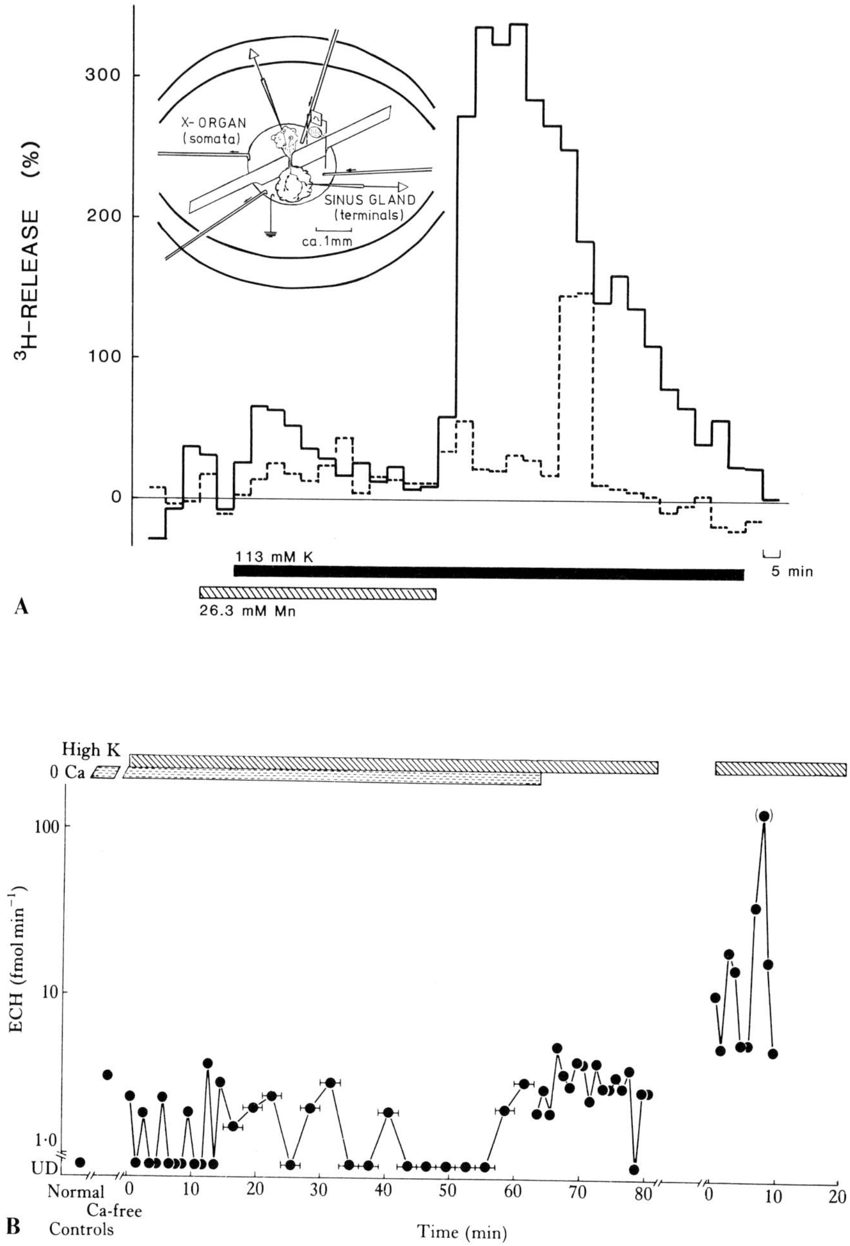

Fig. 7A, B. Calcium dependence of high-K-stimulated secretion: observations relevant to voltage-dependent inactivation (*C. carniflex*). **A** Block of ^{3}H secretion in response to elevated K by Mn. Fractions were collected at 5-min intervals from the axon terminal region (*continuous line*) and somatic region (*dashed line*). The Mn (*hatched bar*) is applied to both the somatic and axon terminal region, while the elevated K (*solid bar*) is restricted to the axon terminal region. Release expressed as in Fig. 6, radiolabeling as in Fig. 5. Note that upon removal of Mn, secretion begins immediately and is of normal amount and duration (cf. Fig. 6), indicating a lack of voltage-dependent inactivation. *Inset*: diagram of divided

The demonstration that release of RPCH is inhibited following exposure to high-K, Ca-free saline without any hormonal release having occurred establishes that an inactivation mechanism operates, but leaves for discussion a possible additional role of depletion of peptides from the terminal in the rapid decline of the secretory response during high-K (normal-Ca) exposure. When isolated sinus gland preparations were challenged with a series of 10-min pulses of high K with intervening periods of 30 min to 1 h in normal saline (sufficient time for full recovery of intracellularly recorded terminal resting potential), second and subsequent secretory responses were at most 70%, and usually around 20%, of the RPCH released during the first response. By contrast, release during electrical stimulation of the axon tract (trains of five stimuli at 5/s every 10 s), while at about a tenth the rate observable during exposure to high K, continued without decrement for at least 3 h. The amounts of RPCH released by 3 h of electrical stimulation were comparable to those released during three or four 10-min pulses of high K (ca. 300 fmol). However, this amount is less than 2% of the total RPCH stored in the sinus gland. Limitation of the amount of hormonal material that can be released by stimulation to a small part of the total stored has been the general observation in neurosecretory systems. This has led to the suggestion of a "readily releasable pool," which is distinguishable from the bulk of stored material (for further discussion see Newcomb et al., this volume). In conclusion, the rapid decline in RPCH release during exposure to high K is directly attributable to a voltage-dependent inactivation, but may also be accelerated by depletion of a readily releasable pool.

The slow decline of release rates of biosynthetically radiolabeled peptides from the sinus gland during high-K perfusion may reflect depletion of the radiolabeled pool. Autoradiographic studies of XOSGs following various pulse-chase regimes (E. Stuenkel and E. Gillary, unpublished) provide convincing pictures of radiolabeled material that is transported to the sinus gland being concentrated at first (at 14–24 h) in terminals abutting the internal blood spaces. Figure 1 B illustrates a preparation given a 5-h pulse of ^{3}H-leucine (X-organ only exposed) followed by a 19-h chase, and subsequently utilized in one of the release studies. Comparison of the amounts of the peptides $<10\,000$ M_r present in high-K perfusates of such preparations with the amounts present in the sinus gland suggests that there may be a preferential release of more completely processed material (Newcomb et al. 1985). Whether the decline in release of radiolabeled material reflects a decline in total peptide hormone release or merely in radiolabeled hormone release remains undetermined. However, the generality of the observation that only a limited proportion of stored material can be released, mentioned previously, makes it likely that secretion of all peptides declines. The $t_{1/2}$ of 47 min

chamber. (From Stuenkel 1985). **B** Suppression of RPCH secretion in response to high K by removal of Ca. Fractions were collected at 1-min intervals and bioassayed. A period of 20 min perfusion in nominally Ca-free saline preceded the introduction of 193 m*M* K in Ca-free saline at time 0. Note lack of secretory response. Note, also, lack of response upon reintroduction of Ca (25 m*M*) at 60 min, suggesting occurrence of voltage-dependent inactivation. After an hour of perfusion with normal saline, the switch to high-K perfusion (at second time 0) produces a typical secretory response. (From Cooke and Haylett 1984)

is somewhat longer than that observed for release of oxytocin from the rat neurohypophysis (ca. 30 min, Nordmann 1976), for example. It represents one of the best-sustained secretory performances thus far observed.

3.4 Secretory Characteristics of the Neurosecretory Somata

The routing of secretory material to particular membrane domains of secretory cells is a topic of considerable interest (e.g., Palade 1975; Blobel 1980; Kelly 1985). Even in non-neural secretory cells, where secretion across the plasma membrane is requisite, directionality is frequently found (e.g., secretion occurs from the apical but not the basolateral membrane). In neurosecretory cells the movement of secretory products along axons and their accumulation in axon terminal structures provides a clear representation of directionality and points to the importance of the terminal structures in secretion. In this regard it is not surprising that with a few exceptions (Loh et al. 1975; Bie and Thorn 1967), secretion from peptidergic neurosecretory cell bodies has been little studied. The presence in the XOSG of an extensive collateral arbor (Fig. 1 C; Andrew and Saleuddin 1978; Cooke and Stuenkel 1985) where the X-organ cells might synapse onto other neuronal collaterals and of fully processed neurosecretory material resident within the somata (Stuenkel 1983, 1986) suggests that collaterals or somata might be sites of release. A voltage-dependent Ca entry process is present in at least some of the somata as evidenced by the dual Na and Ca dependence of somatic action potentials in somata that are invaded by the action potential (see above). Historical evidence for somatic secretion is based on continued molt inhibition (due to an XOSG hormone) subsequent to ablation of the sinus gland if the X-organ is left intact (Passano 1953).

Utilizing the divided chamber in which somata and collaterals are separated from terminals and separately perfused, the release of both RPCH and biosynthetically ^{3}H-labeled material from each region was assessed in response to elevation of saline $[K]_o$ (Fig. 6; Stuenkel 1985). No release of RPCH bioactivity was detected in perfusate from the chamber including the somata and collateral region. However, a slight transient increase in ^{3}H release was observed and suggests that release from peptidergic neurosecretory somata or collaterals cannot be entirely excluded. The stimulation of label efflux lasted ca. 3 min and exhibited a ca. twofold increase from prestimulation efflux levels. This represented less than 4% of the total amount of stimulated efflux observed from the terminals of the same preparations similarly tested. Expressing the stimulated efflux as a percentage of the estimated total hormone within the somata and terminals (Stuenkel 1983) would suggest that a significant fraction, albeit a small absolute amount, of the somatic material is available for release. The average membrane depolarization in response to application of elevated $[K]_o$ to the soma is somewhat less (average value of -26 mV for 113 mM $[K]_o$ than that observed in terminals (-22 mV).

3.5 Electrophysiological Correlates

The onset of the increase in peptide secretion shows a high correlation with simultaneously monitored terminal depolarization (see Fig. 5). Further, under none of the ionic substitutions mentioned above is the rate or extent of the terminal depolarization induced by elevated K noticeably affected. Thus, the reduction in the secretory response resulting from omission of saline Ca or addition of Cd or Mn is not the result of an altered depolarizing response to elevated K. When the perfusate is switched to an elevated K saline, the intracellular recording shows a ramp depolarization of the membrane potential accompanied initially by an increased spontaneous impulse firing rate. As depolarization continues, action potential amplitude decreases, and spiking activity eventually ceases. Terminal membrane potential reaches a steady value within 3 min and remains at the depolarized level (averaging −22 mV for 113 m*M* $[K]_o$) throughout the elevated K application. Concurrent with the terminal depolarization is a decrease in terminal input resistance to about one-half which is maintained throughout the elevated K pulse. A delay observed between the onset of K-induced depolarization and that of increased efflux is suggested to result from delays both in chamber turnover and in diffusion of label from sinuses within the neurohemal organ. Return to saline of normal $[K]_o$ results in a repolarization of membrane potential which is slower than the depolarization occurring upon the introduction of the high-K saline. There is a return of spontaneous spiking activity after 10–20 min. For elevated K pulses of less than 20 min, efflux of label declines in parallel with repolarization of the terminal, distinctly lagging behind the restoration of normal-K saline, indicating that it is depolarization, and not the presence of excess K itself, that is important to secretion. The effects of the ionic substitutions on action potentials are consistent with the presence of Ca- and Na-mediated components of the terminal action potentials as discussed.

4 Summary and Perspectives

Work reviewed here shows the XOSG conforms fully to predictions of the stimulus-secretion coupling hypothesis proposed over 20 years ago from studies of the neuromuscular junction (Katz and Miledi 1967), mammalian adrenal medulla (Douglas and Rubin 1963) and neurohypophysis (Douglas and Poisner 1964 a, b). For neural systems it proposes that membrane depolarization resulting from the arrival of action potentials at axon terminals leads to calcium entry which directly triggers, by an unknown mechanism, exocytotic release of secretory material. Support for this hypothesis from observations on the XOSG can be summarized as follows:

1. The secretory rate can be increased by direct electrical stimulation of propagated impulse activity or by membrane depolarization evoked by increased $[K]_o$, but these stimuli are only effective in the presence of extracellular Ca.

2. Simultaneous measurement of elevated K-evoked changes in membrane potential and secretion show secretion to be correlated with membrane depolarization.
3. Ionic blockers of Ca channels affect neither the rate nor extent of the K-induced depolarization, but are effective in blocking peptide secretion.
4. Terminals exhibit overshooting, dual Na-, Ca-mediated action potentials and are enriched relative to axons in voltage-responsive Ca channels.

As in many neurosecretory systems, impulse activity can occur in bursts with terminal impulses often exhibiting spike broadening. At presynaptic terminals of the squid stellate ganglion synapse, increased impulse duration results in additional Ca entry and enhanced transmitter release (Llinás et al. 1981 a, b). It is thus tempting to speculate that bursting may lead to spike broadening at the terminals of the neurohypophysis, since bursting is known to facilitate peptide secretion (Dutton and Dyball 1979; Bicknell et al. 1982). We may also speculate that it facilitates hormone release from the crab sinus gland, and look forward to the availability of more sensitive and quantitative assays to test this suggestion. Efforts to intimately correlate changes in electrophysiological responses with secretory output face limitations inherent to neurohormonal secretion. The response to peptide neurohormones is generally slow, often involving receptor-agonist-initiated biochemical cascades, compared to responses to several non-peptide transmitters which directly produce a conductance change in the closely opposed postsynaptic membrane. It is thus unlikely that secretory efficacy can be monitored impulse for impulse as it can be at a neuromuscular junction, where the postsynaptic fiber provides an instant bioassay.

The studies on the XOSG have provided an instructive example of hormone-specific differences in secretory mechanisms and their resultant differences in the time course of secretion for the different hormones. Thus, we find that RPCH is released in a brief pulse during maintained depolarization, whereas hormones derived from a different prohormone, such as CHH, can be continuously released while depolarization continues. While our knowledge of hormonal function is very incomplete, we can suggest that these differences reflect physiological roles, requiring occasional release or sustained release respectively. Our observations point to the presence or absence of voltage-dependent inactivation of voltage-dependent Ca channels as the cause of the difference in secretory response. Several distinct Ca channel types in mammalian dorsal root ganglion neurons (Nowycky et al. 1985), cardiac muscle (Nilius et al. 1985) and other preparations (Matteson and Armstrong 1986) have been described that show differences in voltage activation, single-channel conductance and inactivation properties. Clearly, quantitative and qualitative differences in ionic channel types are observed among neurons as a group and may, as suggested here, extend to Ca channels at nerve terminals. In support of this hypothesis, release of the neurotransmitter, substance P, from dorsal root ganglion neurons is sensitive to dihydropyridine, while norepinephrine release from sympathetic neurons shows resistance to this type of drug (Perney et al. 1986). Characterization of nerve terminal Ca channels at the single-channel level has previously been restricted by their relative inaccessibility for electrophysiological study. The recent development of terminal preparations allowing patch clamp analysis from the XOSG (Lemos et al. 1986) and the neurohypophysial system (Mason and Dyball 1986; Lemos and Nordmann 1986) now allows this question to be addressed directly.

The burgeoning evidence for a role of changes in $[Ca]_i$ in regulating cascades of biochemical processes leads to questions about the consequences of differences among neurons in the types and distribution of Ca channels. Assuming, as our data suggest, that axon terminals are diverse with respect to properties of their Ca channels and that this diversity accounts for differences in the kinetics of secretion, do differences in properties of the Ca channels lead to subsequent effects on intracellular Ca-dependent processes? What is the significance of the presence of impulse invasion, and, with it, of Ca channels in the somata of some but not all of the crab X-organ neurons? It is tempting to speculate that impulse-mediated Ca entry might participate in regulating such processes as rates of gene transcription or of translation of prohormone from message, or its incorporation into granules, or the rate of granule transport to release sites. There is a paucity of information about whether, and, if so, how the supply of hormone to release sites is matched to secretory demand. The presence of large amounts of hormone in neurohemal organs and the inability of acute secretory stimuli to cause release of more than a fraction of the stored material suggests that regulation may not need to be finely tuned.

The tight coupling of membrane potential, impulse activity and Ca to secretion also lends importance to studies of substances which may modify these parameters, namely neurotransmitters and hormones. The literature reviewed above clearly demonstrates that impulse frequency, membrane potential and secretion in the XOSG system are affected by neurotransmitter activation of receptors. The cellular processes through which these agents act to exert their effects on the XOSG, subsequent to receptor binding, have not been defined and are clearly areas needing further investigation. A number of intracellular signals arising from receptor occupation have been described. Many of these operate via activation of protein kinases such as cAMP-dependent, cGMP-dependent, Ca-calmodulin-dependent kinases or protein kinase C (review: Reichardt and Kelly 1983). Best characterized are neurotransmitters that act through cAMP-dependent protein kinase to phosphorylate ionic channels with a resultant modification of channel behavior (Levitan 1985). For example, β-adrenergic stimulation of mammalian cardiac cells produces an increase in the slow inward Ca current that is believed to result from phosphorylation of a Ca channel via cAMP-dependent protein kinase (reviews: Reuter 1983; Sperelakis 1985). Another receptor-linked mechanism is evidenced by noradrenaline and GABA effects on chick dorsal root ganglion neurons (Dunlap and Fishbach 1978; Holz et al. 1986) and by acetylcholine effects on cardiac muscle (Pfaffinger et al. 1985; Breitwieser and Szabo 1985) in which a unique GTP-binding protein (N or G protein) that does not utilize the cAMP-dependent protein kinase cascade causes both suppression of Ca channels and activation of a specific set of K channels. Recently, inhibition of neurotransmitter release by opioid peptides has been proposed to involve regulation of voltage-dependent Ca channels by the GTP-binding protein G_o (Hescheler et al. 1987). In addition, some neurotransmitters and hormones activate a receptor-linked phospholipase C which leads to the generation of diacylglycerol and inositol (1,4,5)-trisphosphate (IP3). Diacylglycerol, together with Ca and phospholipids, is a potent activator of protein kinase C. This kinase has been implicated in the regulation of Ca, K and Cl channels, and therefore neuronal excitability, in preparations which include both invertebrates and vertebrates (review: Kaczmarek 1987). The ramifications of activation of this receptor type for Ca-dependent secretion are extended when one considers the cogeneration with diacylglycerol of IP3 and, more recently, inositol (1,3,4,5)-tetraphosphate, derived by phosphorylation of IP3. These are messengers involved in the release of Ca from intracellular stores (Streb et al. 1983) and regulation of plasma membrane Ca channels (Irvine and Moore 1986) respectively.

In a hormone-secreting system, such as the XOSG, which is known to exert control over long-term processes like growth, gonad maturation and limb regeneration, as well as over shorter-term homeostatic responses, we would expect to find that the interplay of blood-borne substances and transmitters will include influences of kinds such as those just mentioned. Analysis for such effects has not yet begun. The complexity and potential for precise regulation involved in second messenger and effector systems would be enhanced several-fold if interaction and feedback regulation between several of these systems occurs, as suggested by increasing amounts of evidence. It therefore appears likely that the interaction of multiple transmitters and hormones impinging on secretory cells, such as the XOSG, will result in complex integrated electrical and secretory responses. Dissection of these cellular processes and interactions is of great importance in moving toward understanding the correlation of electrical and secretory activity and of its regulation.

Acknowledgments. We thank our collaborators whose unpublished as well as published work and day-to-day discussions have contributed greatly to the understanding of the crab XOSG specifically, as well as to the general understanding of neurosecretory mechanisms. They include: E. Gillary (light- and electron-microscopic autoradiography), M. Goldstone (histology and technical support), B. Haylett (RPCH secretion, histology and technical support), J. Lemos (patch clamping), M. Nagano (regional intracellular recordings and pharmacology), R. Newcomb (peptide isolation and characterization), J. Nordmann (physiology of isolated terminals), and T. Weatherby (electron-microscopy). We are grateful to P. Ruben for editorial suggestions and C. Kosaki for preparation of the manuscript.

References

Abramowitz AA, Hisaw FL, Papandrea DN (1944) The occurrence of a diabetogenic factor in the eyestalk of crustaceans. Biol Bull 86:1–5

Adiyodi R (1985) Reproduction and its control. In: Bliss DE, Mantel LH (eds) The biology of Crustacea, vol 9. Academic, New York, pp 147–215

Andrew RD (1983) Neurosecretory pathways supplying the neurohemal organs in Crustacea. In: Gupta AP (ed) Neurohemal organs of Arthropoda. Thomas, Springfield, pp 90–117

Andrew RD, Saleuddin AS (1978) Structure and innervation of a crustacean neurosecretory cell. Can J Zool 56:423–430

Andrew RD, Saleuddin AS (1979) Two-dimensional gel electrophoresis of neurosecretory polypeptides in crustacean eyestalk. J Comp Physiol 134:303–313

Andrew RD, Orchard I, Saleuddin AS (1978) Structural re-evaluation of the neurosecretory system in the crayfish eyestalk. Cell Tissue Res 190:235–246

Bicknell R, Flint J, Leng APF, Sheldrick EL (1982) Phasic pattern of electrical stimulation enhances oxytocin secretion from the isolated neurohypophysis. Neurosci Lett 30:47–50

Bie P, Thorn NA (1967) In vitro studies of the release mechanism for vasopressin in rats. II. Studies of the possible release of hormone from hypothalamic tissue. Acta Endocrinol (Copenh) 56:139–145

Bliss DE (1951) Metabolic effects of sinus gland or eyestalk removal in the land crab, *Gecarcinus lateralis*. Anat Rec 111:502–503

Bliss DE, Welsh JH (1952) The neurosecretory system of brachyuran Crustacea. Biol Bull 103:157–169

Blobel G (1980) Intracellular protein topogenesis. Proc Natl Acad Sci USA 77:1496–1500

Breitwieser GE, Szabo G (1985) Uncoupling of cardiac muscarinic and B-adrenergic receptors from ion channels by a guanine nucleotide analogue. Nature 317:538–540

Brown FA, Cunningham O (1939) Influence of the sinus gland of crustaceans on normal viability and ecdysis. Biol Bull 77:104–114

Bunt A, Ashby E (1967) Ultrastructure of the sinus gland of the crayfish *Procambarus clarkii*. Gen Comp Physiol 9:334–342

Bunt A, Ashby E (1968) Ultrastructural changes in the crayfish sinus gland following electrical stimulation. Gen Comp Endocrinol 10:376–382

Chaigneau J (1983) Neurohemal organs in Crustacea. In: Gupta AP (ed) Neurohemal organs of Arthropoda. Thomas, Springfield, pp 53–89

Chang ES, Bruce MJ, Newcomb RW (1987) Purification and amino acid composition of a peptide with molt-inhibiting activity from the lobster, *Homarus americanus*. Gen Comp Endocrinol 65:56–64

Cooke IM (1985) Electrophysiological characterization of peptidergic neurosecretory terminals. J Exp Biol 118:1–35

Cooke IM, Haylett BA (1984) Ionic dependence of secretory and electrical activity evoked by elevated K^+ in a peptidergic neurosecretory system. J Exp Biol 113:289–321

Cooke IM, Stuenkel EL (1985) Electrophysiology of invertebrate neurosecretory cells. In: Poisner AM, Trifaro J (eds) The electrophysiology of the secretory cell. Elsevier, Amsterdam, pp 115–164

Cooke IM, Sullivan RE (1982) Hormones and neurosecretion. In: Atwood H, Sandeman D (eds) The biology of Crustacea. Academic, New York, pp 205–290

Cooke IM, Haylett BA, Weatherby TM (1977) Electrically elicited neurosecretory and electrical responses of the isolated crab sinus gland in normal and reduced calcium salines. J Exp Biol 70:125–149

Douglas WW, Poisner AM (1964 a) Stimulus-secretion coupling in a neurosecretory organ: the role of calcium in the release of vasopressin from the neurohypophysis. J Physiol (Lond) 172:1–18

Douglas WW, Poisner AM (1964 b) Calcium movements in the neurohypophysis of the rat and its relation to the release of vasopressin. J Physiol (Lond) 172:19 30

Douglas WW, Rubin RP (1963) The mechanism of catecholamine release from the adrenal medulla and the role of calcium in stimulus-secretion coupling. J Physiol (Lond) 167:288–310

Dunlap K, Fischbach GD (1978) Neurotransmitters decrease the calcium component of sensory neurone action potentials. Nature 276:837–839

Dutton A, Dyball REJ (1979) Phasic firing enhances vasopressin release from the rat neurohypophysis. J Physiol (Lond) 290:433–440

Edgington DR, Stuart AE (1979) Calcium channels in the high resistivity axona membrane of photoreceptors of the giant barnacle. J Physiol (Lond) 294:433–445

Fernlund P (1976) Structure of a light-adapting hormone from the shrimp, *Pandalus borealis*. Biochim Biophys Acta 439:17–25

Fernlund P, Josefsson L (1972) Crustacean color-change hormone: amino acid sequence and chemical synthesis. Science 177:173–175

Fingerman M (1985) The physiology and pharmacology of crustacean chromatophores. Am Zool 25:233–252

Gabe M (1966) Neurosecretion. Pergamon, Oxford, p 872

Garcia U, Aréchiga H (1986) GABAergic input to crustacean neurosecretory cells. Soc Neurosci Abstr 12:243

Garcia U, Onetti C, Valdiosera RF (1985) Calcium currents in the secretory neuron soma of the X-organ of the crayfish. Soc Neurosci Abstr 11:520

Glantz RM, Kirk MD, Arechiga H (1983) Light input to crustacean neurosecretory cells. Brain Res 265:307–311

Gorman A, Thomas MV (1978) Changes in the intracellular concentration of free calcium ions in a pace-maker neurone, measured with the metallochromic indicator dye Arsenazo III. J Physiol (Lond) 275:357–376

Hamill OP, Marty A, Neher E, Sakmann B, Sigworth FJ (1981) Improved patch-clamp techniques for high resolution current recording from cells and cell-free membrane patches. Pflugers Arch 391:85–100

Hanström B (1931) Neue Untersuchungen über Sinnesorgane und Nervensysteme der Crustaceen. I. Z Morphol Ökol Tiere 23:80–236

Hescheler J, Rosenthal W, Trautwein W, Schultz G (1987) The GTP-binding protein, Go, regulates neuronal calcium channels. Nature 325:445–446

Holz GG, Rane SG, Dunlap K (1986) GTP-binding proteins mediate transmitter inhibition of voltage-dependent calcium channels. Nature 319:670–672

Huberman A, Aguilar M (1986) A neurosecretory hyperglycemic hormone from the sinus gland of the Mexican crayfish *Procambarus bouvieri*. I. Purification and biochemical characterization of the most abundant form of the hormone. Comp Biochem Physiol [B] 85:197–204

Irvine RF, Moor RM (1986) Micro-injection of inositol 1,3,4,5-tetrakisphosphate activates sea urchin eggs by a mechanism dependent on external Ca^{2+}. Biochem J 240:917–920

Iwasaki S, Satow Y (1969) Spontaneous grouped discharge of secretory neuron soma in X-organ of crayfish, *Procambarus clarkii*. J Physiol Soc Jpn 31:629–630

Iwasaki S, Satow Y (1971) Sodium- and calcium-dependent spike potentials in the secretory neuron soma of the X-organ of the crayfish. J Gen Physiol 57:216–238

Jaros PP (1978) Tracing of neurosecretory neurons in crayfish optic ganglia by cobalt iontophoresis. Cell Tissue Res 194:297–302

Jaros PP (1979) Immunocytochemical demonstration of the neurosecretory X-organ complex in the eyestalk of the crab *Carcinus maenas*. Histochemistry 63:303–310

Kaczmarek LK (1987) The role of protein kinase C in the regulation of ion channels and neurotransmitter release. Trends Neurosci 10:30–34

Katz B, Miledi R (1967) The timing of calcium action during neuromuscular transmission. J Physiol (Lond) 189:535–544

Katz B, Miledi R (1969a) Tetrodotoxin-resistant electrical activity in presynaptic terminals. J Physiol (Lond) 203:459–487

Katz B, Miledi R (1969b) Spontaneous and evoked activity of motor nerve endings in calcium Ringer. J Physiol (Lond) 203:689–706

Keller R (1983) Biochemistry and specificity of the neurohemal hormones in Crustacea. In: Gupta AP (ed) Neurohemal organs of Arthropoda. Thomas, Springfield, pp 118–148

Keller R, Kegel G (1984) Studies on crustacean eyestalk neuropeptides by use of high performance liquid chromatography. In: Hoffmann J, Porchet M (eds) Biosynthesis, metabolism and mode of action of invertebrate hormones. Springer, Berlin Heidelberg New York, pp 145–154

Keller R, Jaros PP, Kegel G (1985) Crustacean hyperglycemic neuropeptides. Am Zool 25:207–221

Kelly RB (1985) Pathways of protein secretion in eukaryotes. Science 230:25–32

Kleinholz LH (1936) Crustacean eyestalk hormone and retinal pigment migration. Biol Bull 70:159–184

Lemos JR, Nordmann JJ (1986) Ionic channels and hormone release from peptidergic nerve terminals. J Exp Biol 124:53–72

Lemos JR, Nordmann JJ, Cooke IM, Stuenkel EL (1986) Single channels and ionic currents in peptidergic nerve terminals. Nature 319:410–412

Levitan IB (1985) Phosphorylation of ion channels. J Membr Biol 87:177–190

Llinás R, Steinberg IZ, Walton K (1981a) Presynaptic calcium currents in squid giant synapse. Biophys J 33:289–322

Llinás R, Steinberg IZ, Walton K (1981 b) Relationship between presynaptic calcium current and postsynaptic potential in squid giant synapse. Biophys J 33:323–352

Loh Y, Sarne Y, Gainer H (1975) Heterogeneity of proteins synthesized, stored and released by the bag cells of *Aplysia californica*. J Comp Physiol 100:283–295

Mangerich S, Keller R, Dircksen H (1986) Immunocytochemical identification of structures containing putative red pigment-concentrating hormone in two species of decapod crustaceans. Cell Tissue Res 245:377–386

Martin G, Keller R, Kegel G, Besee G, Jaros P (1984) The hyperglycemic neuropeptide of the terrestrial isopod, *Porcellio dilatatus*. I: isolation and characterization. Gen Comp Endocrinol 55:208–216

Mason W, Dyball R (1986) Single ion channel activity in peptidergic nerve terminals of the isolated rat neurohypophysis related to stimulation of neural stalk axons. Brain Res 383:279–286

Matteson DR, Armstrong CM (1986) Properties of two types of calcium channels in clonal pituitary cells. J Gen Physiol 87:161–182

Mattson M (1986) New insights into neuroendocrine regulation of the crustacean molt cycle. Zool Sci 3:733–744

Nagano M (1983) Effects of 5HT and GABA on spontaneous electrical activity of a peptide neurosecretory system. J Physiol Soc Jpn 45:418

Nagano M (1986 a) Heterogeneity of neurons in the crustacean X-organ as revealed by intracellular recording and injection of horseradish peroxidase. Brain Res 362:379–383

Nagano M (1986 b) Regional inhibitory effects of 5HT and GABA on the spontaneous electrical activity of a crab neurosecretory system. Biomed Res 7:267–277

Nagano M, Cooke IM (1987) Comparison of electrical responses of terminals, axons, and somata of a peptidergic neurosecretory system. J Neurosci 7:634–648

Newcomb R (1983) Peptides in the sinus gland of the land crab *Cardisoma carnifex*: isolation and amino acid analysis. J Comp Physiol [B] 153:207–221

Newcomb R (1987) Amino acid sequences of neuropeptides in the sinus gland of the land crab *Cardisoma carnifex*: a novel neuropeptide proteolysis site. J Neurochem 49/2:574–583

Newcomb R, Stuenkel EL, Cooke IM (1985) Characterization, biosynthesis and release of neuropeptides from the X-organ sinus gland system of the crab *Cardisoma carnifex*. Am Zool 25:157–171

Nilius B, Hess P, Lansman JB, Tsien RW (1985) A novel type of cardiac calcium channel in ventricular cells. Nature 316:443–446

Niwa A, Kawai N (1982) Tetrodotoxin-resistant propagating action potentials in presynaptic axon of the lobster. J Neurophysiol 47:353–361

Nordmann JJ (1976) Evidence for calcium inactivation during hormone release in the rat neurohypophysis. J Exp Biol 65:669–683

Nordmann JJ, Weatherby TM, Haylett BA (1986) Ultrastructural changes in isolated peptidergic nerve terminals induced by digitonin permeabilization and K^+ stimulation in the sinus gland of the crab, *Cardisoma carnifex*. Cell Tissue Res 246:365–371

Nowycky MC, Fox AP, Tsien RW (1985) Three types of neuronal calcium channels with different calcium agonist sensitivity. Nature 316:440–443

Obaid AL, Orkand RK, Gainer H, Salzberg BM (1985) Active calcium responses recorded optically from nerve terminals of the frog neurohypophysis. J Gen Physiol 85:481–489

Palade G (1975) Intracellular aspects of the process of protein synthesis. Science 189:347–358

Passano LM (1951) The X-organ-sinus gland neurosecretory system in crabs. Anat Rec 111:502

Passano LM (1953) Neurosecretory control of molting in crabs by the X-organ-sinus gland complex. Physiol Comp Oecol 3:155–189

Perney TM, Hirning LD, Leeman SE, Miller RJ (1986) Multiple calcium channels mediate neurotransmitter release from peripheral neurons. Proc Natl Acad Sci USA 83:6656–6659

Pfaffinger PJ, Martin JM, Hunter DD, Nathenson NN, Hille B (1985) GTP-binding proteins couple cardiac muscarinic receptors to a K channel. Nature 317:536–538

Potter DD (1956) Observations on the neurosecretory system of portunid crabs. PhD thesis, Harvard University

Potter DD (1958) Observations on the neurosecretory system of Portunid crabs. In: Bargmann W, Hanström B, Scharrer E, Scharrer B (eds) Zweites Internationales Symposium über Neurosekretion. Springer, Berlin Heidelberg New York, pp 113–118

Quackenbush LS, Fingerman M (1984) Regulation of neurohormone release in the fiddler crab, *Uca pugilator*: effects of gamma-aminobutyric acid, octopamine, met-enkephalin, and beta-endorphin. Comp Biochem Physiol [C] 79:77–84

Rao KR, Riehm JP, Zahnow CA, Kleinholz LH, Tarr GE, Johnson L, Norton S, Landau M, Semmes OJ, Sattleberg M, Jorenby WH, Hintz MF (1985) Characterization of a pigment-dispersing hormone in eyestalks of the fiddler crab *Uca pugilator*. Proc Natl Acad Sci USA 82:5319–5322

Rehm M (1959) Observation on the localisation and chemical constitution of neurosecretory material in nerve terminals in *Carcinus maenas*. Acta Histochem (Jena) 7:88–106

Reichardt LF, Kelly RB (1983) A molecular description of nerve terminal function. Annu Rev Biochem 52:871–926

Reuter H (1983) Calcium channel modulation by neurotransmitters, enzymes and drugs. Nature 301:569–574

Ruben P, Cooke I (1987) Comparison of cation channels in isolated and in situ peptidergic neurosecretory terminals. Biophys J 51:250a

Ruben P, Thompson S (1984) Rapid recovery from K current inactivation on membrane hyperpolarization in molluscan neurons. J Gen Physiol 84:861–875

Scudamore HH (1947) The influence of the sinus glands upon molting and associated changes in the crayfish. Physiol Zool 20:187–208

Shivers R (1976) Exocytosis of neurosecretory granules from the crustacean sinus gland in freeze-fracture. J Morphol 150:227–252

Silverthorn SU (1975) Neurosecretion in the sinus gland of the fiddler crab, *Uca pugnax*. Cell Tissue Res 165:129–133

Skinner D (1985) Interacting factors in the control of the crustacean molt cycle. Am Zool 25:275–284

Sperelakis N (1985) Phosphorylation hypothesis of the myocardial slow channels and control of Ca^{2+} influx. In: Zipes DP, Jalife J (eds) Cardiac electrophysiology and arrhythmias. Grune and Stratton, New York, pp 123–135

Streb H, Irvine RF, Berridge MJ, Schulz I (1983) Release of Ca^{2+} from a nonmitochondrial intracellular store in pancreatic acinar cells by inositol-1,4,5-trisphosphate. Nature 306:67–69

Stuenkel EL (1983) Biosynthesis and axonal transport of proteins and identified peptide hormones in the X-organ sinus gland neurosecretory system. J Comp Physiol [B] 207:191–205

Stuenkel EL (1985) Simultaneous monitoring of electrical and secretory activity in peptidergic neurosecretory terminals of the crab. J Physiol (Lond) 359:163–187

Stuenkel EL (1986) A common precursor to two major crab neurosecretory peptides. Peptides 7:397–406

Valdiosera R, Onetti C, Garcia U (1986) Calcium-activated inward current in neurosecretory cell bodies. Biophys J 49:368a

Van Herp F, Van Buggenum HJM (1979) Immunocytochemical localization of hyperglycemic hormone (HGH) in the neurosecretory system of the eyestalk of the crayfish *Astacus leptodactylus*. Experientia 35:1527–1529

Weatherby TM (1981) An ultrastructural study of the sinus gland of the crab, *Cardisoma carnifex*. Cell Tissue Res 220:293–312

Weatherby TM, Haylett BA (1985) Ultrastructural changes associated with K^+-evoked peptide secretion from a neurohemal organ of the crab, *Cardisoma carnifex*. Cell Tissue Res 242:67–73

Webster SG, Keller R (1986) Purification, characterisation and amino acid composition of the putative moult-inhibiting hormone (MIH) of *Carcinus maenas* (Crustacea, Decapoda). J Comp Physiol [B] 156:617–624

Welsh JH (1941) The sinus glands and 24-hour cycles of retinal pigment migration in the crayfish. J Exp Zool 86:35–49

Changes in Information Content with Physiological History in Peptidergic Secretory Systems

R. W. Newcomb, D. K. Hartline and I. M. Cooke

Contents

1 Introduction

This review seeks to focus attention on the potential complexity of the information conveyed by the release of chemicals during the synaptic or secretory activity of neurons. The importance of peptides in the control of neural function is underscored by the growing research in four different areas: (a) co-localization of peptides with classical neurotransmitters (Lundberg and Hökfelt 1983; Lloyd et al. 1987); (b) demonstration of peptidergic neurons in all parts of the central nervous systems of vertebrate and invertebrate species by immunohistochemical and biochemical approaches (e.g., Swanson and Sawchenko 1983; Siwicki et al. 1987; Kaldany et al. 1985); (c) cases of classical neurosecretory cells (e.g., those of the vertebrate hypothalamus, Swanson and Kuypers 1980) which do not have their processes restricted to neurohemal organs (e.g., the neurohypophysis), but participate in widespread interactions within the central nervous system; and (d) a spec-

Békésy Laboratory of Neurobiology, University of Hawaii, Honolulu, Hawaii 96822

Current Topics in Neuroendocrinology, Vol. 9

trum of activities ranging from neurotransmitter to neurohormonal processes and their involvement in complex behaviors (Koob and Bloom 1982). Further, in all known instances, those neurons known to secrete peptides as either the major or a co-localized product never secrete a single peptide, but rather a mixture of peptides.

It has now been demonstrated that several co-released peptides can have a distinct yet complementary biological activity on several different targets, supporting the suggestion that such a mixture of peptides can coordinate complex endocrine or behavioral responses (Mains et al. 1977; Scheller et al. 1983; Sossin et al. 1987). Moreover, it has recently been demonstrated that peptide mixtures can have biological effects on particular cells which are different from the summed effects of the individual peptides (Helsop et al. 1986; Elliot and Goodfriend 1986). Variations in neuropeptide amounts in released mixtures may thus produce effects on target cells which interact in ways yet to be explored in detail.

The generality and similarity of peptide hormone production mechanisms observed in diverse systems and animals (White et al. 1985; Lynch and Snyder 1986; Johnson 1987) point to the potential significance of co-release of peptides from single neurons. The initial product of ribosomal synthesis provides a preprohormone. A signal sequence directs the preprohormone into the endoplasmic reticulum, where removal of the signal sequence provides a prohormone. The prohormone may undergo some initial proteolysis and side-chain modification in the Golgi apparatus before being packaged, together with proteolytic and side-chain modifying enzymes, into membrane-bound granules (secretory granules).

Further processing of the contents of the secretory granule then occurs during transport and storage of the granule prior to release of the contents by exocytosis at specific sites (Burford and Pickering 1973; Orci et al. 1987). In diverse neural systems (including rat neural lobes, crab sinus gland, and sea hare bag cells: see below and Newcomb and Scheller 1987), the rates at which some of the processing reactions occur are slow relative to the life span of granules, so that the processing does not go to completion. The result is a highly complex mixture of more and less completely processed products, with intermediates resulting from incomplete reactions always present. An immediate consequence following from rates of prohormone cleavage that are slow relative to granule turnover is that the relative proportions of products in secretory granules will differ with the age of the granule. The actual products released as a result of the processing of complex prohormones have yet to be defined. A consequence is that the true biological properties of secreted peptide mixtures are not yet known.

It thus becomes relevant to know the age of granules at sites of release. To know this, we need to understand the pathways and rates of granule transport within the often highly complex shape of individual neurons. Several lines of evidence suggest for the neurohypophysis (Heap et al. 1975; Chapman et al. 1982; Nordmann 1985) and the crab sinus gland (E. Stuenkel and E. Gillary, unpublished work) neurohemal organs that the newest granules are transported first to release sites and later to storage areas. The age of granules undergoing release – and hence the peptides and the relative proportions released – will differ from those in the bulk neurohemal organ. From this we would predict that changes in the relative proportions of the various peptide intermediates and products will occur with changes in secretory performance. The work reviewed below documents such changes resulting from altered secretory demands in the rat neurohypophysis (Newcomb and Nordmann 1987).

From such considerations it follows that if we are to characterize the properties of peptidergic neurosecretion we must not only know the biosynthetic processing pathways, but also the activities, specificities and kinetics of each of the processing enzymes co-packaged with the prohormone into granules. Furthermore, in order to know the extent of processing that has occurred, we must know the age of the granules undergoing release. This requires knowledge of the rates and routes of transport of granules in relation to the neuronal dimensions of the release and storage sites, and of the history of secretory output.

This review describes an approach to the problem of determining the chemical output of a peptidergic neuron under differing regimes of secretory demand, attempting to account for the combined effects of chemical processing reactions and granule transport kinetics. The processing situation is so complex that it is doubtful that a given set of measures of a single parameter (for example, peptide amounts in lysates) could be used to specify all of the important parameters determining peptide output. What can be done is to recombine a diverse series of experimental data, each directly or indirectly specifying one or several of the parameters needed, and from these data attempt to generate an "hypothesis" (i.e., a quantitative model) for the peptide output properties of a cell. The behavior of a particular model can be compared with the actual response of the cellular system to experimental perturbation, in order to test the validity of a particular "hypothesis." If the model proves successful, it can itself be used to predict results of further experimental tests, which can then be used to modify or substantiate the model. Given that there is a certain degree of confidence in the model, it may be used to make cautious predictions regarding the properties of more complex systems. Examples of the application of such models at two different levels of experimental sophistication are provided in Sects. 2.3 and 3.2.

Quantitative data, obtained by high-performance liquid chromatography (HPLC), on the amounts of all peptides present in individual neurohemal organs obtained from rat neurohypophyses (Newcomb and Nordmann 1987) and crab sinus glands (Newcomb 1987 and unpublished work) are combined with available or assumed data on the kinetics of chemical processing and of granule transport in order to construct and test models that predict peptide composition under a number of conditions. The models provide a number of experimentally testable predictions, which could lead to confirmation of the model or to its further refinement or modification. We also discuss some interesting kinetic properties of some simple neuropeptide processing/secretory granule transport situations.

2 Processing of Prohormone to Peptides

In this section we focus on the kinetics of enzymatic cleavage of a prohormone into peptide fragments. The situation is considered theoretically first, giving rise to a specific model describing the changes in concentration of various peptides over time. Variations of the model, which simulate some different possible biological causes of variations in neuropeptide product distribution, are briefly discussed. We then present experimental data on processing in the crab sinus gland, and compare the data with model predictions.

2.1 Quantitative Relationship Among Peptides Derived from a Prohormone

The first issue to be addressed is how to describe mathematically the proteolytic cleavage of a prohormone containing many potential cleavage sites. In order to mathematically specify peptides derived from a common prohormone, we will use a terminology based on the final products of the completely processed prohormone. These correspond to segments of the prohormone, which can be numbered consecutively from the amino terminus. Intermediates are named by specifying the first and last segments they contain (Fig. 1; $P_{i,i}$ is shortened to P_i). Cleavage sites are designated by the segment on their amino-terminal side (i.e., *site i* is to the right of *segment i* in the figures). For computational purposes, each distinct intermediate can be represented as a mathematical "compartment" containing a certain amount of material. A given compartment (intermediate) is kinetically linked by unidirectional first-order rate constants to compartments representing single-cleavage site precursors as inputs and those representing single-site cleavage products as outputs (Fig. 1, inset). Additional compartments can be formally introduced to fit side-chain or terminal modifications into this process. The kinetic decay problem can be viewed as specifying the flux of material through the

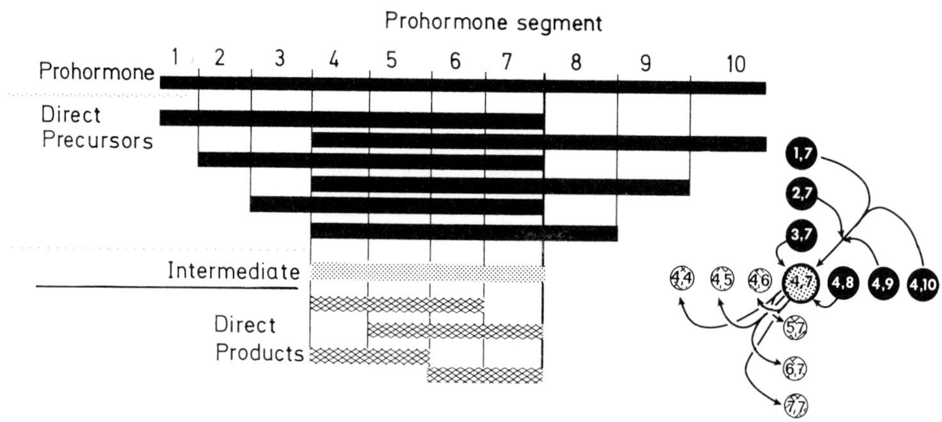

Fig. 1. Diagram of the potential direct precursors and products for an intermediate in the proteolytic processing of a prohormone. Potential direct precursors are those prohormone fragments which terminate at one end of the intermediate and extend over its other end. Potential direct products are those fragments which terminate at one end of the intermediate and do not contain one or more peptide segments on the opposite end of the intermediate. In the modeling of the prohormone decay problem, the amount of each intermediate at a given time increment is calculated from its previous amount, amounts of the direct precursors, rates of cleavage of these precursors, and rates of cleavage of the intermediate. *Inset*, diagram of the compartmental flux structure of the model program used to simulate the processing schema shown

compartments. The unidirectional rates of transfer of material between these compartments are equivalent to the rates of proteolytic cleavage. General texts on the properties of such compartmental models are available (Carson et al. 1983; Godfrey 1983).

The rate of change in the amount of any given peptide fragment is the sum of all rates of cleavage at the carboxyl terminus of peptides ending at its amino terminus, plus the rates of cleavage at the amino terminus of peptides ending at its carboxyl terminus, minus the rates of all internal cleavage reactions (see Fig. 1 for a schematic relating to the particular intermediate designated in our terminology 4, 7). The general situation can be represented by:

$$
\begin{aligned}
dP_{i,j}/dt = & \sum_{m=1}^{i-1} K_{m,j,i-1}\,P_{m,j} && \text{cleavage at site } i-1 \text{ of precursors ending at } j \\
& + \sum_{m=j+1}^{N+1} K_{i,m,j}\,P_{i,m} && \text{cleavage at site } j \text{ of precursors beginning at } i \\
& - \sum_{m=i}^{j-1} K_{i,j,m}\,P_{i,j} && \text{internal cleavage of peptide } P_{i,j}
\end{aligned} \tag{1}
$$

where $P_{a,b}$ represents a peptide containing segments a through b inclusive, and $K_{a,b,c}$ represents the first-order rate constant of cleavage of $P_{a,b}$ at site c (e.g., in Fig. 1, the intermediate singled out is $P_{4,7}$ and the four cleavage products are $P_{4,6}$, $P_{5,7}$, $P_{4,5}$ and $P_{6,7}$. These are formed from $P_{4,7}$ with rate constants $K_{4,7,6}$, $K_{4,7,4}$, $K_{4,7,5}$ and $K_{4,7,5}$, respectively).

2.2 Models of Peptide-Processing Kinetics

2.2.1 General Model

The generalized prohormone-processing situation is easily simulated by using a digital computer to numerically solve Eq. 1 for all peptides $P_{i,j}$. Other factors of biological or analytical importance can be added by simple alterations of the programs. These include synthesis of precursor, release of products, movement of processing reactions through different regions of the cell, decay of enzyme activities, and variable activities of multiple enzymes. For a single homogeneous cell region such as a terminal in a steady-state situation (ss), with input due only to precursor synthesis, S, and loss due only to processing (Eq. 1) and release (governed by a first-order rate constant, R), all time derivatives are zero, hence:

$$
\underset{i,j \neq 1,N+1}{P_{i,j}(ss)} = \frac{\sum_{m=1}^{i-1} K_{m,j,i-1}\,P_{m,j}(ss) + \sum_{m=j+1}^{N+1} K_{i,m,j}\,P_{i,m}(ss)}{R + \sum_{m=i}^{j-1}} \tag{2}
$$

$$
P_{1,N+1}(ss) = \frac{S}{R + \sum_{m=1}^{N} K_{1,N+1,m}}
$$

A computer program calculating these values directly can be used to assess the effects of variation of processing and release rate constants on steady-state peptide quantities.

2.2.2 Model Runs for a Three-Site Example

The effects of various potentially biologically important processing situations on a simple processing scheme are shown in Fig. 2. In this figure, the lower part diagrams the situation being considered, and the plots above show the changes in peptide content obtained. Four situations are considered: (A) decay over time of a unit amount of prohormone; (B) prohormone decay with processing enzyme inactivation; (C) steady-state terminal with balanced but variable synthesis and release; (D) steady-state terminal with processing rate varied.

Situation A represents the decay of a unit amount of prohormone having three cleavages sites, with cleavage rate constants of 0.33, 0.66, and 1.0 day^{-1} at sites, 1, 2, and 3 from the amino terminus, respectively (Eq. 1 with initial amounts of $P_{i,j} = 0$ except $P_{1,4} = 1$). Peptides produced from the prohormone by a single cleavage rise with a non zero initial slope; those requiring two cleavages have a zero initial slope. Intermediates requiring one cleavage for generation tend to have greater peak abundances than those requiring two.

Situation B is the same as that in A, but with the cleavage activity at the third site decaying with a rate constant of 1.0 day^{-1}. This simulates a simple case of a biological situation which could be caused by a number of factors, including (a) a cascade of multiple processing enzymes which activate and/or inactivate each other, (b) a changing environment within the secretory granule, and (c) passage of the processing reactions through different cellular regions which might exhibit different enzyme activities. Regardless of the mechanism, the problem is very similar. The simple case of enzyme inactivation considered in Fig. 2 B has the interesting effect of stabilizing intermediates containing the affected cleavage site, but there is little effect on intermediates which do not contain this cleavage site.

Situation C involves the same set of cleavage rate constants as A, but in a homogeneous terminal with synthesis balanced by release (Eq. 2). The peptide composition of the terminal is graphed as a function of the release rate constant (R). This simulates variations in peptide content caused by variations in secretory granule turnover times. If the release rate is low, the mixture is dominated by final

Fig. 2 A–D. An example of prohormone decay situation and the effects of some biologically important variations. **A** Simple three-site cleavage situation. Cleavage rate constants are kept the same at a given site on different peptides, but are varied from 0.33 to 0.66 to 1.0 day^{-1} on progressive cleavage sites from the amino terminus (*bottom*). Time courses for the changes in amounts of the individual peptides are given in the *upper two panels*. **B–D** Variations added to this set of cleavage rate constants. **B** Effects of selective decay of the activity of the third-site cleavage rate according to the first-order rate constant of 1.0 day^{-1}. **C** Variations in peptide content at steady state in a homogeneous compartment with peptide amounts plotted as a function of the release rate constant (see text). **D** Effects of scaling the rate constant at the third site from 0 to $10\times$ in a homogeneous compartment at equilibrium

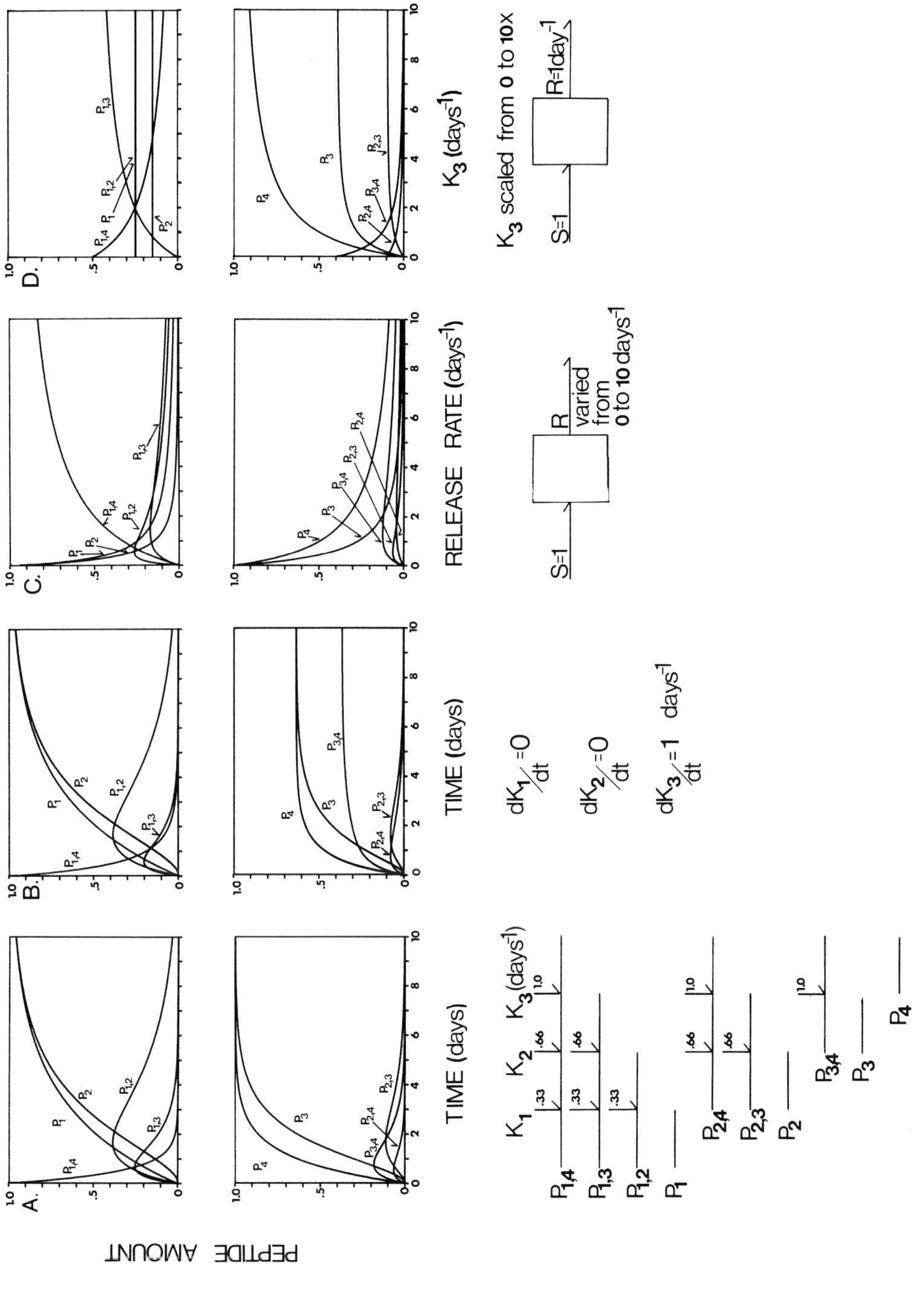
A.
B.
C.
D.
PEPTIDE AMOUNT
TIME (days)
TIME (days)
RELEASE RATE (days^{-1})
K_3 (days^{-1})
K_1 K_2 K_3(days^{-1})
$dK_1/dt = 0$
$dK_2/dt = 0$
$dK_3/dt = 1$ days^{-1}
S=1
R varied from 0 to 10 days^{-1}
K_3 scaled from 0 to 10x
S=1
R=1day^{-1}

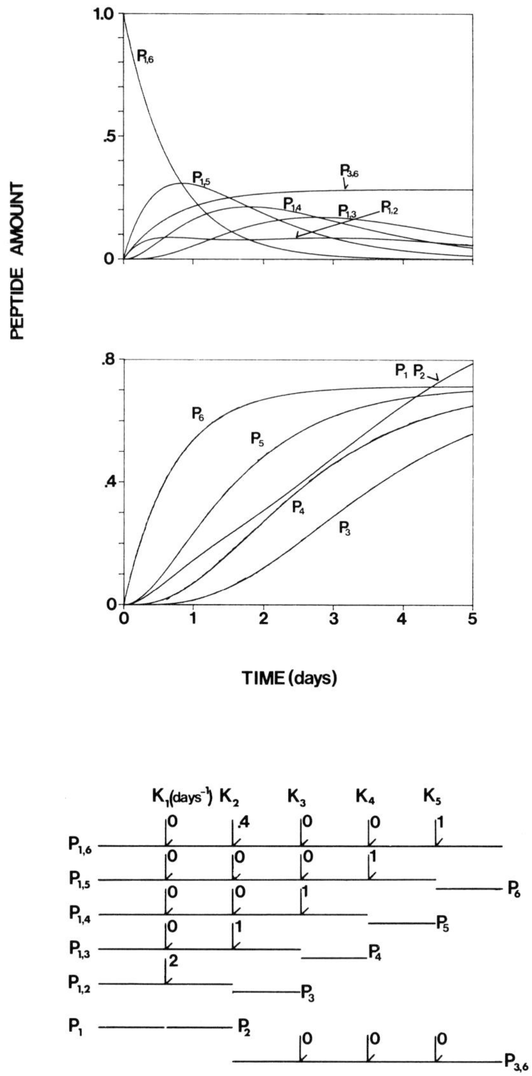

Fig. 3A

Fig. 3 A, B. Different extremes of prohormone processing kinetics. Two five-site cleavage situations are shown. **A** Two aspects of the case where cleavage rate constants differ widely at different sites and at the same site on peptides of different lengths. The sequential passage of a series of intermediates through a single pathway is only obtained when all cleavage sites except one are zero, and when this single "active" cleavage sites changes location on succesive intermediates. This situation is simulated for $P_{1,5}$, $P_{1,4}$, and $P_{1,3}$. If a single cleavage on the prohormone, $P_{1,6}$, is added at the site generating the final intermediate, $P_{1,2}$, a damped oscillation in the amounts of this final intermediate can be simulated. **B** All cleavage rates equal. This results in the production of significant amounts of all possible intermediates and products. Further, this situation results in a large number of pathways in the generation of any product peptide

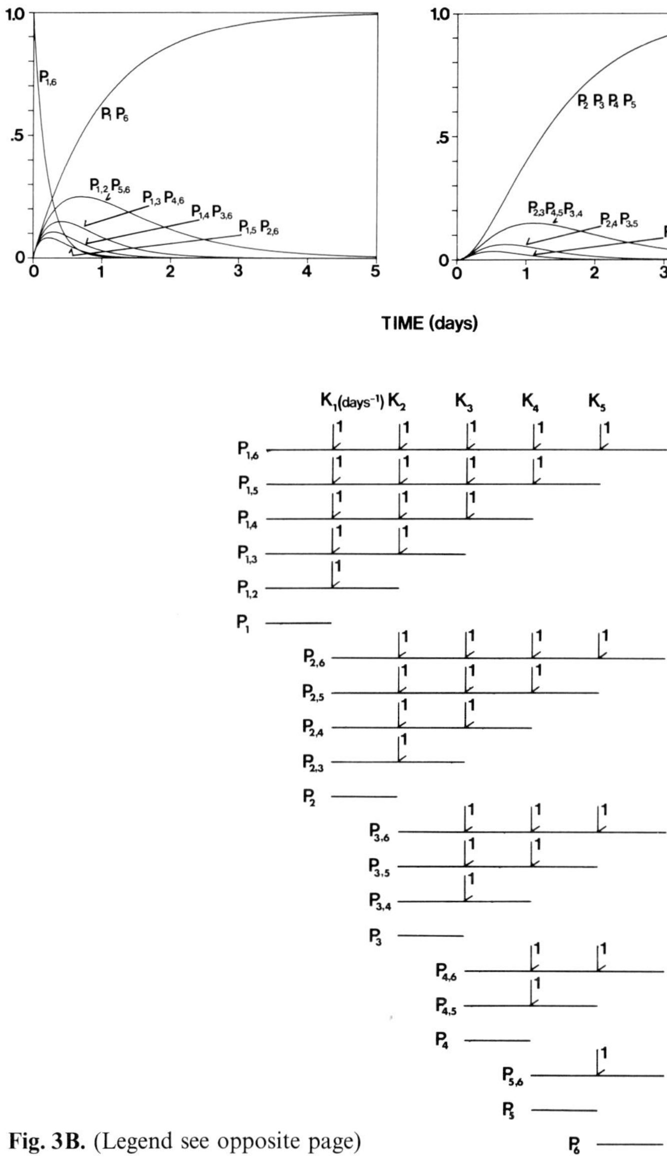

Fig. 3B. (Legend see opposite page)

products. If it is high, the precursor dominates. For each intermediate there is an optimal release rate which maximizes its concentration in the mixture.

Situation D is similar to C, but with peptide composition varied by changing the relative enzyme activity at site 3. This simulates the effect of variations in relative activities of multiple processing enzymes with different specificities. As with the enzyme inactivation situation, there is little effect on intermediates not containing the cleavage site.

Both enzyme inactivation (situation B) and reduction of enzyme activity at a particular site (situation D) can have the interesting effect of stabilizing otherwise unstable intermediates in older granules. This results in more complex product distributions in older granules and in intermediates having biological activity being present in a number of stabilized forms. As we will show below, variations in release rates and variations in relative enzyme activities can both result in qualitatively similar variations in steady-state peptide content, but with very different sets of cleavage rate constants (see below under simulation of sinus gland peptide content).

The selectivity of the effects of varying enzyme activity or enzyme inactivation rates on enhancing or depressing relative quantities of different prohormone fragments is interesting. These mechanisms might conceivably be used to select between different stable and/or unstable product mixtures obtained from a given prohormone for release by the cell. In general, variations in enzyme inactivation (Fig. 2 B), variations in secretory granule turnover times (Fig. 2 C), and variations in enzyme activities and/or specificities (Fig. 2 D) all must be considered as possible causes of the differences in the product mixture obtained from a given prohormone.

2.2.3 Model Runs Involving Length-Dependent Cleavage Rates

Further insight into potential consequences of multisite processing schemes can be gained by considering two extremes: (1) one in which all cleavages proceed at nearly equal rates with these rates independent of peptide length, and (2) one in which cleavages proceed at very different rates with the cleavage rate at a given site very dependent on peptide length. Examples of these situations are illustrated in Fig. 3. The equal rate situation (Fig. 3 B) is interesting in that it results in a larger number of different molecular species being present in a given secretory granule at any given time. This situation also results in a larger multiplicity of pathways involved in the generation of any particular species. The unequal rate situation, by contrast (Fig. 3 A), involves simple and well-ordered changes in peptide content leading to large differences in the peptide content of secretory granules of different ages. In the extreme case, a chain of intermediates is generated, each derived from the one preceding in the sequence, and with each proteolytic event also yielding a final product peptide. In Fig. 3 A, peptides $P_{1,5}$, $P_{1,4}$, and $P_{1,3}$ together with peptides P_5, P_4, and P_3 follow this scheme.

We find that the greatest variation in mixtures of product peptides is obtained when the two situations are combined. Fig. 3 A shows the situation in which rates of cleavage at sites 2 and 5 on the prohormone, $P_{1,6}$, are made nearly equal. All other cleavage rate constants are made zero except those at the carboxyl end of intermediates derived from $P_{1,5}$. Cleavage of the prohormone generates $P_{1,2}$ and $P_{1,5}$ in amounts proportional to the ratio of the cleavage rate constants. $P_{1,2}$ is rapidly generated and rapidly cleaved to P_1 and P_2, but the cleavage rate constant at site 1 is zero on other peptides containing this site. The series of intermediates $P_{1,5}$, $P_{1,4}$, and $P_{1,3}$ provides an alternate pathway for the generation of $P_{1,2}$, but only after an initial lag. The net effect is to channel $P_{1,2}$ through two alternative biosynthetic pathways of different time courses. This yields a damped oscillation in the amount of this peptide, and results in the long-term presence of the unstable peptide $P_{1,2}$.

2.3 Application of the Model to a Neurohemal Organ

The sinus gland of the land crab *Cardisoma carnifex* provides a good example of a prohormone-processing situation in which both intermediates and final products are present in and can be released from nerve terminals. Here, one peptide with two internal cleavage sites provides a situation simple enough to be experimentally tractable, but complex enough for modeling studies to have contributed substantially to understanding. We first review the sinus gland preparation, then discuss its modeling.

2.3.1 The Crab Eyestalk Neurosecretory System

The X-organ – sinus gland system of decapod crustacea is of considerable value in a comparative approach to understanding how anatomical and biochemical properties interact to define the chemical output of a peptidergic neuron. The system can be dissected intact with discrete cell body, nerve, and axon terminal regions, then subjected to a variety of anatomical, physiological, and biochemical studies (see Stuenkel and Cooke, this volume; Cooke 1977, 1985; Weatherby 1981; Stuenkel 1983, 1985, 1986; Newcomb 1983, 1987; Newcomb et al. 1985; Lemos et al. 1986; Nordmann et al. 1986; Nagano and Cooke 1987).

Comprehensive characterization of the peptide content of the sinus gland of the crab *C. carnifex* (Newcomb 1983) showed a simple and well-defined set of peptides. Amino acid sequence analyses showed one group of peptides, labeled C through I, to result from incomplete proteolytic reactions at two sites on peptide H (Newcomb 1987). The amino acid sequences of these peptides are summarized in Fig. 4. Also present in significant quantities were two peptides with hyperglycemic activity (crustacean hyperglycemic hormones, or CHHs; Keller and Wunderer 1978) labeled J and L, and a peptide peak of related composition, K. Crustacean molt-inhibiting hormones (MIH; Webster and Keller 1986; Chang et al. 1987) are of similar composition to CHHs, and that of the crab *Carcinus maenas* (Webster and Keller 1986) is very similar to that of K. Molecular weights of MIHs and CHHs have not been precisely defined. A single major precursor in the X-organ has been demonstrated (Stuenkel 1986), and this potentially encodes all the peptides C through L. In the course of processing, this single major precursor undergoes a series of shifts in its isoelectric point, at least some of which precede proteolysis to product peptides (Stuenkel 1986). Since the primary structure of the prohormone is not known, the kinetics of the initial proteolytic events are difficult to interpret.

Although the analysis developed here may in time be applied to the entire series of peptides, we will focus only on the C through I series. HPLC analysis of material in the sinus gland after [^{3}H]leucine labeling of the X-organ shows that peptide H is synthesized before its fragments (Stuenkel 1983). The coexistence of all possible fragments of peptide H in the sinus gland (Fig. 4) shows that multiple

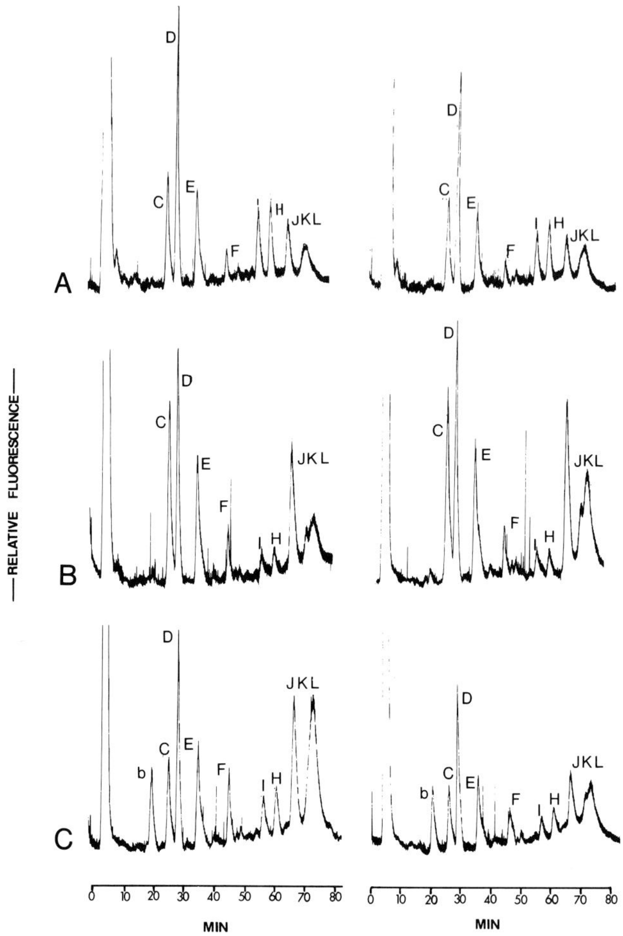

PEPTIDE	
H	RSADGFGRMESLLTSLRGSAESPAALGEASAAHPLE
I	RSADGFGRMESLLTSL
F	LLTSLRGSAESPAALGEASAAHPLE
E	LLTSL
C	RSADGFGRME
D	GSAESPAALGEASAAHPLE

Fig. 4 A–C. Sample chromatograms of single sinus glands showing variations in peptide content among animals and duplication of peptide content between contralateral sinus glands. **A–C** indicate chromatograms of single sinus glands from different animals, with the *left* and *right* for each showing chromatograms of the contralateral sinus glands. A summary of the peptide sequences (Newcomb 1987) is shown in the *lower part* of the figure.

biosynthetic pathways are involved in the generation of at least one of the final products.

2.3.2 Peptide Content of Single Sinus Glands

Given the observation of incomplete proteolytic cleavage of the H peptide, experiments were undertaken to investigate whether these might proceed to different extents in sinus glands from different animals. Such differences were observed (Newcomb et al. 1985; R. Newcomb, unpublished data). By dissecting the sinus gland away from the surrounding eyestalk tissue, a preparation consisting primarily of peptidergic nerve terminals is obtained. Direct quantitation of all peptides in single sinus glands by HPLC is easily accomplished. Figure 4 shows chromatograms of peptides obtained from the two sinus glands of a given animal as compared with those from different animals. What is striking is that the relative peak heights from each of the peptides are very similar in the right and left sinus glands of the same animal, but show a distinctly different pattern of peak heights in each animal. Further, a single peptide "b" is present in significant quantity in about 15% of the crabs and absent from the remainder (Fig. 4, animal C). Peptide b turns out to represent a modified form of C (see below). Analysis of variance comparing peptide ratios between contralateral sinus glands to those between sinus glands from different animals showed that the differences in b through I peptide content between animals are highly significant ($p < .001$ for peptides b, C, D, I and H relative to E; $p = .05$ for peptide F relative to E).

Control experiments showing that peptides and measured peptide ratios were not artifactual included (a) showing the stability of radiolabeled peptide H in lysates (Stuenkel 1983), (b) showing that the proteolysis that did occur under conditions specifically designed to allow artifactual proteolysis (room-temperature distilled-water lysates of sinus gland) yielded only a slow and specific degradation of peptides C and E, with the other peptides remaining stable, (c) showing that 0.1 *N* HCl extracts were completely stable and that such extracts were identical to 100 °C H_2O extracts of the contralateral sinus glands, and (d) showing that partially extracted sinus glands showed identical b through H peptide ratios when compared to contralateral sinus glands completely extracted by several homogenizations.

The combined observations from pulse-chase analyses (Stuenkel 1983, 1986), peptide isolation and sequencing (Newcomb 1983, 1987), and quantitative measurements (R. Newcomb, unpublished data) support the following schema of proteolytic processing in the sinus gland. Proteolysis of peptide H occurs on a time

---

Here, boxed amino acids are those removed in the processing of peptide H, which takes place in the sinus gland secretory granules. Note the presence of peptide b in animal **C**, and its absence in animals **A** and **B**. HPLC elution was with a 90-min gradient of 5%–95% methanol in 0.05 *M* sodium phosphate, pH 6.2, using a 10-mm particle diameter octadecyl-silica column (Bio-Rad; 250 × 4.0 mm). Detection is by on-line reaction of the HPLC eluant with fluorescamine. With the extraction by sonication used here, variations in extraction efficiency influence the measurement of amounts of peptides J, K, and L, but not the b through I peptides

scale of weeks and occurs to different extents in different animals, but with the extent of proteolysis and all-or-none generation of peptide b tightly coupled in contralateral sinus glands. The amino acid sequences show that the cleavages at the different sites almost certainly require at least two enzymes, one acting at a single basic residue (as observed in many peptidergic systems), and another recognizing the sequence Glu-Ser-Leu (Newcomb 1987), a previously undescribed specificity in neuropeptide processing. Several related questions emerge. First, how are the variations in peptide content of the sinus gland related to potential variations in the composition of released peptides, and do such variations result in differences in the physiological response to secretion from the sinus gland? Second, what physical processes are ultimately responsible for changes in stored and secreted peptide content?

2.3.3 Stoichiometric Analysis of Sinus Gland Peptide Content

Quantitative analysis of the variable peptide contents has been useful in substantiating the biosynthetic pathways and, in conjunction with the models, in suggesting underlying mechanisms for the variations. To obtain quantitative data on peptide amounts, standard curves were prepared by isolating the individual peptides, determining amounts by quantitative amino acid analyses, and then determining the peak area per unit amount with the method described in Fig. 4. Data on peptide quantities in single sinus glands from 20 animals were obtained. There is a natural variation in peptide quantities in sinus glands from different animals. To remove this factor from subsequent analysis, peptide quantities were normalized to a constant amount (230 pmol, which is the average for the study) of processed H per sinus gland; that is, the amount of H which would have been present to account for the amounts of the cleavage products observed according to the stoichiometric equations.

The data on peptide quantities were first analyzed according to the stoichiometry of processing peptide H, that is – using brackets to designate mole quantities – the differences [C]–[F] and [D]–[I] should equal [E]. Regression analysis of the stoichiometric equalities (Fig. 5A) showed highly significant relationships. Further, multiple regression analysis showed that both variables ([C] and [F], and [D] and [I]) make equal and highly significant contributions to the individual regression fits. These analyses strongly substantiate the inferences from the amino acid sequences and pulse-chase kinetics that the greater part of the H peptide fragment biosynthesis occurs via peptide H as an intermediate. However, the re-

Fig. 5A, B. Quantitative relationships between peptide amounts in single sinus glands. **A** Plots of peptide amounts according to stoichiometric relationships predicted from the amino acid sequences of the C through I peptides. These predict that [D]–[I] and [C]–[F] should equal [E]. The data on peptide amounts are normalized to a constant amount of processed peptide H, as described in the text. In the plot of [C]–[F] vs [E] the values obtained for those sinus glands containing C are shown with this peptide either considered equivalent (◎), or not (○), to peptide b in the stoichiometric equality. **B** Plots of normalized amounts of the individual peptides against normalized amounts of peptide H. These relationships are not due to stoichiometry, and are simulated by various kinetic processes in Fig. 6

A

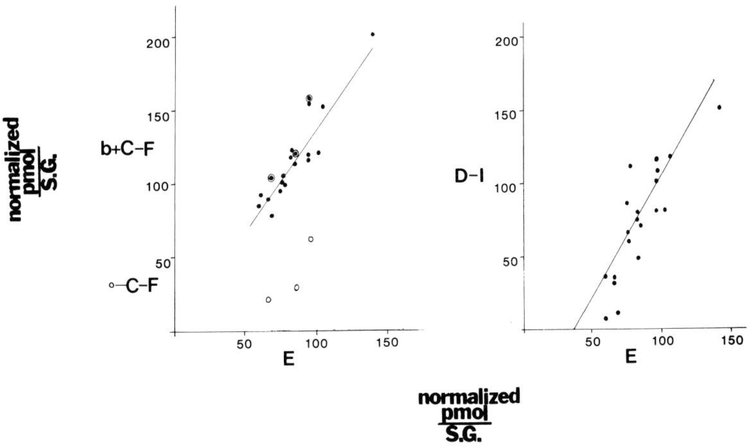
normalized
pmol
S.G.
b+C−F
C−F
D−I
E
E
normalized
pmol
S.G.

B

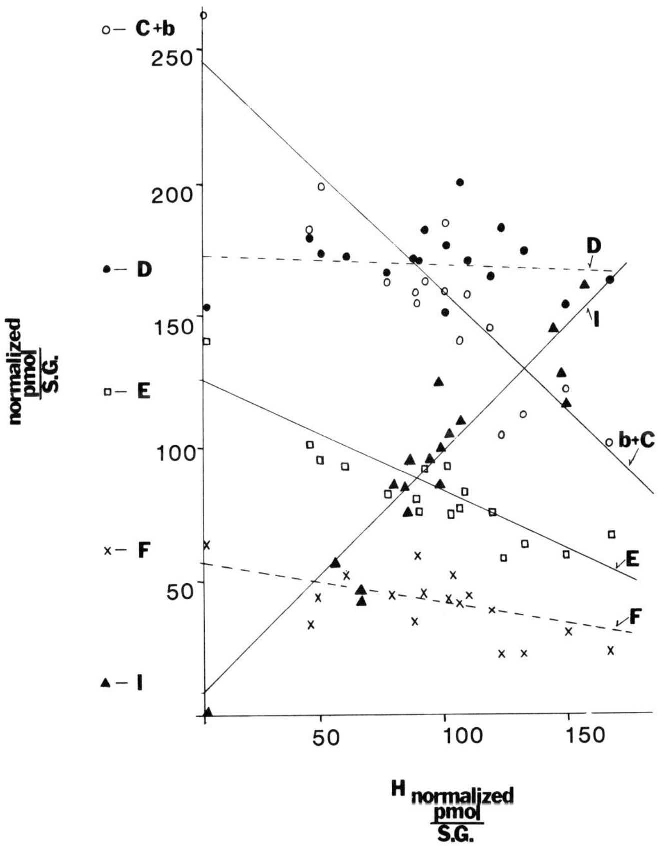
C+b
D
E
F
I
normalized
pmol
S.G.
D
I
b+C
E
F
H normalized
pmol
S.G.

gressions through the stoichiometric relationships (slopes of 1.4 and 1.7) do not have the expected slopes of 1, and are indicative of some other process contributing to the measured peptide amounts. Specific degradation of peptides C and E in distilled water lysates of sinus glands suggests that similar degradation might occur in the secretory granules. This would account for the deviations from the theoretical slopes but not the deviation from a zero intercept observed with the plot of [D]–[I] vs [E].

An interesting application of the stoichiometric analysis is obtained with peptide b. If this peptide is not considered equivalent to peptide C in those animals which contain this peptide, then values for the [C]–[F] = [E] stoichiometric equality fall well outside the normal range. If the two are considered equivalent, then the values are well within the normal range (Fig. 5A). This observation can be considered direct evidence of a structural relationship between peptides C and b. The mechanisms related to the all-or-none appearance of peptide b, and the precise duplication of its relative amounts in contralateral structures should be of considerable interest.

2.3.4 Stoichiometry-Independent Relations in Sinus Gland

Although much of the variation in quantities of particular peptides can be related to variations in stoichiometrically related peptides, the overall source of variation of this family of peptides among different sinus glands is not clear. The puzzle is made still more intriguing by the finding of stoichiometrically independent relations between each of the fragments and their biosynthetic precursor (H). This is shown in Fig. 5B. Here, normalized [H] peptide fragments in single sinus glands are plotted as functions of normalized quantities of H. Significant regression lines ($p < .05$) are obtained for all peptides except peptide F ($p = .05$) and peptide D (close to zero slope). There is no reason to expect amounts of a precursor peptide to be related to those of its products by stoichiometry, hence relationships such as these must be due to kinetic processes. Inspection of Fig. 5B shows that with decreasing amounts of precursor H, there are increasing amounts of at least the final products C and E, which would be expected if different lengths of exposure to the processing enzymes were responsible. However, as we saw with the theoretical model runs, there may be several other ways of accounting for varying ratios of peptides in the mixture. The models may thus help gain insight into the processes explaining the observed relationships between precursor and product peptides.

Fig. 6. Simulation of relationships between single sinus gland peptide amounts and peptide H amounts according to different possible kinetic situations. The figure shows plots of peptide amounts vs the relevant variable (*top*); how these plots translate into plots of normalized peptide amounts vs normalized peptide H amounts (*center*); and a summary of the situation being simulated (*bottom*). These are: **I**, simulation of the decay of peptide H; **II**, decay of peptide H with inactivation of the conversion rates at the second site from the amino terminus (see Fig. 4); **III**, steady-state amounts in a homogeneous compartment with different release rates; and **IV**, steady-state amounts in a homogeneous compartment, with peptide amounts expressed as a function of the relative enzyme activity as the first site from the amino terminus

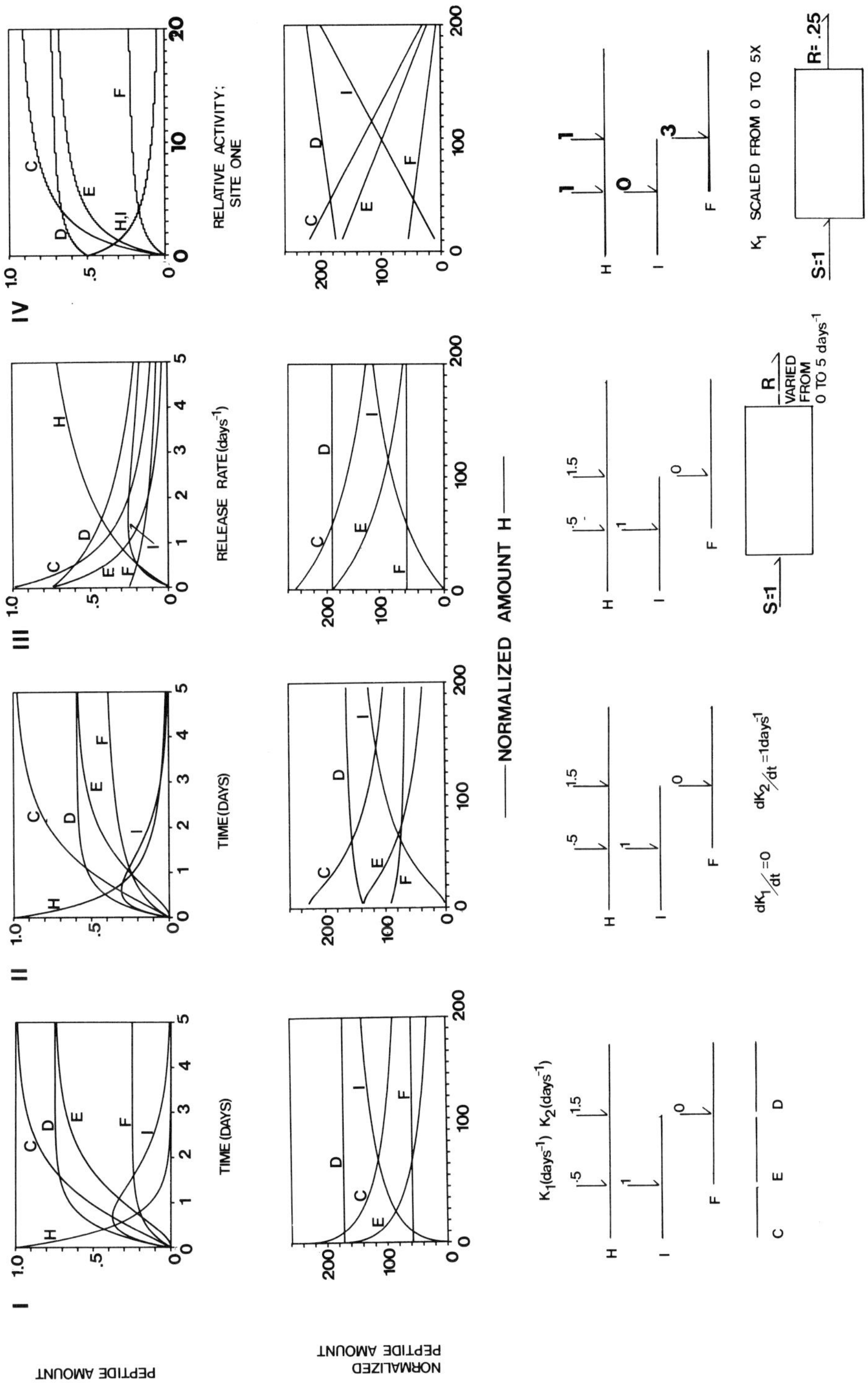

I
II
III
IV
PEPTIDE AMOUNT
NORMALIZED PEPTIDE AMOUNT
TIME (DAYS)
TIME(DAYS)
RELEASE RATE(days-1)
RELATIVE ACTIVITY; SITE ONE
NORMALIZED AMOUNT H
K1(days-1) K2(days-1)
dK1/dt =0
dK2/dt =1days-1
S:1
R
VARIED FROM 0 TO 5 days-1
K1 SCALED FROM 0 TO 5X
R=.25

2.3.5 Modeling Sinus Gland Peptide Ratios

The approach is to derive plots of products vs normalized precursor from model runs similar to those shown in Fig. 2. Parameters for the model are adjusted until the situation in Fig. 5 B is approximated. This provides a demonstration of sufficiency for the particular mechanism simulated by the model as an explanation for the relationships in Fig. 5 B. Where different explanations are found to be sufficient, the values of the parameters used to fit the experimental data can be used to devise experimental tests of the proposed schemes.

The following kinetic models were tested for their ability to simulate the observed relationships (Fig. 6).

Model I: changes in [H] were produced by decay of a pulse of H.

Model II: changes in [H] were produced by changing the rate of inactivation of an enzyme active at a single site on H.

Model III: the sinus gland was represented by a single homogeneous compartment in steady state, with differences in [H] produced by variations in release rates.

Model IV: the sinus gland was represented as a homogeneous compartment in steady state with differences in [H] produced by varying relative enzyme activity at the two sites on H.

In Fig. 6, runs for each model are shown which fit the qualitative aspects of the experimental data. In this figure, each kinetic situation is summarized in the lower part. Peptide quantities are shown as functions of the relevant variable in the row of graphs in the top. The center row shows these as normalized peptide amounts plotted as a function of normalized precursor amounts. Better quantitative fits are possible, but rate constants have been kept identical in models I–III to allow better comparison of the different cases. It is seen that each situation allows qualitative matching of the data to variation in peptide quantities. Although model IV is the only one which gives strictly linear relationships similar to the regression lines in Fig. 5 B, in practice it is not likely that we could tell whether the curvature present in various plots is present in the experimental data. Differences in the rates of cleavage at the different sites needed to fit the experimental data suggest concrete experimental tests for underlying mechanisms. In a model requiring differences in granule age (models I–III), the relative magnitudes of the cleavage rates must be as indicated in the figure to produce the slopes and relative ordering of peptides seen in the experimental plots of Fig. 5 B. Further, a zero slope for peptide F requires this peptide to be stable in the secretory granules. A downward slope implies inactivation of the activity generating this peptide.

The model invoking variations in relative enzyme activities (model IV) uses a very different set of rate constants to produce the same plots of [peptide] vs [H]. Further, this explanation requires that any activity variations be at site 1 and also that peptide I (instead of F) be stable in secretory granules. Thus, different physical situations potentially responsible for the variations in sinus gland peptide content are associated with markedly different kinetics of the processing of peptide H. Long-term pulse-chase analyses similar to that in Stuenkel (1983) could give the individual cleavage rates, and these should suggest a mechanism for variations in sinus gland peptide content.

3 Effects of Cellular Compartmentation and Transport on Peptide Quantities

The processing models presented in the previous section simulate prohormone decay in a single homogeneous cell region. In this section, we consider a nonhomogeneous cell and the consequences of differing granule transport rates and pathways. Neurons may have accumulations of secretory granules in cell bodies, at multiple sites along an axon, and at different areas near a given release site (Nordmann 1977; Weatherby 1981). If processing reactions are slow or incomplete, the age distribution of secretory granules at a release site will determine the peptide mixture actually secreted. Theoretical considerations leading to an explicit model will be presented first, and then this model will be applied to data from the rat neurohypophysis.

3.1 Modeling Considerations

To aid in the analysis of the overall processing situation, we constructed a generalized "granules" model representing different cell regions as mathematical compartments. Neurosecretory granules are permitted to "diffuse" between the different compartments, simulating transport and diffusion processes. In addition, granules may be released from specified compartments and new granules may be synthesized into specified compartments. Newly synthesized granules contain a precursor "A," which is processed to a form "B." This compartmental model is capable of simulating secretory granule age distributions under many variations of synthesis and release conditions.

Granules are represented by three one-dimensional arrays storing the compartment assignment, the birth date, and the amount of unprocessed peptide ("A"). Time is quantized (Euler integration). At each time increment for each compartment, the number of new granules added is calculated from the current synthesis rate, and that number of empty granule slots is filled with compartment assignment, birth time, and initial peptide content. Granules already assigned to compartments are selected randomly for inclusion in the allotment to be transferred to other compartments. The number of granules moving into a particular compartment is proportional to the concentration of granules in the compartment of origin and the coefficient of intercompartmental "diffusion" (transport) out of the compartment. The amount of unprocessed peptide is decremented according to first-order kinetics, the rate constant of which can in turn be decremented according to a first-order enzyme-inactivation scheme. One extra compartment with no back-diffusion serves for granule release. As granules are released, their ages and contents are tallied, and their array space is returned to the unassigned pool. For processing schemes more complex than the simple decay of a precursor, the distribution of secretory granule ages for any given cellular compartment can be combined with the results of prohormone decay simulation (Eq. 1) as a function of age, in order to generate the product distribution for that compartment.

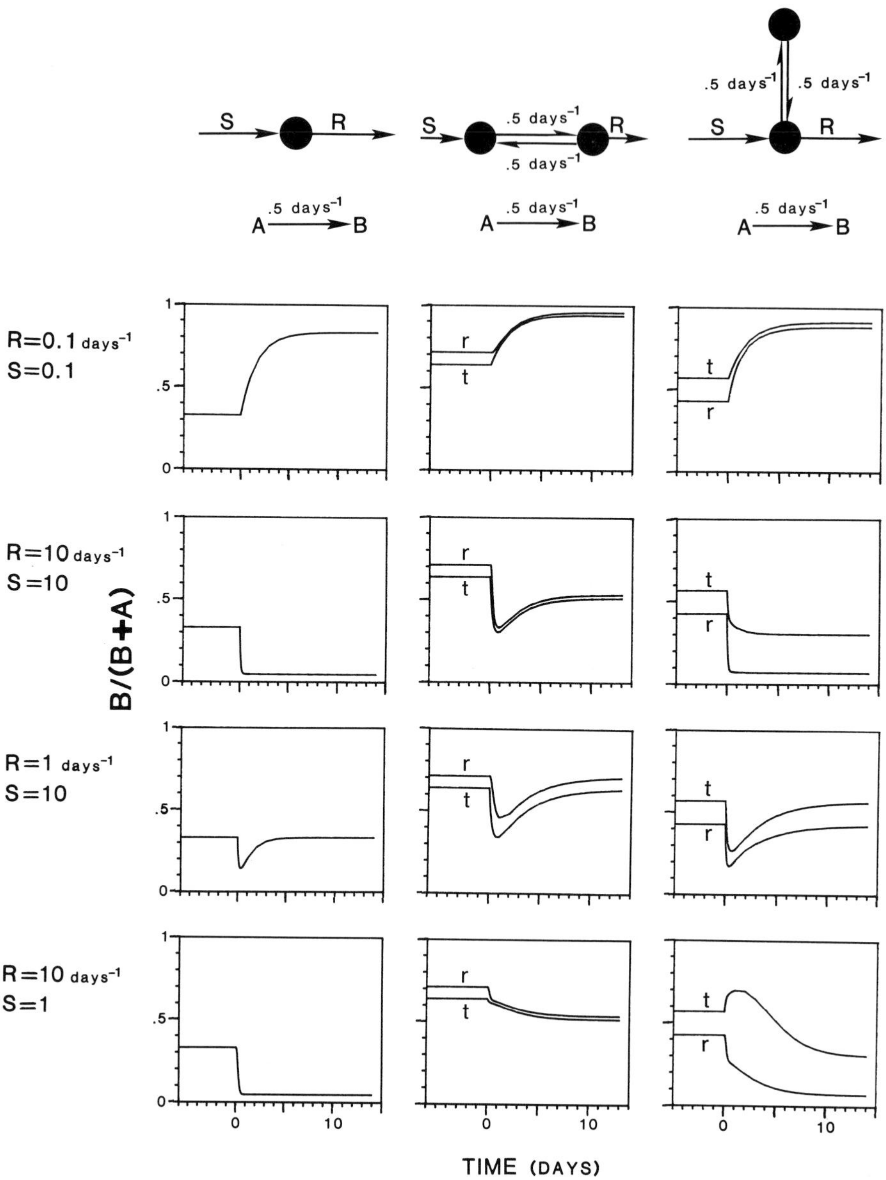

Fig. 7. Effect of compartmentation on changes in peptide content with changes away from equilibrium synthesis (*S*) and release rates (*R*). A bulk diffusional compartmental model incorporating a simple "A to B processing" reaction with first-order diffusional kinetics was used. The models, diagrammed at the *top* of the figure, were equilibrated to a release rate constant of one day^{-1} and step tenfold increases or decreases in release and/or synthesis rates simulated; the particular changes in the modeled *R* and *S* are indicated at the *left*. The response of the terminal (*t*) and released (*r*) peptide content are expressed as the proportion of product B to total B+A. Equal compartment volumes, rate constants for intercompartmental transfer of material of 0.5 day^{-1}, and a rate constant for the A to B conversion of 0.5 day^{-1} were used for the simulations

Figure 7 illustrates the potentially important role that cellular compartmentation can have in determining the changes in peptide content secreted with changes in secretion rates. Here a simple first-order precursor to product conversion (A to B) is considered for three different compartment geometries (schematics at top). The figure shows changes in the proportion of product to total peptide (B/[B+A]) in the terminal (t) vs release (r) in response to tenfold increments in release and/or synthesis. Alterations with changing conditions in B/(B+A) depend strongly on the geometry of compartmental arrangements. The different response types seen here can be compared to measured B/(B+A) for real secretory structures, thus giving some idea of what types of cellular compartmentation might be present.

3.2 Application of the Model to the Rat Neurohypophysis

Owing to the significant body of data available, the neural lobe of the rat pituitary provides an excellent opportunity for testing the uses of a quantitative model to explain released and stored peptide content in terms of a comprehensive set of physical parameters. These include (a) accurate measures of rates of prohormone and peptide processing (Burford and Pickering 1973; Russel et al. 1981); (b) measures of the rate of secretory granule turnover (Burford and Pickering 1973); (c) measures of volumes of axonal compartments both near and distant from release sites and of secretory granule densities in those compartments (Nordmann 1977); and (d) a variety of studies suggesting (but not demonstrating) geometrical arrangements of axonal compartments and approximate pathways of secretory granule movements (Sachs and Haller 1968; Heap et al. 1975; Nordmann 1985; Chapman et al. 1982). These data provide parameters for the model just described. Below we describe the measurement of peptide quantities in several physiological experiments, and then present some results of simulating them with the model.

3.2.1 Review of Rat Neurohypophysis Peptide-Processing Data

The mammalian hypothalamic-neurohypophysial system of peptidergic secretory neurons includes terminals at the median eminence, which release peptides to the portal blood system of piutary, as well as the system of terminals constituting the neural lobe of pituitary (releasing oxytocin, vasopressin, and associated neurophysins to the systemic circulation). In the studies discussed here, the neural lobe has been isolated and the median eminence removed.

In the neural lobe of the male Wistar rat, the pro-oxytocin and provasopressin molecules are subjected to rapid cleavages such that, on arrival at the neural lobe, secretory granules contain oxytocin and its associated intact neurophysin, or vasopressin and its associated intact neurophysin together with one or several forms of the associated glycopeptide (Burford and Pickering 1973; Russel et al. 1981). The oxytocin neurophysin (OT-Np or "A") is subjected in the neural lobe to a slow proteolysis to the form lacking the carboxyl terminal glutamate residue (OT-Np′ or "B"; Burford and Pickering 1973; Newcomb and Nordmann 1987;

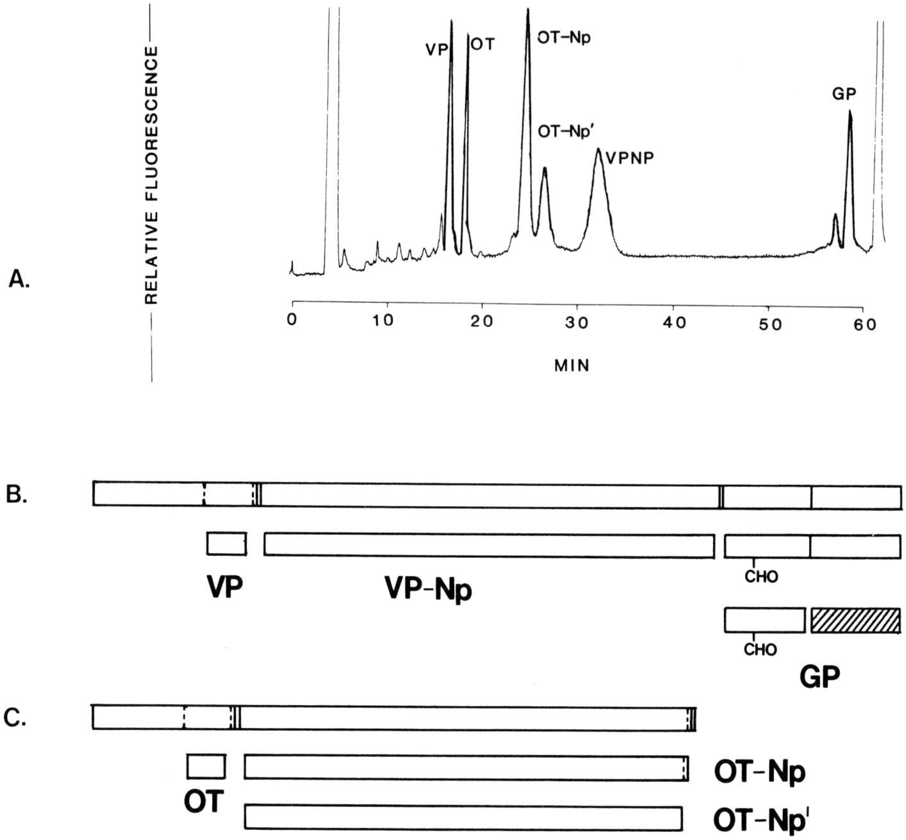

Fig. 8 A–C. HPLC analysis of neural lobe peptide content. **A** Chromatogram obtained from three neural lobes from 28- to 32-day-old male Wistar rats. **B** A summary of peak identities with fragments of the provasopressin molecule, and **C** with fragments of the pro-oxytocin molecule. The majority of the minor peaks arise from small quantities of adhering intermediate lobe. *Solid vertical lines* on the prohormone schematic represent basic residues removed in proteolytic processing, while *dashed vertical lines* represent other amino acids removed in processing (Ivell and Richter 1984, see also text). The *cross-hatched* carboxyl terminal fragment of the glycopeptide was not identified with certainty here. Total peptide amounts are about the same as for single neural lobes from the 60-day-old rats used for analysis of the effects of perturbation of secretion rates, but proportionally more of the oxytocin neurophysin is in the uncleaved form (OT-Np). Separation and detection was as with the sinus gland peptides, but using an octylsilica column and a slightly more complex gradient. *VP*, vasopressin; *VP-Np*, vasopressin neurophysin; *GP*, glycopeptide; *OT*, oxytocin; *OT-Np*, oxytocin neurophysin; *OT-Np′*, oxytocin neurophysin less the carboxyl terminal residue

diagram in Fig. 8). Preliminary observations on other rat species indicate that species differences may exist. We will call the ratio of product to total peptide, OT-Np′/(OT-Np+OT-Np′), or B/(B+A), the "processing ratio." The conversion occurs on the same time scale as the secretory granule turnover (Burford and Pickering 1973), so the processing ratio is sensitive to changes in secretory granule turnover times. All aspects of neural lobe processing and secretory granule movement kinetics come to be reflected in this processing ratio. The ratio, therefore, is useful in testing the validity of the models.

As with the sinus gland, an HPLC separation with quantitation by post-column fluorescamine derivatization was used to determine amounts of the peptides in single neural lobes (Newcomb and Nordmann 1987). Peptide identities and purity were demonstrated by amino acid analysis, carboxypeptidase Y digestion, gel electrophoresis, and in the case of the glycopeptide, Edman degradation and gel filtration. As with the sinus gland, appropriate studies demonstrated stability of the extracts and provided assurance that the measurements represented in vivo amounts. Figure 8 shows a sample chromatogram of neural lobe lysates and summarizes the identify of the individual peaks.

This procedure was used to determine quantities of A and B in single neural lobes in the following situations (Newcomb and Nordmann 1987):

1. Dehydration Experiments. Rats were deprived of water for 5 days, followed by resupply of normal drinking water. In the early stages of the dehydration, an increase in the B/(B+A) ratio occurred; the opposite occurred with rehydration (Fig. 11).

2. Chronic Osmotic Stress. Rats were given drinking water with 1.5% NaCl for 20 days. Results showed that material stored in the neural lobe reached a new

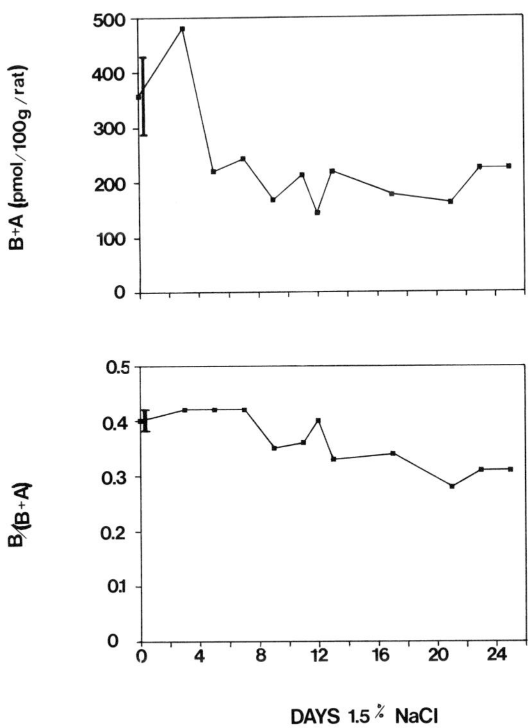

Fig. 9. Changes in oxytocin neurophysin amounts (*top*) and processing ratio B/(A+B) (*bottom*) in single neural lobes with chronic administration of drinking water with 1.5% NaCl. Neurophysin amounts are determined by peak areas as compared to standard curves preparated from the isolated peptides. The standard error of the mean is indicated for controls ($n=9$). Other points are single determinations

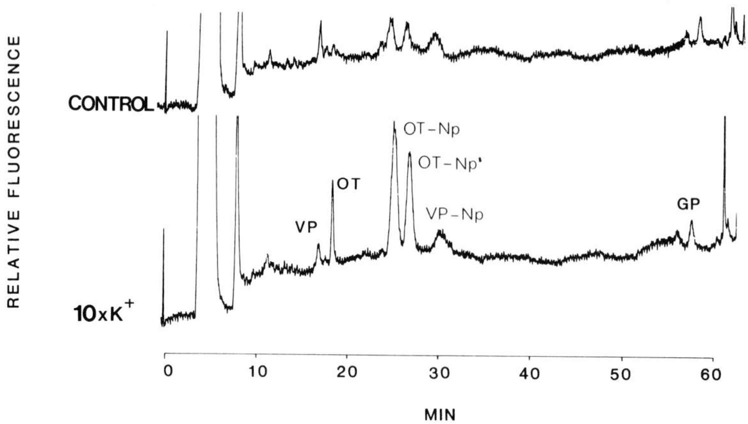

Fig. 10. Representative chromatograms of perfusates of 20 neural lobes from 60- to 70-day-old male Wistar rats with control and tenfold K^+ salines. The *lower trace* is the fourth tenfold K^+ pulse and shows 400 pmol of total oxytocin neurophysin. The processing ratio for the oxytocin neurophysin in the release is very close to that in the bulk neural lobe, indicating that secretory granules exposed to release by this stimulus are not of a very different age from the bulk population (Newcomb and Nordmann 1987). The control is the preceding wash with normal saline

stable or semistable state. Total peptide content decreased to half the initial value over 5 days and remained at this level for at least 20 days (Fig. 9). B/B+A showed a delayed decline followed by a stable lower value over the 20-day period. This would be consistent with the suggestion that the maintained secretory demand initially decreases the granule population while an increasing turnover rate decreases the average age of the population of granules in the neurohemal structure.

3. Age. In rats of increasing ages, a progressive increase in processing ratio was noted. For example, B/(B+A) was about 0.32 in rats of 28–32 days (Fig. 8), and about 0.39 in 60- to 70-day-old rats (Figs. 9–11). This observation is consistent with an increasing average age of the overall secretory granule population in older rats.

4. Potassium-Induced Release. Quantitative analysis of the peptides released by stimulation of the neural lobe with tenfold normal potassium showed the processing ratio to be close to that of the bulk tissue homogenate (Fig. 10). In interpreting this observation it must be considered that tenfold K^+ may not release the identical granule population released by axonally mediated activity.

The observations on the peptide-processing ratio and the changes it shows with a variety of secretory regimes and with animal age allow realistic testing of an overall model of the neural lobe processing situation.

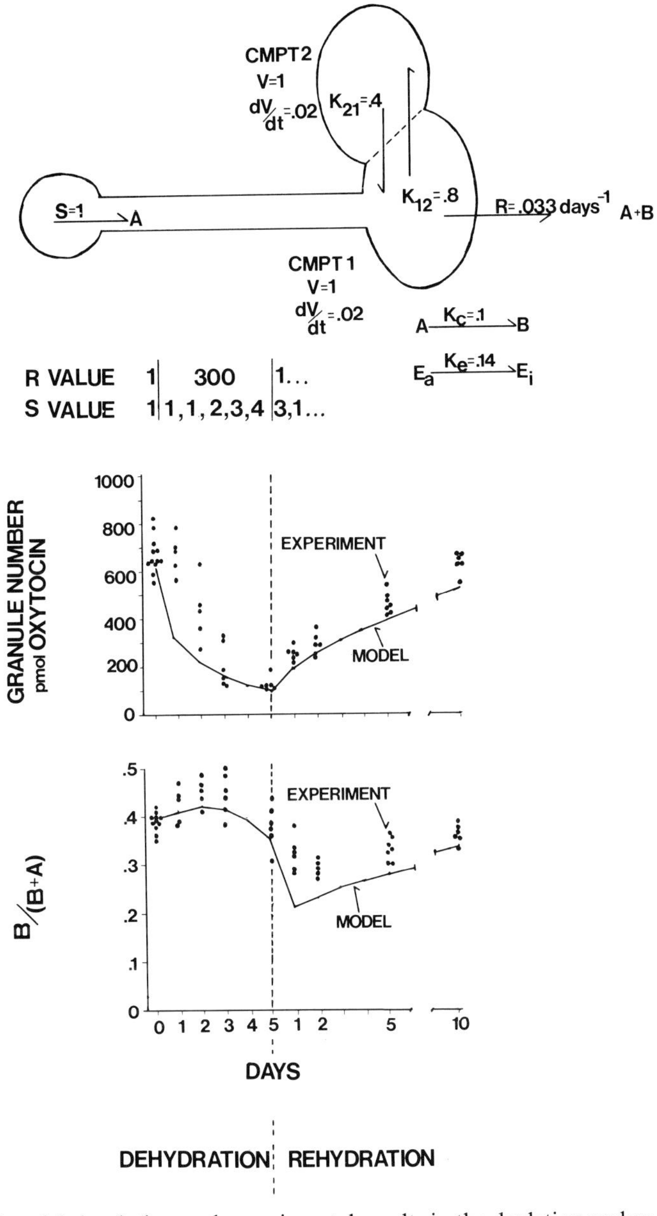

Fig. 11. Comparison of model simulation and experimental results in the depletion and replenishment of the neural lobe peptide content induced by dehydration and rehydration. The *top* part of the figure summarizes the neural lobe model. Values for synthesis (S), release (R), compartment volumes (V), rates of change of compartment volumes (dV/dt), rates of granule transfer between compartments (K_{12} and K_{21}), conversion of the oxytocin neurophysin (K_c), and inactivation of this conversion rate (K_e), are given. Units for rate constants are reciprocal days. The *center panel* shows total oxytocin content in single neural lobes with dehydration and rehydration (*points*), and the results of the model (*solid line*). The *lower panel* shows the same for the processing ratio for the oxytocin neurophysin. In the experiment, rats of approximately 60 days of age are deprived of water for 5 days

3.2.2 Simulation of Peptide Processing in the Neural Lobe

We turn now to the granules model introduced above. The following model parameters were set from experimental data.

1. The rate of the A to B conversion and the rate of decay of the conversion rate were derived from pulse-chase data (Burford and Pickering 1973).
2. The relative volumes of compartments near and distant from release sites were taken from Nordmann (1977).
3. The overall turnover rate of the model and, in particular, the value of the release rate constant were derived from the experimentally measured secretory granule turnover time (Burford and Pickering 1973).
4. Diffusion from the storage compartment (Cmpt 1, Fig. 11) into the release compartment was assumed to be the limiting factor in dehydration-induced depletion, so its rate constant was derived from depletion rates taken from Jones and Pickering (1969).
5. The relative magnitudes of the inter-compartment flux rate constants were set from relative volumetric densities of the secretory granules in the two compartments (taken from Nordmann 1977).

A widely accepted picture of neural lobe compartmentation has emerged from observations by several groups (see Heap et al. 1975; Chapman et al. 1982 for discussion; Burford et al. 1973 for an early model). As a first approximation, it is thought that newly synthesized material is preferentially made available for release in axonal endings, followed by some degree of removal to axonal swellings. This situation could be represented by two compartments, one for storage (representing swellings) and one for release (representing endings). We investigated first the general behavior of different types of simple compartmental models under the conditions of the dehydration-rehydration experiment, that is, a large increase in release followed by a return to normal values. We found that the simple two-compartment model with synthesis and release into and out of the same compartment yielded the type of behavior seen in the dehydration experiment (see Fig. 7), with other schemes containing an isolated compartment showing this behavior to a lesser extent. Attempts to obtain quantitative agreement with various three-compartment models incorporating the neural lobe experimental data were unsuccessful, while quantitative agreement was found with the two-compartment model having the isolated side compartment. The model for the neural lobe found to be reasonably consistent with available experimental data is summarized in the top part of Fig. 11. This model fits a simple anatomical picture of nearly equivalent populations of axonal endings and side compartments.

The neural lobe model was tested with the measured B/(B+A) values in rats of different ages and at different stages of dehydration and rehydration. It was also tested for its ability to simulate released vs stored B/(B+A) ratios. Because a model including growth of the lobe with age of the rat is more realistic, we incorporated growth into the model. In the absence of experimental data, the simple assumption of a volume increase in direct proportion to that of the rat (2% of day 20 volume per day) was made; synthesis, release and intercompartmental flux rates were scaled accordingly.

In simulating the dehydration-rehydration experiment, an abrupt increase in release-rate constant (R) was assumed during dehydration, with an abrupt return to normal upon restoration of water. In order to give a good fit to the experimentally observed drop in the oxytocin neurophysin amounts (top graph, Fig. 11) and the initial increase in B/(B+A) (lower graph), a large initial increase in release (300× in Fig. 11) was required, which rapidly emptied the release compartment. Experimental values for changes in synthesis rates are not available. Measurements of prohormone mRNA levels in the hypothalamic neuronal somata (Sherman et al. 1986) show an increase with dehydration, but the relation between these levels and synthesis cannot be predicted exactly (for example, Welsh et al. 1985). Any effect in the neural lobe would be seen after a lag of about 1 day. Increasing synthesis in the model (a gradual increase to 4× is shown in Fig. 11) does give a reasonable fit for B/(B+A). More importantly, increased synthesis is required to produce low B/(B+A) values close to those seen experimentally at the end of the dehydration-rehydration regime. For a good fit of the rehydration points after 1 day, synthesis needs to be rapidly returned to normal, otherwise B/(B+A) values remain low.

Overall, the properties of the system as incorporated in the model result in a reasonable, though not exact, fit by the model of the experimentally observed changes in the oxytocin neurophysin forms during the dehydration-rehydration experiment (Fig. 11). The model further predicts values of B/(B+A) of 0.39 in the whole terminal and of 0.35 in the release for a 61-day-old rat, in agreement with the experimental data (Newcomb and Nordmann 1987; Figs. 10 and 11). The model thus forms a tentative hypothesis for a complicated, yet apparently straightforward situation. The model can now be used to generate predictions about the behavior of the neural lobe during other experimental manipulations. These predictions may then be used to further test the model.

4 Discussion

The problem of determining the precise chemical output of a peptidergic neuron is of obvious importance to our understanding the information content and potential biological role of peptidergic neurotransmission. In particular, if we are to investigate the potential importance of mixtures of peptides and variations of these mixtures, we need to know the quantitative amounts of the peptides contained in and released from neurons and the factors which affect these. The direct investigation of this problem is rendered difficult by anatomical and chemical complexity. The approach which we have presented here is to take a series of measurements of parameters determining the output of neurosecretory systems and to reconstruct from it a predicted output. The validity of models produced this way is tested by comparing their predictions against experimental observations of perturbations of the secretory system.

In the case of the sinus gland, a variety of important parameters remain to be determined. Here several models are capable of simulating the observed variations in peptide content. They allow us to test complex hypotheses for sufficiency in explaining experimental data. In the case of the neural lobe, the models are reasonably successful in accounting for the data on the composition of the peptide mixture stored in the neural lobe and released from it. The preliminary conclusion from the neural lobe modeling is that, even though complex changes of composition during experimental manipulation are predicted, the overall processing/compartmentation situation can be reduced to a limited number of kinetically simple physical processes; it is the interaction of these processes which accounts for any observed complexity. A most valuable feature of the present model is that it allows tentative assignment of particular mechanisms as actual causes of variations in peptide content. Such assignments are not yet possible for other peptidergic secretory systems, in which not all factors in the processing situation are quantitatively accounted for.

The successful use of certain types of experimental data in the construction of the neural lobe model indicates that similar studies will be a useful starting point in attempting quantitative descriptions of peptide output from more complex systems. To summarize, the information required was: (a) a precise analysis of the kinetics of the processing situation and of secretory granule lifetimes (Burford and Pickering 1973); (b) quantitative measures of relative volumes of axonal compartments near and away from release sites, and of secretory granule densities in these compartments (Nordmann 1977); and (c) a series of measures of amounts of all peptides with growth, depletion, and replenishment of peptide amounts (Jones and Pickering 1969; Newcomb and Nordmann 1987). These studies have been very straight-forward to apply to the neural lobe and, with a little ingenuity, should be just as directly applicable to more complex systems.

It is tempting to speculate that interactions between processing kinetics and compartmentation properties have evolved to give particular changes in the proportions and amounts of secreted peptide forms in response to biologically important changes in neural activity. In this regard, similarities and differences in the responses of neurohemal organs having different simple compartmentation schemes to differences in synthesis and release rates (Fig. 7) should be noted. The neural lobe response to dehydration is essentially that of the lower right panel of this figure. Here, the rate of change to a new, stable released-peptide content in response to an increased release rate is slowed by the flux of material out of the side compartment. The addition of inactivation of the oxytocin neurophysin conversion rate to this compartmentation scheme ensures that changes in released proportions of the two neurophysins during the depletion of the neural lobe are rather small. One possible functional role for the properties of secretory granule movements and peptide-processing kinetics in the neural lobe is that they have evolved to stabilize the presence of multiple cleavage fragments in nearly equal amounts, and thus to increase the number of different chemicals which can reliably be used under varying conditions. An interesting test of this idea would be to look for an increase in the A-to-B conversion rate in rats after several weeks of drinking water with 2% NaCl. Under these conditions the neural lobe is depleted of peptides (Jones and Pickering 1969), with new material, synthesized at an increased rate (Majzoub et al. 1983), rapidly passing though the neural lobe. Under such conditions, the only way the animal could obtain both forms of the oxytocin neurophysins for hormonal signalling would be to increase the conversion rate. Coordinated regulation of prohormone and processing enzyme synthesis has been reported (Millington et al. 1986), and it will be of interest to use the neural lobe model to determine the effect on secretory output.

The alternative to stabilization of multiple forms of a given peptide in nearly equal amounts would be for the early and late members of a prohormone processing pathway to be used independently. We do know that larger forms of opiate peptides are active (for example, opiates E and F; Lewis and Stern 1983), and that their receptor selectivities and in vivo stabilities are often different from those of the smaller active opiate peptides which they contain. A highly active secretory system will have faster secretory granule turnover times and a tendency to secrete larger forms, with the opposite true for a less active system. The forms of the peptides secreted may convey information on the overall activity of the secreting cell to the target cells, and it is interesting to try to predict how the distribution of forms secreted will vary with secretory activity.

Toward this end, we can use the models to investigate the interactions of varying cellular compartmentation properties with more complex processing schemes. We have as yet no experimental data with which to compare results, but the neural lobe model does give some indication of the interesting behavior likely to

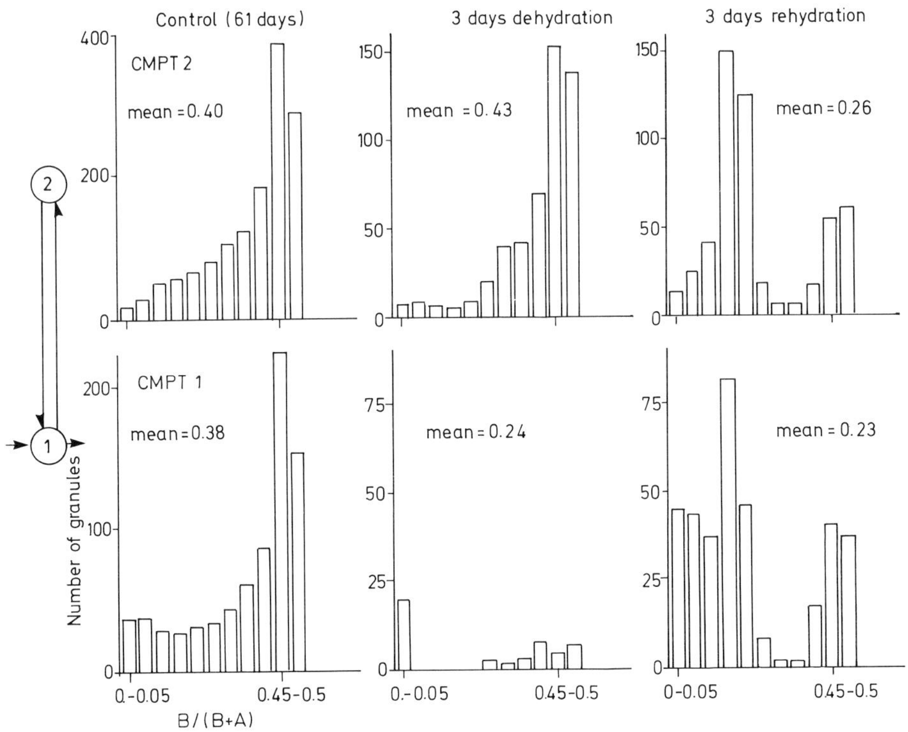

Fig. 12. Simulated distributions of processing ratio for the oxytocin neurophysin in neural lobe axon terminals (compartment 1) and swellings (compartment 2) with dehydration and rehydration. Simulation was carried out with the "granules" model described in the text, with the parameters used to fit the experimental data as given in Fig. 11

emerge. Figure 12 shows distributions of granules of different maturity (i.e., having different oxytocin neurophysin processing ratios) in release and storage compartments during dehydration and rehydration. The age distribution during the dehydration-rehydration regime (not illustrated) shows a large amount of very new material mixed in with a broad spectrum of older material which diffuses from the side compartment. This older material is almost all at a B/(B+A) value of 0.5; without inactivation of the processing rate, it would be close to 1.0 (that is, all B). It is seen that the neural lobe type of compartmentation results in a distinct bimodal distribution of precursor and product in released material under depletion and replenishment regimes. Therefore, if the neural lobe model is to be used to predict what mixture of released peptides is relevant in testing for a distinct physiological role, it would be a mixture of very early intermediates with the final products. This mixture would typify the output of a secretory structure similar to the neural lobe undergoing large changes in synthesis and release rates.

With more complex processing, as in Figs. 2 and 3, differences in secretory granule age distributions with differences in secretory activity will translate into marked differences in the forms of neuropeptides. With multiple active peptides derived from one prohormone coordinating a complex physiological response (as, for example, in control of egg-laying behavior by the *Aplysia* bag cell peptides, Scheller et al. 1983), the overall biological effect of changes in secreted peptide forms may be quite significant. The interaction of different types of cellular compartmentation with complex processing kinetics will make it difficult to predict what changes in secreted peptide amounts will occur without actual experimental determination. Further, especially in heterogeneous cell populations, multiple mechanisms affecting released peptide content may occur. A model systems approach might provide an analytical tool. Our ability to successfully simulate the available data on variations in peptide amounts in the sinus gland and neural lobe shows that quite precise descriptions of peptide outputs under varying conditions can be obtained. The approach should thus be applicable to the kinetic analysis of released peptide mixtures in suitable model systems expressing complex multifunctional prohormones. In addition to neuronal systems, classical endocrine cells exhibit proteolytic processing of prohormones that commonly does not proceed to completion. For example, this has been shown in the anterior lobe of the pituitary with the pro-opiomelanocortin molecule (Mains and Eipper 1981), in the endocrine pancreas with the precursor for pancreatic eicosapeptide (Nielsen et al. 1986), in the pancreas and intestine with preproglucagon (Mojsov et al. 1986), and in the adrenal medulla with the proenkephalin molecule (Lewis and Stern 1983; Fleminger et al. 1984). Approaches similar to the ones described here should be applicable to such cases.

With new evidence that mixtures of peptides can have effects unpredicted from their individual effects (see Sect. 1) it becomes important to know with precision the amounts of all peptides and other active substances being released and reaching the target cells. Our simulation studies show that selective variations in the relative amounts of neuropeptides derived from a given prohormone could be caused equally well by variations in degrees of enzyme inactivation, variation in rates of secretory granule turnover, and variations in activities of multiple enzymes (Fig. 6). These mechanisms are shown capable of yielding stable (Figs. 3

and 6) and unstable (Fig. 11) peptide contents in the sinus gland and neural lobe. We except these three types of mechanisms of peptide content variation to dominate in dictating variations in the mixture of peptides acting over short times and distances after release from a peptidergic neuron. Elucidation of the actual mechanism requires an understanding of the entire cellular situation, including processing kinetics, and rates and pathways of secretory granule movements. Neuropeptides are often not stable after release (reviews: Douglass et al. 1984; Loh et al. 1984; Lynch and Snyder 1986; McKelvy and Blumberg 1986; Draznin et al. 1985; Murthy et al. 1986), and effects of processes occurring after release will need to be accounted for in cases of tonic release and action at a distance.

While there is growing general awareness of the pervasive and crucial participation of peptides in the coordination of neural, endocrine, and physiological activities of animals, the capabilities of individual peptidergic cells for chemical signalling are yet to be widely appreciated. Methods of analysis described here should contribute to increased understanding of their capabilities for responding to changed demands as well as of the mechanisms underlying such responses.

Acknowledgments. Not only the data reviewed but the ideas developed in this chapter have benefitted from the contributions of our collaborators, among which we would particularly like to mention J. J. Nordmann, E. L. Stuenkel, and R. Scheller. We are grateful to C. Evans and D. Gassie for helpful suggestions on the manuscript, to B. Tomiyasu for assistance with the figures, and to C. Kosaki for preparation of the manuscript. Work in the authors' laboratories was supported by NIH grants NS24739 to R.N., NS15314 to D.H., and NS15453 to I.C., NSF grant BNS84-04459 to I.C., and grants from the Research Council (University of Hawaii) and University of Hawaii Foundation.

References

Burford GD, Pickering BT (1973) Intra-axonal transport and turnover of neurophysins in the rat. Biochem J 136:1047–1052

Burford GD, Clifford CW, Jones CW, Pickering BT (1973) A model for the passage of the neurohypophyseal hormones and their related proteins through the rat neurohypophysis. Biochem J 136:1053–1058

Carson ER, Cobelli C, Finkelstein L (1983) The mathematical modeling of metabolic and endocrine systems. Wiley, New York

Chang ES, Bruce MJ, Newcomb RW (1987) Purification and amino acid composition of a peptide with molt-inhibiting activity from the lobster, *Homarus americanus*. Gen Comp Endocrinol 65:56–64

Chapman DB, Morris JF, Valtin H (1982) How do granules distribute between nerve endings and nerve swellings in the neural lobe? Evidence from Brattleboro rats. In: Baertschi AJ, Dreifuss JJ (eds) Neuroendocrinology of vasopressin, corticotropin and opiomelanocortins. Academic, London, pp 1–10

Cooke IM (1977) Electrical activity of neurosecretory terminals and control of peptide hormone release. In: Farner DS, Lederis K (eds) Peptides in neurobiology. Plenum, New York

Cooke IM (1985) Electrophysiological characterization of peptidergic neurosecretory terminals. J Exp Biol 118:1–35

Douglass J, Civelli O, Herbert E (1984) Polyprotein gene expression: generation of diversity of neuroendocrine peptides. Annu Rev Biochem 53:665–715

Draznin B, Sherman N, Sussman K, Dahl R, Vatter A (1985) Internalization and cellular processing of somatostatin in primary culture of rat anterior pituitary cells. Endocrinology 117:960–965

Elliot ME, Goodfriend MD (1986) Atrial natriuretic peptide inhibits protein phosphorylation stimulated by angiotensin II in bovine adrenal glomerulosa cells. Biochem Biophys Res Commun 140:814–820

Fleminger G, Lahm H, Udenfriend S (1984) Changes in rat adrenal catecholamines and proenkephalin metabolism after denervation. Proc Natl Acad Sci USA 81:3587–3590

Godfrey K (1983) Compartmental models and their applications. Academic, London

Heap PF, Jones CW, Morris JF, Pickering BT (1975) Movement of neurosecretory product through the anatomical compartments of the neural lobe of the pituitary gland. Cell Tiss Res 156:483–497

Helsop JP, Blakeley DM, Brown KD, Irvine RF, Berridge MJ (1986) Effects of bombesin and insulin on inositol (1,4,5)triphosphate and inositol (1,3,4)triphosphate formation in Swiss 3T3 cells. Cell 47:703–709

Ivell R, Richter D (1984) Structure and comparison of the oxytocin and vasopressin genes from the rat. Proc Natl Acad Sci USA 81:2006–2010

Johnson RG Jr (ed) (1987) Cellular and molecular biology of hormone- and neurotransmitter-containing secretory vesicles. Ann NY Acad Sci 493:590

Jones CW, Pickering BT (1969) Comparison of effects of water deprivation and sodium chloride imbibition on the hormone content of the neurohypophysis of the rat. J Physiol (Lond) 203:449–458

Kaldany R-R, Campanelli JT, Schaefer M, Shyamala M, Scheller RH (1985) Low molecular weight proteins of *Aplysia* neurosecretory cells. Peptides 6:445–449

Keller R, Wunderer G (1978) Purification and amino acid composition of the neurosecretory hyperglycemic hormone from the sinus gland of the shore crab, *Carcinus maenus*. Gen Comp Endocrinol 34:328–335

Koob G, Bloom F (1982) Behavioral effects of neuropeptides: endorphin and vasopressin. Annu Rev Physiol 44:571–582

Lemos JR, Nordmann JJ, Cooke IM, Stuenkel EL (1986) Single channels and ionic currents in peptidergic nerve terminals. Nature 319:410–412

Lewis RV, Stern AS (1983) Biosynthesis of the enkephalins and enkephalin-containing polypeptides. Annu Rev Pharmacol Toxicol 23:353–372

Lloyd PE, Frankfurt M, Stevens P, Kupferman I, Weiss KR (1987) Biochemical and immunocytological localization of the neuropeptides FMRFamide, SCP_A, SCP_B, to neurons involved in the regulation of feeding in *Aplysia*. J Neurosci 7:1123–1132

Loh YP, Brownstein MJ, Gainer H (1984) Proteolysis in neuropeptide processing and other neural functions. Annu Rev Neurosci 7:189–222

Lundberg JM, Hökfelt T (1983) Coexistence of peptides and classical neurotransmitters. Trends Neurosci 6:325–333

Lynch DR, Snyder S (1986) Neuropeptides: multiple molecular forms, metabolic pathways, and receptors. Annu Rev Biochem 55:773–799

Mains RE, Eipper BA (1981) Differences in the post-translational processing of β-endorphin in rat anterior and intermediate pituitary. J Biol Chem 256:5683–5688

Mains R, Eipper B, Ling N (1977) Common precursor to corticotropins and endorphins. Proc Natl Acad Sci USA 74:3014–3018

Majzoub JA, Rich A, Boom J, Habener JF (1983) Vasopressin and oxytocin mRNA regulation in the rat assessed by hybridization with synthetic oligonucleotides. J Biol Chem 258:14061–14064

McKelvy JF, Blumberg S (1986) Inactivation and metabolism of neuropeptides. Annu Rev Neurosci 9:415–434

Milington WR, O'Donohue TL, Chappell MC, Roberts JL, Mueller GP (1986) Coordinate regulation of peptide acetyltransferase activity and pro-opiomelanocortin gene expression in the intermediate lobe of the rat pituitary. Endocrinology 118:2024–2033

Mojsov S, Heinrich G, Wilson IB, Ravazzola M, Orci L, Habener JF (1986) Preproglucagon gene expression in pancreas and intestine diversities at the level of post-translational processing. J Biol Chem 261:11880–11889

Murthy KK, Thibault G, Garcia R, Gutkowska J, Genest J, Cantin M (1986) Degradation of atrial natriuretic factor in the rat. Biochem J 240:461–469

Nagano M, Cooke IM (1987) Comparison of electrical responses of terminals, axons, and somata of a peptidergic neurosecretory system. J Neurosci 7:634–648

Nielsen HV, Gether U, Schwartz TW (1986) Cat pancreatic eicosapeptide and its biosynthetic intermediate: conservation of a monobasic processing site. Biochem J 240:69–74

Newcomb R (1983) Peptides in the sinus gland of *Cardisoma carnifex*: isolation and amino acid analysis. J Comp Physiol [B] 153:207–221

Newcomb R (1987) The amino acid sequences of neuropeptides in the sinus gland of the land crab *Cardisoma carnifex*: a novel neuropeptide proteolysis site. J Neurochem 49:574–583

Newcomb R, Nordmann JJ (1987) Quantitative HPLC and analysis of rat neurophysin metabolism. Neurochem Int 11:229–240

Newcomb R, Scheller RH (1987) Proteolytic processing of the *Aplysia* egg-laying hormone and R3–14 neuropeptide precursors. J Neurosci 7:854–863

Newcomb R, Stuenkel EL, Cooke IM (1985) Characterization, biosynthesis and release of neuropeptides from the X-organ sinus gland system of the crab *Cardisoma carnifex*. Am Zool 25:157–171

Nordmann JJ (1977) Ultrastructural morphometry of the rat neurohypophysis. J Anat 132:213–218

Nordmann JJ (1985) Hormone content and movement of neurosecretory granules in the rat neural lobe during and after dehydration. Neuroendocrinology 40:25–32

Nordmann JJ, Weatherby TM, Haylett BA (1986) Ultrastructural changes in peptidergic nerve terminals induced by digitonin permeabilization and K+ stimulation in the sinus gland of the crab, *Cardisoma carnifex*. Cell Tiss Res 246365–371

Orci L, Ravazzola M, Storch MJ, Anderson RGW, Vassali J-D, Perrelet A (1987) Proteolytic maturation of insulin is a post-Golgi event which occurs in acidifying clathrin-coated secretory vesicles. Cell 49:865–868

Russel JT, Brownstein MJ, Gainer H (1981) Time course of appearance and release of ^{35}S cysteine labelled neurophysins and peptides in the neurohypophysis. Brain Res 205:299–311

Sachs H, Haller E (1968) Further studies on the capacity of the neurohypophysis to release vasopressin. Endocrinology 76:251–262

Scheller RH, Jackson JF, McKallister LB, Rothman BS, Mayeri E, Axel R (1983) A single gene encodes multiple neuropeptides mediating a stereotyped behavior. Cell 32:7–22

Sherman GT, McKelvy JF, Watson SJ (1986) Vasopressin mRNA regulation in individual hypothalamic nuclei: a northern and in-situ hybridization analysis. J Neursci 6:1685–1694

Siwicki K, Beltz B, Kravitz E (1987) Proctolin in identified serotonergic, dopaminergic, and cholinergic neurons in the lobster, *Homarus americanus*. J Neurosci 7:522–532

Sossin W, Kirk M, Scheller R (1987) Peptidergic modulation of neuronal circuitry controlling feeding in *Aplysia*. J Neurosci 7:671–681

Stuenkel EL (1983) Biosynthesis and axonal transport of proteins and identified peptide hormones in the X-organ sinus gland neurosecretory system. J Comp Physiol B 153:191–205

Stuenkel EL (1985) Simultaneous monitoring of electrical and secretory activity in peptidergic neurosecretory terminals of the crab. J Physiol (Lond) 359:163–187

Stuenkel EL (1986) A common precursor to two major crab neurosecretory polypeptides. Peptides 7:397–406

Swanson L, Kuypers H (1980) The paraventricular nucleus of the hypothalamus: cytoarchitectonic subdivisions and the organization of projections to the pituitary, dorsal vagal complex and spinal cord as demonstrated by retrograde fluorescence double-labeling methods. J Comp Neurol 194:555–570

Swanson L, Sawchenko P (1983) Hypothalamic integration: organization of the paraventricular and supraoptic nuclei. Annu Rev Neurosci 6:269–324

Weatherby TM (1981) Ultrastructure of the sinus gland of the crab *Cardisoma carnifex*. Cell Tiss Res 220:293–312

Webster SB, Keller R (1986) Purification, characterization and amino acid composition of the putative molt-inhibiting hormone (MIH) of *Carcinus maenus* (Crustacea, Decapoda). J Comp Physiol [B] 157:617–624

Welsh M, Nielsen DA, MacKrell AJ, Steiner DF (1985) Control of insulin gene expression in pancreatic B cells and in an insulin-producing cell line, RIN-5F cells: II regulation of insulin mRNA stability. J Biol Chem 260:13590–13594

White JK, Stewart K, Krause J, McKelvy J (1985) Biochemistry of peptide-secreting neurons. Physiol Rev 65:553–606

Insect Neuropeptides

A. THORPE and H. DUVE

Contents

1 Introduction

The term "neurosecretion" was originally used in the pioneering studies of Ernst and Bertha Scharrer to characterise the activities of neurons that contained electron-dense granules about 400 nm in diameter. For a considerable time afterwards it was thought that such "neurosecretory" neurons were special variants of the "authentic" or "ordinary" neurons that contained small synaptic vesicles. Gradually, however, it was shown that almost every neuron terminal contained at least some "large-cored vesicles" in addition to the small vesicles. Following the work of Bargmann (1966) in which the term "peptidergic neuron" was coined specifically for neurons containing elementary granules that terminated synapti-

School of Biological Sciences, Queen Mary College, University of London, Mile End Road, London El 4NS, UK

Current Topics in Neuroendocrinology, Vol. 9

cally on the pituitary intermediate lobe cells, it has subsequently become recognised that most, if not all, neurons are more or less peptidergic (Fujita 1985).

Concomitant with the increasing awareness of the presence of peptidergic neurons has come the recognition that earlier distinctions made between the nervous and endocrine systems are more artificial than real. Thus, certain neurons of the central and/or peripheral nervous system have been shown to manufacture peptides previously considered to be the secretory products of specific endocrine cells. In particular, regulatory peptides of the gastrointestinal (GI) tract of vertebrates such as cholecystokinin (CCK) and vasoactive intestinal peptide (VIP) are now known to occur in the nervous system, and conversely, newly identified neuropeptides such as the enkephalins and neurotensin have been demonstrated at other sites within the body, including the GI tract. This dual occurrence of certain of the regulatory peptides within the nervous and GI tissues has led to the introduction of the term "brain-gut peptides". The rejection of the traditional distinctions made between the nervous and endocrine systems has led to a consideration of the brain as a real "endocrine" organ (Motta 1980).

Peptidergic neurons are now known to contain within their secretory granules a complex variety of substances, including the regulatory peptides themselves (often with other co-synthesised products cleaved from a common precursor molecule which may or may not be co-released); bioactive monoamines and/or acetylcholine; ATP and/or other adenine nucleotides; "carrier" proteins; enzymes for the conversion of amines (e.g. dopamine-β-hydroxylase) and for the processing and cleavage of peptides (e.g. various carboxy- and endopeptidases); glycosaminoglycans; and metallic ions, especially Ca^{2+}.

Although the original discoveries of peptidergic neurons were made in both invertebrates (e.g. *pars intercerebralis/corpus cardiacum* of insects) and vertebrates (hypothalamo-hypophysial complex of mammals), it is understandable that subsequently, with a few exceptions, the significant advances in our knowledge of neuropeptide biology have come from mammalian studies. Thus, within mammals we now recognise the existence of a wide variety of neuropeptides identified, however, from only a small range of species. For many of these substances the complete amino acid sequence is known, together with that of the precursor molecule and the nucleotide sequence of the gene encoding it. To varying degrees, for each identified mammalian peptide, we also have knowledge of precursor processing, post-translational modifications, formation of co-synthesised products, storage in secretion granules, intracellular peptide turnover, secretion mechanisms, specific control of secretion, processing and degradation in the blood, peptide recognition by receptors at target tissues, identity and characterisation of specific receptor molecules, mechanism of action, biological function and, for certain peptides of man, abnormalities in disease.

Our knowledge of the neuropeptides of invertebrates is generally much more fragmentary, despite the fact that they undoubtedly exercise control over the major life processes of these animals in much the same way as they do in vertebrates.

From the vast number of different insects (over 85000 species), a few, selected primarily because of their economic importance, have attracted detailed attention with respect to the neuroendocrine system, and these studies have led to a basic understanding of the ways in which hormones are able to affect developmental, growth and maturation processes. Much of the rapid progress in these areas of fundamental research has, however, been made in partial ignorance of the extensive neuropeptide repertoire possessed by insects. Thus, although insect neuroendocrinologists were among the first to recognise the existence of neuropeptides and their involvement in fundamental physiological processes (e.g. the "brain hormone" of Kopec 1922), nevertheless the diversity of these substances was (and still is) largely unknown. In a similar way, the many excellent insect neurophysiological research programmes have concentrated almost entirely on the classical non-peptidergic neurotransmitter substances. It can be seen from this that one of the major challenges confronting modern insect neurochemical and neurophysiological research is that of developing our knowledge of the neuropeptides at least to the levels currently attained in mammalian research. Thus, it is necessary to know the full extent to which neuropeptides exist in the insect nervous system and to isolate and characterise the molecules. We also need to localise the peptides to specific neurons, trace their pathways within the CNS, elucidate the stimuli necessary for their secretion, and develop an understanding of their mechanisms of action and their roles in physiology, metabolism and behaviour.

As testimony to the interest in insect neuroendocrinology, several excellent volumes dealing comprehensively with the subject have recently been published (see for example Raabe 1982; Downer and Laufer 1983; Kerkut and Gilbert 1985).

In this chapter it is the intention to review some of the general problems of insect neuropeptide research and to examine more closely specific areas of the authors' interest in the localisation, isolation and characterisation of peptides related to those that have hitherto been recognised only in vertebrates. One of the issues that will be discussed is the extent to which conservation of key functional amino acid sequences may have occurred during evolution.

2 Categories of Insect Neuropeptides

For present purposes the insect neuropeptides have been categorised as follows:

A. Peptides, the structure and physiological role of which have been identified. Monitored in bioassay. (See Table 1.)
B. Peptides, the physiological role of which has been established. Structure either unknown or only partially known. Monitored in Bioassay. (See Table 2.)
C. Peptides, the presence of which has been identified by immunological means [either radioimmunoassay (RIA) of tissue extracts or immunocytochemistry (ICC) applied to insect tissues] with antibodies and/or antisera raised against the biologically active peptides of vertebrates. Structure either unknown or incompletely known. Physiological role identified only in a few cases. (See Table 3.)

In the majority of instances within the various categories of peptides, the generalised term (e.g. "eclosion hormone") has been used. This is a matter of pure convenience, however, since it is clear that with such a large number of different species of insects, of which only a small fraction have actually been investigated, we may not always be dealing with a generalized and widespread molecule of universal significance, but rather with a variant that may have evolved to suit the highly specialised requirements of a particular species. This is perhaps more likely to be true for peptides regulating, for example, specialised aspects of a life cycle or unusual types of reproductive behaviour. However, even with identified peptides that control particular aspects of metabolism, e.g. the adipokinetic hormone that is known to control lipid mobilisation, we are beginning to recognise complete families of peptides with individual species variations.

Furthermore, although the allocation of insect peptides into the separate categories designated in this chapter indicates a uniqueness within one particular group, nevertheless one of the points that will emerge from the present account is a certain amount of overlap of categories as identified amino acid sequences become assigned to peptides previously identified only by their known physiological function(s). Thus, the insulin-like structure newly discovered for the prothoracicotropic hormone of *Bombyx* could not have been deduced with reference to the physiological role the peptide has in the initiation of ecdysone release.

2.1 Methods Used to Identify and Characterise Insect Neuropeptides

2.1.1 Physiological Experimentation

The existence of most of the insect hormones, including the neurohormones (neuropeptides), has been established by physiological studies, many of which have subsequently come to be regarded as "classical". Particularly useful have been experiments in which components of the neuroendocrine system including the entire brain or parts of it (median or lateral neurosecretory cells of the pars intercerebralis), corpus cardiacum or corpus allatum have been removed, with or without reimplantation. Such studies have led to the recognition that key physiological activities are controlled by neurohormonal factors released from these organs into the haemolymph. Likewise, experiments involving parabiosis and ligation have added greatly to our knowledge of the endocrine control of insect physiology. (For a general discussion of these experiments the reader is referred to Highnam and Hill 1977.)

2.1.2 The Problems of Size and Tissue Distribution

Undoubtedly a major problem in characterising the neuropeptides of insects lies in the small size of the organisms. This unavoidable difficulty is compounded by the fact that the biologically active molecules are produced usually by only a few cells which are frequently dispersed throughout the nervous system.

A major effort is necessary, therefore, to procure sufficient material with which to begin the process of peptide purification. As will be seen, such efforts may include the rearing of insects on an almost commercial scale and the collection from these animals of enriched sources of the molecules such as heads or specific ganglia. Recombinant DNA techniques may offer some short cuts in the future, but currently the significant advances are still being made with the methods of standard peptide chemistry.

For those involved in neuropeptide research the historical precedents seen in the successful elucidation of the molecular structure of the two other major classes of insect hormones, the ecdysteroids and the juvenile hormones, are inspirational. Thus, although ecdysone, unlike most of the neuropeptides, is conveniently confined to one or two individual organs (the prothoracic glands of larvae and pupae and the adult ovaries), nevertheless the definitive studies of this hormone were carried out using massive amounts of starting material. The steroid structure of ecdysone was determined from 250 mg hormone purified from no less than 1000 kg (dry weight) of the pupae of the silkworm *Bombyx mori* (Karlson et al. 1965; Huber and Hoppe 1965).

Juvenile hormone (JH) is also produced in a discrete endocrine organ, the corpus allatum, a fact that has proved useful for purposes of both physiological and chemical study. However, it was its presence in surprisingly large quantities (microgram amounts!) in the abdominal tissues of the adult male *Cecropia* moth (Williams 1956) that led to the elucidation of the structure of JH (Roller et al. 1969).

2.1.3 The Monitoring of Neuropeptides During Purification: Bioassay vs Radioimmunoassay

Of vital importance in any purification study is the means by which the purified substance is identified and monitored throughout the isolation procedures. The existence of peptides listed under categories A and B has been recognised by the physiological processes over which they are believed to exert a controlling influence, and for workers engaged in the purification of these molecules it has been necessary to devise a bioassay centred upon this specific area of physiology. The necessary criteria for a successful bioassay are specificity, sensitivity and speed and/or ease of operation. Unfortunately these are not easy criteria to achieve, and success in the field of neuropeptide biochemistry has often been hampered by the difficulties presented by the bioassay. Examples of successes and failures will be given below as individual neuropeptides are discussed.

For the peptides listed in category C, the vast majority of which may be conveniently termed "vertebrate-type", a bioassay is not possible, since at the moment we have almost no knowledge of the physiological roles they have in the insect. This is not too surprising, since for certain of the vertebrate neuropeptide counterparts, e.g. cholecystokinin (CCK8), we are uncertain as to function. The radioimmunoassay of peptides is certainly a method that can be developed to give speed and sensitivity. The problem of specificity, however, as with bioassay, can be considerable. As Rehfeld (1982) has pointed out, an antibody is always specific in that binding sites are always directed against a particular amino acid structure of some three to six residues. The point is whether or not the RIA itself is specific, i.e. whether or not the part of the antigen recognised by the antibody occurs in other antigens that are otherwise dissimilar. The use of a series of sequence-specific RIAs with antibodies directed against different parts of the same molecule is an extremely useful research tool in that it diminishes the likelihood of non-specific effects. Studies of the vertebrate-type peptides of insects carried out in our own laboratory have made use of this safeguard whenever possible, and examples will be given later.

2.1.4 The Cellular Localisation of Neuropeptides and the Identification of Neuronal Pathways

It has proved extremely difficult to identify the precise cellular sources of insect neuropeptides. As an example, the cells producing the "brain hormone" (now known as the prothoracicotropic hormone, PTTH) have only recently been identified, despite the fact that the existence of the hormone itself was proposed by Kopec as early as 1922 (Kopec 1922).

Formerly, physiological methods were used to identify the sources of peptides (such as PTTH). These included surgical lesioning of the brain, or the severance of particular nerve tracts with a resultant physiological effect dependent upon the removal of the source of the active principle. Such methods usually point only to a particular region or a group of cells, however, and not to individual neurons. One notable exception is the demonstration of the cells that produce PTTH in the pupal brain of *Manduca sexta*, which have been identified by Agui et al. (1979). Thus, two neurosecretory cells, one in each of the lateral protocerebral areas, have been isolated and their content assayed in vitro for PTTH activity in the prothoracic gland/ecdysone release bioassay (Bollenbacher et al. 1980).

The immunochemical methods that have been largely responsible for many of the rapid advances in neuropeptide research in mammals have recently been adopted for use in insects. Antibodies raised against the insect peptides whose structure has been elucidated (notably proctolin, adipokinetic hormone and PTTH) have been used in standard immunocytochemical procedure on a variety of insects to demonstrate the cellular sources of these peptides (see the relevant sections). A large number of cytological studies have also been carried out with antisera raised against many of the vertebrate biologically-active peptides. The results of these studies have suggested the presence of insect peptides that are related to those of vertebrates, at least in as much as they share common antigenic determinants. These results have often been interpreted – perhaps too freely by some authors – as indicating the presence of a closely related molecule. Our approach has been to use the ICC studies as a preliminary stage in the identification of insect neuropeptides. Positive results here have led to the introduction of biochemical studies aimed at purifying and characterising the peptides and hence ascertaining their precise degree of relatedness to the vertebrate molecules.

Nevertheless, despite possible limitations of the ICC method, studies of this type have revealed the amazing complexity and richness of the peptidergic neurosecretory system within the nervous system of insects. As neuronal markers we have been able to use vertebrate peptide antisera to trace complete neuronal pathways in a way that was formerly only possible with the more non-specific silver stains, fluorescent dyes or horseradish peroxidase methods of marking. Linked to electron microscopy, it has also been possible to use ICC to detect specific nerve terminals and even to distinguish between peptides contained in different granules within the same terminals (Duve et al. 1988).

Some of the recent trends in neuropeptide research will now be discussed with reference to a range of peptides selected from the three different categories. Where possible, reference will be made to stimulus-secretion coupling, although for many of the insect neuropeptides rather little is known about this subject.

3 Category A Peptides

Category A peptides are shown in Table 1.

3.1 Adipokinetic Hormone

An active principle from the corpus cardiacum (CC) that controls lipid utilization during flight of the desert locust *Schistocerca gregaria* was termed the "adipokinetic hormone" (AKH) by Mayer and Candy (1969). A similar factor from the corpus cardiacum of the migratory locust, *Locusta migratoria*, was also postulated by Beenakkers (1969).

It was later shown that AKH is released from the cells of the glandular lobe of the corpus cardiacum shortly after the start of flight (Goldsworthy et al. 1972). It is moved in the haemolymph (a) to the fat body where it promotes triglyceride breakdown to specific diglycerides via cyclic AMP mechanisms, and (b) to the flight muscle where it stimulates fatty acid oxidation and suppresses carbohydrate oxidation. In this way the diglycerides are utilized to provide the energy for prolonged flight. Although very little information is generally available concerning the regulatory mechanisms governing the release of neurohormones either from individual neurosecretory cells per se or from neurohaemal organs, nevertheless, for AKH a few of the details are beginning to emerge. Thus, it has been suggested that the initial stimulus for the release of AKH at the onset of flight could be a lowering of haemolymph trehalose at this time since injection of trehalose prevents the rise in lipid levels normally induced by flight (Houben and Beenakkers 1973).

At the cellular level of control, Orchard and Loughton (1981 a) have shown that axons in nervus corpora cardiaca II (NCC II), which are known to synapse with the glandular cells of the corpora cardiaca (Rademakers 1977), when stimulated electrically, result in the release of hyperlipemic hormone. They have, furthermore, studied the pharmacology of the synapse between the NCC II axons and the glandular cells and shown it to be aminergic, with the evidence suggesting that the transmitter is octopamine (Orchard and Loughton 1981 b).

The fact that the adipokinetic hormone is present in large quantities in a discrete neurohaemal organ, the corpus cardiacum, has enabled purification methods to be developed that result in the isolation of the pure peptide in a straightforward, rapid manner. This is in contrast to the more widely distributed neuropeptides such as proctolin and many of the vertebrate-type peptides to be discussed later.

Table 1. Category A peptides

Trivial name (and abbreviated form)	Structure	Species from which peptide has been isolated	Tissue source for extraction and purification	Identified sites of production	Function	Reference
Proctolin	H-RYLPT-OH	*Periplaneta americana*	Whole animals (125 kg)	Throughout the CNS	Myotropic peptide, neurotransmitter	Brown (1975)
Adipokinetic hormone (AKH)						
a) AKH I	pELNFTPNWGT amide	*Locusta migratoria*	Corpora cardiaca (3000)	Glandular lobe of CC	Lipid mobilisation	Stone et al. (1976)
b) AKH I	pELNFTPNWGT amide	*Schistocerca gregaria*	Corpora cardiaca (3000)	Glandular lobe of CC	Lipid mobilisation	Cheeseman et al. (1977)
c) AKH II-L	pELNFSAGW amide	*L. migratoria*	Corpora cardiaca (3000)	Glandular lobe of CC	Lipid mobilisation	Siegert et al. (1985); also Gäde et al. (1986)
d) AKH II-S	pELNFSTGW amide	*S. gregaria*	Corpora cardiaca (3000)	Glandular lobe of CC	Lipid mobilisation	Carlsen et al. (1979); Gäde et al. (1986)
e) AKH	pELTFTSSWG amide	*Manduca sexta*	Corpora cardiaca (3000)	Glandular lobe of CC	Lipid mobilisation	Zeigler et al. (1985)
f) AKH	pELTFTSSWG amide	*Heliothis zea*	Brain–suboesophageal ganglion–corpora cardiaca–corpora allata complexes (2200)	Glandular lobe of CC	Lipid mobilisation	Jaffe et al. (1986)
Cardioacceleratory peptides						
a) CC-1	pEVNFSPNW amide	*P. americana*	Corpora cardiaca–corpora allata (4000)	CC	Cardioacceleratory and hyperglycaemic activity	Scarborough et al. (1984)

Table 1 (continued)

Trivial name (and abbreviated form)	Structure	Species from which peptide has been isolated	Tissue source for extraction and purification	Identified sites of production	Function	Reference
b) CC-2	pELTFTPNW amide	*P. americana*	Corpora cardiaca–corpora allata (4000)	CC	Cardioacceleratory and hyperglycaemic activity	Scarborough et al. (1984)
Prothoracicotropic hormone						
(4K-PTTH-II)	(A chain) H-GIVDE CCLRPCSVDVLL SYC-OH	*Bombyx mori*	Heads of adult males (648 000)	NSC of pars inter-cerebralis	Stimulatory on release of ecdysone from prothoracic glands	Nagasawa et al. (1984, 1986)
	(B chain) pEQPQA VHTYCGRHLARTL ADLCWEAGVD-OH					
Leucosulfakinins						
LSK-I	EQFEDYGHMRF amide	*Leucophaea maderae*	Heads of adults (3000)	Brain and CC	Myotropic peptide (on cockroach hindgut)	Nachman et al. (1986a)
LSK-II	pESDDYGHMRF amide	*Leucophaea maderae*	Heads of adults (3000)	Brain and CC	Myotropic peptide (on cockroach hindgut)	Nachman et al. (1986b)

For sequence determination studies (Stone et al. 1976), batches of 500 glandular lobes from adult locusts were disrupted by ultrasonication in methanol which was then removed under a stream of nitrogen. Distilled water was added to the residue and the resulting suspension added to a column of G-75-50 glass beads. The column was eluted with distilled water and the absorbance of the effluent monitored at 206 nm. AKH activity was determined by means of bioassay (see below). Hormonally active functions were pooled and water removed by rotary evaporation under reduced pressure at 50 °C. Methanol was then added to the residue and the methanolic extract containing the hormone was subjected to silica gel thin-layer chromatography. The silica gel, containing AKH activity, was the scraped off the glass plate, mixed with methanol and later recovered as pure AKH hormone by centrifugation of the silica gel substrate and evaporation of the methanol. Such a procedure is reported to give a 50% yield which comprises 50–100 nmol AKH from 500 glandular lobes of *Locusta* and 100–125 nmol from 500 glandular lobes of *Schistocerca*.

A variation of this method of extraction was developed by Cheeseman et al. (1977), who used a Sephadex LH-20 column eluted with 80% methanol, followed by thin-layer cellulose two-dimensional chromatography.

As with all peptide extraction and isolation procedures, a sensitive, specific means of assay is essential and for AKH, the lipid-mobilizing response of the hormone when injected into the haemolymph of locusts has been adopted (Goldsworthy et al. 1972).

The samples are dissolved in insect saline to give a 20-μl injection volume which is administered to the locust between the third and fourth abdominal sterna. Samples of haemolymph (5 μl) are withdrawn from a small puncture made in the arthroidal membrane at the base of the hind leg and changes in total lipid concentration are measured at various time intervals and compared with each other and with preinjection values. The changes in total lipid reflect, in effect, the increasing diglyceride concentration, as this is the principal mobilisation product. Dose-response curves with a near-linear initial portion, followed by a gradual flattening out of the curve at higher doses show that the hormone-receptor response is saturable. Furthermore, the time taken for lipid levels to reach initial values has been shown to be dependent upon the dose of AKH injected, suggesting that the system responsible for removing the hormone from the haemolymph (sited in the Malpighian tubules?) is also saturable.

The chemical identity of AKH was elucidated by Stone et al. (1976) from material extracted from 3000 *corpora cardiaca* (approx. 750 nmol). The peptide was known to be heat-stable when hydrolysed in acid and to yield at least 2 molecules of aspartic acid, two threonine, one glutamic acid, one proline, one glycine, one leucine and one phenylalanine molecule. However, when purified material was subjected to the Edman degradation procedure, it was discovered that the N-terminus of AKH is blocked. The peptide was therefore digested with the bacterial protease thermolysin, which produced two fragments. The C-terminal fragment was partially sequenced using the dansyl-Edman procedure and that of the N-terminal fragment determined in part following digestion with a carboxypeptidase. Mass spectrometry was used to confirm the structures of both the thermolytic fragments and the intact hormone, with the result that AKH was finally characterised as pyrrolidone carboxylic acid (PCA) Leu-Asn-Phe-Thr-Pro-Asn-Trp-Gly-Thr-NH_2.

In addition to its occurrence in the glandular lobes of the *corpora cardiaca* of locusts, it has subsequently been suggested that the peptide (or a closely related substance) may occur in a population of peptidergic neurons within the nervous system (Schooneveld et al. 1983). As stated in the Introduction, the occurrence of biologically active peptides in different cell types at different locations within the body is well known from vertebrate studies, and it is entirely to be expected that a similar situation will occur in invertebrates. The finding of an AKH-like peptide in the nervous system and also in embryological stages of the locust, during which time flight could not possibly occur, introduces many more questions as to the possible functions of the material. We certainly can no longer expect the single peptide, single source, single action idea to stand up to close scrutiny, and studies on the multifunctional influence of individual peptides on a variety of biological activities are likely to provide insect physiologists with a rich vein of research material over the next few years.

3.2 Proctolin

Proctolin, the myotropic pentapeptide, H-Arg-Tyr-Leu-Pro-Thr-OH, was the first insect neuropeptide to be identified (Brown and Starratt 1975; Starratt and Brown 1975). The peptide causes contractions of the slow striated muscles of the gut of *Periplaneta americana*, the species in which it was originally discovered. Subsequently, it has been shown to be widely distributed in the Insecta and to have effects at low thresholds (10^{-9} *M*) on different types of muscles such as the heart of *Periplaneta* (Miller 1979) and the leg muscle of locusts (Piek and Mantel 1977).

As evidenced by ICC studies, proctolin-containing neurons are both numerous and widespread within the nervous system of insects such as *P. americana* (Eckert et al. 1981; Bishop et al. 1981; Bishop and O'Shea 1982), the Colorado potato beetle *Leptinotarsa decemlineata* (Veenstra et al. 1985a), and *Calliphora vomitoria* (Duve and Thorpe, unpublished observations). Proctolinergic nerve fibres are equally widely distributed and are especially numerous, for example, in the dorsocaudal neuropil of the terminal ganglion of *Periplaneta*, where, according to Agricola et al. (1985), they give rise to presynaptic terminals. These studies suggest that proctolin functions as a neurotransmitter or neuromodulator within the CNS in addition to its role in the periphery, as evidenced by the account of proctolinergic terminals on the musculature of the fore- and hindgut, on the vas deferens and on certain segmental muscles of the Colorado potato beetle (Veenstra et al. 1985a).

Proctolin was isolated initially from the viscera of the cockbroach *P. americana*, a tissue containing relatively high levels of the peptide (Brown 1967). In the later definitive study by Brown and Starratt (1975) whole cockroaches were used [125 kg fresh weight (125000 insects) yielded 180 μg pure proctolin]. This "heroic" study exemplifies other attempts currently in progress, in our laboratory and elsewhere, to isolate and characterise peptides that are known to have a wide distribution within the insect body, e.g. CCK-like peptides of *Calliphora* (Duve and Thorpe 1984a; Duve et al. 1985) and is in direct contrast to the studies of other peptides that have a more specific and limited tissue distribution, e.g. AKH isolated from the glandular lobe of the *corpora cardiaca* and prothoracicotropic hormone, known to occur in a small number of neurosecretory cells in the brain and isolated from an enriched source of heads only (see below).

The main problems in using a great quantity of impure insect tissue as the start material for extraction is, of course, that the degree of purification required is compounded by the many unwanted proteins, peptides and troublesome lipids and pigments. Furthermore, a variety of enzymes are released into the extraction fluid and these have the potential for breaking down the peptide to be identified. It is possible to counteract this disadvantage by low-temperature extraction procedures, by the use of acidified extracting fluid or by the addition of enzyme inhibitors such as Trasylol. The methods used for the isolation of proctolin are given in the original paper (Brown and Starrat 1975) and will not be reviewed here.

One point of major concern, however, in all peptide purification studies is the means by which the peptide is to be monitored through the various steps of the isolation process. In the case of proctolin and several other insect peptides to be discussed here, a bioassay has been developed for this purpose.

The proctolin bioassays have been described as "sensitive, convenient and relatively rapid", three prerequisites in the development of any assay. At its most simple the assay relies upon the isolation of the proctodeum of *P. americana* without its nerve supply, which is then suspended in a suitable organ bath of known volume. The test sample (proctolin in varying stages of purification) is applied and the proctodeal contractions are recorded isotonically. After relaxation, the preparation can be returned to baseline values within a short time, in preparation for the next test sample.

In addition to the bioassay criteria listed above, specificity of action is another to which paramount importance must be attached. For proctolin, this can present a real problem in that insects possess a number of myotropic neuropeptides, including the recently identified leucosulfakinins (see below).

3.3 Prothoracicotropic Hormone

The complete structure of the prothoracicotropic hormone (PTTH) of *Bombyx mori* was reported by Nagasawa and his colleagues (1986) following an initial publication in which the first 19 amino acid residues of the A chain were identified (Nagasawa et al. 1984). There are at least three forms of the hormone in *Bombyx*, and the one that has been identified has been designated 4K-PTTH-II. Remarkably, the structure of the peptide resembles vertebrate insulin in many important features. Thus, there are two non-identical chains (A and B). The A chain has 20 amino acid residues and the B chain is a mixture of four peptides which display a microheterogeneity in that two consist of 28 residues and the other two of 26 residues. The sequences of the A and B chains are shown in Fig. 1, where they are compared with human insulin and porcine relaxin. The molecule displays a high

A chains

	1 5 10 15 20
4K-PTTH-II	H-Gly-Ile-Val-Asp-Glu-Cys-Cys-Leu-Arg-Pro-Cys-Ser-Val-Asp-Val-Leu-Leu-Ser-Tyr-Cys-OH
Human insulin	H-Gly-Ile-Val-Glu-Gln-Cys-Cys-Thr-Ser-Ile-Cys-Ser-Leu-Tyr-Glu-Leu-Glu-Asn-Tyr-Cys-Asn-OH
Porcine relaxin	H-Arg-Met-Thr-Leu-Ser-Glu-Lys-Cys-Cys-Glu-Val-Gly-Cys-Ile-Arg-Lys-Asp-Ile-Ala-Arg-Leu-Cys-OH

B chains

	1 5 10 15 20
4K-PTTH-II	pGlu-Gln-Pro-Gln-Ala-Val-His-Thr-Tyr-Cys-Gly-Arg-His-Leu-Ala-Arg-Thr-Leu-Ala-Asp-Leu-Cys-
Human insulin	Phe-Val-Asn-Gln-His-Leu-Cys-Gly-Ser-His-Leu-Val-Glu-Ala-Leu-Tyr-Leu-Val-Cys-
Porcine relaxin	pGlu-Ser-Thr-Asn-Asp-Phe-Ile-Lys-Ala-Cys-Gly-Arg-Glu-Leu-Val-Arg-Leu-Trp-Val-Glu-Ile-Cys-

	23 25
4K-PTTH-II	Trp-Glu-Ala-Gly-Val-Asp-OH
Human insulin	Gly-Glu-Arg-Gly-Phe-Phe-Tyr-Thr-Pro-Lys-Thr-OH
Porcine relaxin	Gly-Val-Trp-Ser-OH

Fig. 1. Amino acid sequences of 4K-PTTH-II (bombyxin) from *Bombyx mori* compared with human insulin and porcine relaxin. —, identical residues of PTTH and insulin; ---, identical residues of PTTH and porcine relaxin. (From Nagasawa et al. 1986)

degree of homology with human insulin (18 sequence identities or 40%) and a lesser degree of homology to porcine relaxin (11 sequence identities). Importantly, most of the hydrophobic core residues are identical in PTTH-II and insulins from whatever source. These include A1 Ile, A6 Cys, A11 Cys, A16 Leu, A20 Cys, B11 Leu, B15 Leu and B19 Cys, and this leaves no doubt that PTTH is a member of the insulin family of peptides. Bombyxin, as the peptide has been named (Mizoguchi et al. 1987), has the distinction of being the first invertebrate insulin to be identified and characterised.

The neuropeptide was isolated from a total of 648 000 heads of male adult *Bombyx* (4.86 kg) in a 15-step purification procedure involving heat treatment, fractional precipitations, gel filtrations, ion-exchange chromatography and high-performance liquid chromatography. The yield was about 300 μg/10^6 heads. Reductive alkylation of disulphide bonds of 4K-PTTH-II was found to generate two non-identical peptides referred to as DA and DB. The amino acid sequence of DA was determined by means of automated Edman degradation and the amino acid sequence of DB by Edman degradation of peptide fragments obtained by enzyme digestion.

The data of 4K-PTTH-II suggest that it is a member of the insulin family of peptides. Furthermore, they suggest that the variants within this family probably arose from a common ancestral gene. We have no knowledge of exactly how much closer the insect insulin-related peptide is to this ancestral gene than the mammalian insulin, insulin-like growth factor or relaxin peptides. Indeed, they do not necessarily have to be set at an earlier evolutionary position, since specialisation within the insects has proceeded to the same temporal end point as that within mammals, which means that they are in no way "primitive" organisms. It is clear from the data, however, that the ancestral genes have been highly conserved during evolution.

It is an interesting fact that a number of earlier reports have suggested that insulin-like peptides occur in insects. These studies have been reviewed by Thorpe and Duve (1984). The pattern from several accounts taken from a variety of different insect species is the same. Thus, specific cells within the median neurosecretory groups show immunoreactivity towards bovine or porcine insulin antisera (Duve and Thorpe 1979; Yui et al. 1980; El Salhy et al. 1980; Lavensau et al. 1984). A recent ICC study by Mizoguchi et al. (1987), in which a monoclonal antibody raised against a synthetic decapeptide that corresponds with the N-terminal 1–10 sequence of the bombyxin A chain was tested on the neuroendocrine tissues of *Bombyx*, has shown that bombyxin is produced in four pairs of median neurosecretory cells in the brain. It seems highly probable that these cells correspond exactly with the four pairs of cells identified in *Bombyx* by Yui et al. (1980) as being insulin-immunoreactive. Indeed, a comparative insulin/bombyxin ICC study on *Bombyx* carried out by Ishizaki et al. (1986) confirms that the same cells are reactive to antisera directed against both peptides. As one might expect of the median neurosecretory cells in the brain, bombyxin (insulin)-immunoreactive material can be traced from the perikarya along axons to the *corpora cardiaca* (although it is not present there in any great quantity). Interestingly, bombyxin-immunoreactive material is also found in fibres entering the corpora allata, suggesting a functional relationship with this organ.

If one extrapolates from the ICC studies carried out on *Bombyx* and from the results from other insect species that have been studied with anti-insulin sera, then it could well be argued that the insulin-immunoreactive median neurosecretory cells seen in these species are, in fact, producing a PTTH homologue. In addition to the cytological studies, two biochemical studies on *Manduca* (Tager et al. 1976) and *Calliphora* (Duve et al. 1979) have succeeded in purifying an insulin-immunoreactive peptide from either heads or *corpora cardiaca/corpora allata* complexes. An RIA for vertebrate insulin was used to monitor the peptides in both instances and both studies have also made use of insulin bioassays on the purified material to confirm its insulin-like nature.

As with the results from ICC, it is tempting to speculate that the insect neuropeptides, characterised as insulin-like with reference to immunochemical assay and bioassay, are homologous to the *Bombyx* PTTH (bombyxin). It seems very likely that a molecular species (for sake of argument we will call it insulin) that has had its essential characteristics conserved during the evolutionary period spanning insects to mammals will be found to be common to all species of insects. The question at issue is whether or not the molecules identified in *Calliphora, Manduca* and other insects *is* the homologue or whether there is another, as yet unidentified, insulin-like molecule.

Central to this discussion is the problem of the physiological role of the bombyxin and other insulin-like molecules. The facts about bombyxin itself are somewhat strange in that its actual prothoracicotropic activity, i.e. the ability to induce the prothoracic gland to synthesise and release ecdysone, is not actually manifest in *Bombyx* itself. The bioassay organism is the saturniid moth *Samia cynthia ricini*. Thus, in the pupa-adult metamorphosis step, the peptide fails to provoke development in brain- or head-removed *Bombyx* and the same is true if one considers fourth to fifth instar larval development. Its physiological function in the silk moth *Bombyx*, therefore, remains unclarified, and in this species it is a much higher molecular weight form of PTTH of 22000 daltons that is known to be able to activate the prothoracic gland.

It is also relevant to note that PTTH was originally named by its function in activating the prothoracic glands. Since these degenerate promptly after adult ecdysis, the question arises as to its function in the adult, the stage in the life cycle from which it has been extracted and purified. Since it is produced in the median neurosecretory cells (MNCs) and since the products of these cells are known to have a direct access to the haemolymph via the neurohaemal organ, the corpus cardiacum, then a metabolic role (such as is known for insulin in vertebrates) is certainly not out of the question. According to Ishizaki and Suzuki (1980), it seems likely that the releasing sites of PTTH are widely distributed throughout the surface of the PTTH-producing cells. If this is so, then a neurotransmitter or neuromodulatory role for the peptide, in addition to its neurohormonal role, also seems likely. The stimulus for the secretion of any peptide acting as a neurotransmitter or neuromodulator is likely to be via presynaptic contact with a range of interacting neurons, and this being so we cannot be sure of the *precise* stimulus. For PTTH acting as a neurohormonal molecule released into the haemolymph to make contact with its target organ, the prothoracic glands, however, it *is* possible to identify the stimuli. For one species, *Rhodnius prolixus*, the stimulatory mechanism for PTTH secretion is known to be provided by the expanded state of the abdomen following the intake of a large blood meal. Severing the nerve cord in the prothorax prevents moulting, suggesting that nervous impulses from the stretched abdomen cause the release of PTTH (Wigglesworth 1964). Additional evidence, such as a neuroendocrine reflex, is provided by the observation that the medial neurosecretory cells in the brain remain in an inactive state during larval starvation, whereas within minutes of a blood meal they undergo cytological changes (Steel and Harmsen 1971).

The neural inputs controlling the release of PTTH in continuously feeding insects have not been determined precisely, although several studies have provided evidence of cytological changes in the MNCs after a variety of external and internal stimuli. In *Manduca sexta*, a study by Nijhout and Williams (1974) has shown that once a fifth-instar larva reaches a critical body weight of ca. 5 g, an unidentified process is initiated that takes 24 h to be completed. Once this process has been completed, the brain is rendered incapable of releasing PTTH. The actual release of the neurohormone occurs in a "gated" manner during the next photophase. Thus the secretion of PTTH occurs during a specific portion of the day under a given photoperiod and sets in train the rhythmicity of ecdysis (Truman 1972; Truman and Riddiford 1974). This mechanism in *Manduca* may be seen to be very similar to that described for *Rhodnius*, in that a critical body weight may well be related to a state of body expansion such that proprioceptors in the body wall would initiate nervous impulses to the brain to initiate, via PTTH, the processes in preparation for the next moult.

PTTH is also involved in the mechanism of diapause, a process that is caused by failure of the brain to secrete PTTH and which is terminated by the resecretion of the hormone. In certain insects it would seem that the brain contains a light receptor-effector system with which it operates the termination of diapause (Williams and Adkisson 1964). Neural influences inhibitory to the release of PTTH are thought to reach the brain from elsewhere in the nervous system continuously during diapause (Ishizaki and Suzuki 1980).

There are many interesting problems to be solved in relation to PTTH stimulus-secretion coupling. However, it is clear that different insects make use of their own PTTH variant in different ways, a fact which makes it difficult to generalise on the subject. The sequencing of the *Bombyx* 4K-PTTH-II molecule should enable a more rapid advance to be made in identifying the properties of PTTH, at least in this particular species.

3.4 Leucosulfakinins

Two myotropic sulphated neuropeptides named leucosulfakinin (LSK) I and II have recently been isolated from extracts of 3000 heads of the cockroach *Leucophaea maderae* (Nachman et al. 1986a, b). These are the latest insect neuropeptides to be characterized and they are interesting on account of the structural homologies shown to the vertebrate peptides gastrin, caerulein and, more particularly, cholecystokinin (CCK) (Fig. 2).

As will be seen later, several previous reports of gastrin/CCK-related peptides in a variety of insects have appeared in the literature, in studies based on both ICC

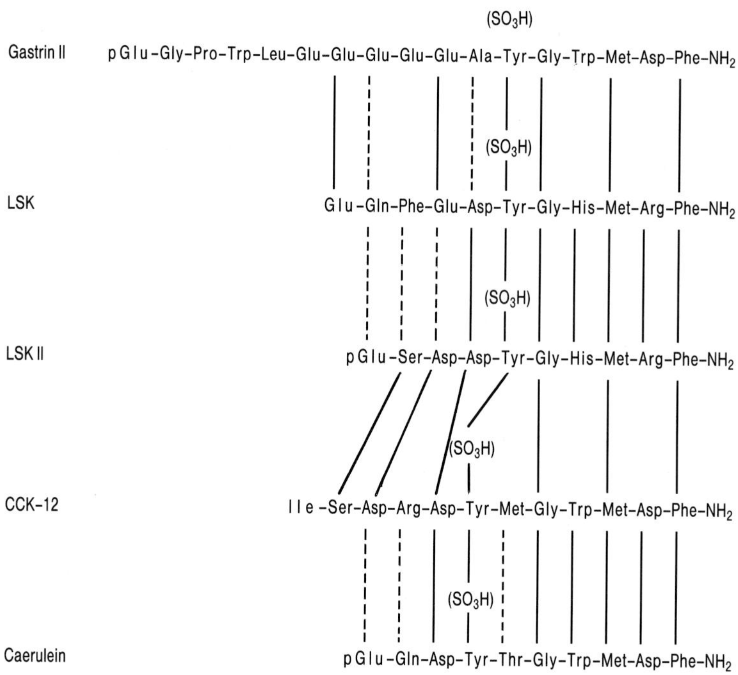

Fig. 2. Amino acid sequences of the leucosulfakinins LSK I and LSK II compared with gastrin II, CCK 12 and caerulein. *Solid lines*, identical amino acids; *dashed lines*, amino acids that could have appeared as a result of single nucleotide changes in the codons. (From Nachman et al. 1986b)

and RIA using gastrin/CCK antisera. The structural analyses of the two peptides from *Leucophaea* gives added support to the view that evolutionary conservation has maintained functionally important peptide sequences.

Gastrin and cholecystokinin share the common C-terminal pentapeptide sequence Gly-Trp-Met-Asp-Phe-NH2. They also contain *O*-sulphated tyrosyl close to the pentapeptide, viz. position 6 in gastrin and position 7 in CCK as counted from the C-terminus. Although activity as a CCK is present in the α-amidated tetrapeptide, it has been shown that the *O*-sulphation of the tyrosine residue enhances the actions of CCK on the contraction of the gall bladder and on the secretion of pancreatic enzymes by a factor of 100 (Amer 1969). Cerebral functions of CCK appear to be less dependent on sulphation (Dodd and Kelly 1981).

The LSKs were extracted by methanol:water:acetic acid (90 : 9 : 1) and purified by a four-step high-performance liquid chromatography procedure. The LSKs were monitored by observing in bioassay the myotropic effect of the fractions. The bioassay measures the changes in frequency or amplitude of spontaneous contractions of the cockroach proctodeum (hindgut). Initial separation yielded five active fractions and one of these, when purified, yielded 1.3 µg of a pure peptide. This was shown to have the primary structure Glu-Gln-Phe-Glu-Asp-Tyr-Gly-His-Met-Arg-Phe (Nachman et al. 1986a). When this sequence was compared with human gastrin I (the nonsulphated form) it was observed that six of the 11 residues were identical. Thus, Glu^1, Glu^4, Tyr^6, Gly^7, Met^9 and Phe^{11} of the LSK sequence matched positions 7, 10, 12, 13, 15 and 17 of human gastrin. Furthermore, this homology has even greater significance, as the sequence differences Gln^2, Asp^5 of LSK and Glu^8, Ala^{11} of gastrin I are possible from single-base substitutions in the respective codons. Fast atom bombardment later showed that the Tyr at position 6 was sulphated, a fact that emphasises the homology with gastrin II, which is identical with gastrin I but has a sulphated tyrosine residue. Nachman and co-workers (1986a, b) conclude from their studies that the sequence homology of LSK-I and gastrin II, together with their analagous biological activity [both are myotropic on smooth muscles of the gut and both stimulate blood (haemolymph) circulation], make it unlikely that their structural convergence is coincidental.

The content of LSK I was calculated to be 0.5 ng/head in *Leucophaea* and the fact that it is present also in the *corpora cardiaca* (Holman et al. 1984), major neurohaemal organs of insects, indicates that it is circulated in the hameolymph as a neurohormonal peptide. The peptide LSK II is related to LSK I by having an identical C-terminal heptapeptide sequence, including the sulphated tyrosine residue at position 6, but it has one residue less (it is a decapeptide) and it is blocked (pGlu) at the N-terminus (Fig. 2) (Nachman et al. 1986b).

The pyroglutamyl residue is a structural feature seen in many biologically active peptides, including the insect AKHs and some vertebrate peptides. It is thought that this may serve the function of protecting the neuropeptide from enzyme degradation during transport in vivo (Gregory et al. 1964). LSK II shows a greater resemblance to CCK and a lesser resemblance to gastrin II than does LSK I.

Residues Asp^3, Gly^6, Met^8 and Phe^{10} are identical to those in the analogous 5, 8, 10 and 12 positions of CCK 12, whilst lateral homologues exist between

Ser^2–Asp^3 and Asp^4–$Tyr(SO_3H)^5$ of LSK II and the corresponding amino acid pairs in positions 2–3 and 5–6 of CCK (see Fig. 2). Intervening residues Arg^4 and Met^7 of CCK prevent direct alignment with the amino acid block Ser-Asp-Asp-Tyr (SO_3H) of LSK II. In addition, sequence differences of $pGlu^1$, Ser^2, Asp^4 of LSK II and Asp^3, Arg^4, Tyr^6, of CCK-12 could arise from single-base substitutions in the respective codons.

As far as the frog skin peptide caerulein is concerned, the $pGlu^1$ of LSK II is identical, and in fact five of the 10 residues in LSK II are identical to those of caerulein.

The presence of the sulphated tyrosine residue in LSK I and LSK II is highly significant when considering homologies with the vertebrate peptides gastrin II and CCK, since this derivatization is relatively uncommon in biologically active peptides. Furthermore, both LSKs contain an aspartic acid residue immediately preceding the Tyr (SO_3H), a feature known to be a component in the recognition site for tyrosyl protein sulphotransferase in CCK and other sulphated peptides.

The structural analysis of the LSKs from *Leucophaea* gives added support to the view that evolutionary conservation has maintained functionally important peptide sequences. Meanwhile, much remains to be discovered about the two peptides, not least of which is their distribution within the CNS and further details concerning their role in physiology. For all peptides with an outlet to the *corpora cardiaca* as suggested here for the LSKs, one can postulate the existence of a type of neuroendocrine reflex, whereby external or internal stimuli trigger neural responses within the CNS which are then translated into hormonal signals.

For the LSKs the act of feeding could provide the initial stimulus leading to their eventual release and functioning in regulating gut motility, the stimulation of the haemolymph circulation and perhaps, also, the enhanced secretion of digestive enzymes and/or salivary output. Such a scenario has direct parallels if one considers the stimulus-secretion coupling mechanisms that operate in the gastrin/CCK endocrine system of mammals.

3.5 The Periplanetins, CC-1 and CC-2

The *corpora cardiaca* are important neurohaemal organs in insects, having both intrinsic glandular cells and also a richly peptidergic neuropil which stores and releases neurosecretory products synthesised in the brain. Previous biochemical studies of cockroach *corpora cardiaca* (homogenates and partially purified fractions) have demonstrated the presence of factors affecting heart rate (Baumann and Gersch 1981) and trehalose levels in the haemolymph (Goldsworthy and Gäde 1983). No sequence data were available for these factors, however, until the recent study by Scarborough et al. (1984), who isolated two octapeptides, each having both cardioacceleratory and hyperglycemic activity, from the cockroach *Periplaneta americana*. The peptides, termed CC-1 and CC-2, appear to represent new members of a family of invertebrate peptides that includes locust adipokinetic hormone and crustacean red-pigment concentrating hormone. One of the peptides (CC-2) also has a restricted sequence homology to the N-terminus of glucagon (Fig. 3).

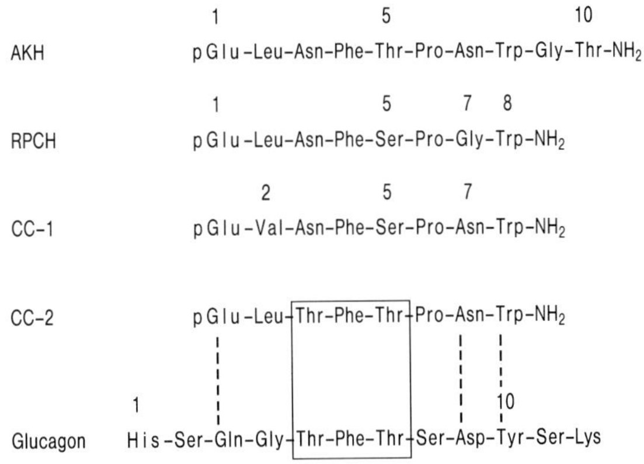

Fig. 3. Primary sequences of adipokinetic hormone (*AKH*), crustacean red pigment-concentrating hormone (*RPCH*) and the periplanetins (*CC-1* and *CC-2*) compared with the N-terminal (1–12) sequence of glucagon. Identical sequences between CC-2 and glucagon are shown *boxed*, and residue differences that could have arisen as a result of single nucleotide changes in the codon are indicated by *dashed lines*. (From Scarborough et al. 1984)

A total of 400 cockroach *corpora cardiaca* were used in the study. Extraction was carried out in 5 *M* acetic acid and the initial step of the purification was carried out either on Sephadex G-25 or by means of a Sep-Pak C18 cartridge (Waters). The prepurified extracts were further purified by gradient elution and reversed-phase high-performance liquid chromatography.

CC-1 is believed "almost certainly" to be the factor originally given the name "neurohormone D" (Baumann and Gersch 1981), and both CC-1 and CC-2 appear to be excellent candidates for factors affecting carbohydrate metabolism and previously named "hyperglycemic factors".

The homology to part of the vertebrate glucagon sequence is of interest in the general context of the growing series of insect/vertebrate peptide comparisons (Duve and Thorpe 1984b) and particularly in that both peptides are hyperglycemic. Perhaps not too much should be made of this finding, however, since the sequence homology is so limited.

4 Category B Peptides

Category B peptides are shown in Table 2.

4.1 Bursicon

Bursicon is the neurohormone responsible in insects for hardening and darkening the cuticle. It was discovered and named by Fraenkel and Hsiao (1962, 1963, 1965) in studies of dipteran species, although similar factors have now been described for other major groups. The evidence that a hormone initiated tanning of the cuticle in blowflies came from the results of classical experiments in which

Table 2. Category B peptides

Trivial names	Physiological function (observed experimental effects)	Species investigated	Sites of occurrence	Tissues used in purification	Amino acid sequence and/ or composition	References
Hypolipaemic hormone	Decreases haemolymph lipid	*Schistocerca Locusta*	Storage lobe of CC	–	–	Orchard and Loughton (1980)
Hyperglycaemic; hypertrehalosaemic; trehalogen	Increased levels of trehalose; glycogenolytic action; phosphorylase-stimulating activity	*Periplaneta americana, Locusta, Carausius, Manduca*	CC	CC	–	Normann and Duve (1969, 1978), Steele (1961, 1963, 1980, 1983), Goldsworthy and Gäde (1983), Holwerda et al. (1977), Gäde (1981)
Hypoglycaemic hormones (factors) (peptides)	Decreased levels of trehalose and glucose	*Calliphora*	Pars intercerebralis MNC/CC	–	–	Duve (1978), Normann (1975)
Diapause hormone						
a) Egg/embryonic	Arrests embryonic development at the germ band formation	*Bombyx mori*	Neurosecretory cells of SOG	Two million male heads	MW between 2000 and 3000 (14 different kinds of amino acids and two different kinds of amino sugars)	Kubota et al. (1976), Isobe and Goto (1980), Yamashita (1983)
b) Larval/pupal	Diapause in larval or pupal stages. Due to an absence of PTTH but also other neuroendocrine factors	*Pieris, Mamestra, Manduca, Heliothis, Ostrinia, Diatraea* and others	Cerebral neurosecretory cells?	–	–	Chippendale (1983)

Table 2 (continued)

Trivial names	Physiological function (observed experimental effects)	Species investigated	Sites of occurrence	Tissues used in purification	Amino acid sequence and/or composition	References
c) Adult	Adult diapause. Mainly controlled by CA but other neuroendocrine factors involved? Via CA?	*Leptinotarsa, Musca, Gyrinus* and others	Cerebral neurosecretory cells?	–	–	de Wilde (1983)
Eclosion hormone	Ensures ecdysis behaviour occurs at an appropriate moment	*Bombyx mori, Manduca sexta* and other Lepidoptera	Pars intercerebralis and CC also TG, AG, and ventral nerve cord	Pharate heads of *Bombyx*	H-SPAIASSY-DAM QI...?	Nagasawa et al. (1985), Reynolds and Truman (1980, 1983), Taghert et al. (1980)
Bursicon	Ensures correct timing of cuticle tanning	*Calliphora, Manduca, Periplaneta, Locusta, Schistocerca, Tenebrio*	Most of CNS	Fly haemolymph and TG; cockroach abdominal ganglia and CC. Whole adults of *Periplaneta*	"Largish peptide" ca. 40000 daltons	Seligman (1980), Reynolds (1983)
Pupariation control factors						
a) Anterior retraction factor (ARF)	Accelerates retraction of anterior segments	*Sarcophaga*	Larval CNS	Larval CNS and haemolymph	"Largish peptide" or protein	Zdarek (1980)
b) Puparium tanning factor (PFT)	Accelerates tanning	*Sarcophaga*	Larval CNS	Larval CNS and haemolymph	"Largish peptide" or protein	Zdarek (1980)

Table 2 (continued)

Trivial names	Physiological function (observed experimental effects)	Species investigated	Sites of occurrence	Tissues used in purification	Amino acid sequence and/ or composition	References
Diuretic hormone	Stimulates fluid secretion by Malpighian tubules	Over 20 species; *Rhodnius*, *Locusta*, *Periplaneta*	Widespread: CNS, brain, CC, TG etc.	SOG in *Locusta*	Composition known for *Locusta*	Proux et al. (1982), Mordue and Morgan (1985), Phillips (1983), Aston and Hughes (1980)
Antidiuretic hormone	Water uptake by rectal sacs	*Locusta*, *Periplaneta*, *Chaoborus* and others	Widespread in CNS, brain, CC, TG etc.	–	–	Gersch (1983), Mordue (1970)
Neurophysins	Similar function to neurophysins of vertebrates, acting as carriers for hormones from neurosecretory cells	*Locusta*	Neurosecretory cells in brain and SOG (also CC)	Brains and CC, SOG	(amino acid composition *Locusta*) estimated MW 11 200	Friedel et al. (1980), Friedel and Loughton (1983), Camier et al. (1980)
Peptidergic cardioaccelerator (neurohormone D)	Heart accelerating	*Periplaneta*	Brain-CC complex also terminal ganglia	CC	Asp_2 Glu_1 Phe_1 Ser_1 Val_1 MW 750–1000	Baumann and Gersch (1981), Krolak et al. (1977)
Chloride transport-stimulating hormone (CTSH)	Control of KCl reabsorption in rectum	*Schistocerca*	CC	Locust CC	MW 8000	Phillips et al. (1980)
Chromactivating factor (a darkening factor)	Rapid pigment movement	*Carausius morosus*, *Gryllus bimaculatus*, *Bombyx mori*	SOG (*not* brain or CC)	6000 TG of *Bombyx* larvae		Hashiguchi et al. (1965)

Table 2 (continued)

Trivial names	Physiological function (observed experimental effects)	Species investigated	Sites of occurrence	Tissues used in purification	Amino acid sequence and/ or composition	References
Melanisation and red coloration hormone (MRCH)	Selective pigment breakdown and synthesis	*Leucania separata*, *Bombyx mori*	Brain-SOG	3000 heads of *Bombyx mori*	–	Suzuki et al. (1976)
Hindgut-stimulating neurohormone		*Leucophaea* *Periplaneta americana*	Brain and CC Head	Brain/head		Holman and Cook (1972)
Factors stimulating proteolytic activity	Reduces intestinal protease activity	*Calliphora*	MNC	–	–	Thomsen and Møller (1963)
Reproductive hormones (peptides)						
a) Egg developmental neurosecretory hormone (EDNH)	Ovarian development (through secretion of ecdysone which then controls fatbody synthesis)	anautogenous mosquitoes (*Aedes* spp.)	Brain and CC		Peptide 6500 daltons	Hanaoka and Hagedorn (1980)
b) Gonadotropic peptidergic head factor (=EDNH?)		Mosquito (*Aedes* spp.)	Heads		Peptide 3500–12000 daltons	Fuchs et al. (1980)
c) Egg maturation factor(s)		*Calliphora*	MNSC (and LNSC?)	–	–	Thomsen (1952), Girardie (1966), Highnam (1962), Lea (1967)

Table 2 (continued)

Trivial names	Physiological function (observed experimental effects)	Species investigated	Sites of occurrence	Tissues used in purification	Amino acid sequence and/ or composition	References
d) Hormones regulating JH production (and hence termination of diapause? and/or stimulation of oogenesis)						
(i) Allatropin	Stimulation of CA	*Locusta*, *Schistocerca*, mosquitoes	MNC			Girardie et al. (1981), Girardie (1983), Mordue (1965)
(ii) Allatostatin	Inhibition of CA	*Locusta*	Pars intercerebralis A_2-NSC			
e) True gonadotrophic effects (on oogenesis)						
(i) Factor initiating vitellogenesis	Preliminary stage of oocyte development	*Tenebrio*	–	–	–	Friedel et al. (1980)
(ii) Factor initiating vitellogenesis	Production and accumulation of yolk in developing oocyte/follicular cells/nurse cells and fat body	*Calliphora*, *Locusta*, *Manduca* and others	Pars intercerebralis and CC (and JH from CA)	Peptide MW 1150		Friedel et al. (1980)
f) Antigonadrophins (oostatic hormone)	Inhibition of vitellogenesis	*Musca*, *Rhodnius*	Ovaries and/or abdominal neurosecretory organs			Liu and Davey (1974), Davey and Kuster (1981)

Table 2 (continued)

Trivial names	Physiological function (observed experimental effects)	Species investigated	Sites of occurrence	Tissues used in purification	Amino acid sequence and/ or composition	References
g) Oviposition						
(i) Myotropins affecting oviduct contractions)	Genital tract contractions	*Rhodnius*, *Locusta*	MNC and CC and throughout CNS			Engelmann (1970)
(ii) Ovulation hormones	Stimulus in mating	*Periplaneta*, *Iphita*	CC, brain			McCaffery (1976), Denlinger et al. (1978)
h) Male maturation						
(i) Sexual behaviour	Regulation of sexual behaviour		Intrinsic cells of CC			Riddiford and Williams (1971)

CC, Corpus cardiacum; CA, corpus allatum; MNC, median neurosecretory cells; LNC, lateral neurosecretory cells; SOG, suboesophageal ganglion; TG, thoracic ganglion; AG, abdominal ganglion

newly emerged specimens were either decapitated (Cottrell 1962) or neck-ligatured (Fraenkel and Hsiao 1962). Such animals failed to tan normally if they were taken only a few minutes after eclosion, whereas if the experiments were delayed, then normal tanning occurred. This suggested that a blood-borne factor produced in the brain initiated the cuticular sclerotization. Proof of this was obtained by injecting the blood from flies undergoing the tanning process normally into decapitated or neck-ligatured specimens and showing that the process was initiated.

Although the original physiological experiments suggested that bursicon was produced in the brain, it is now known that 6–10 times more hormone can be found in the abdominal region of the fused thoracic abdominal ganglion (Fraenkel and Hsiao 1965; Reynolds 1976).

Evidence points to the median neurosecretory cells of the brain and neurosecretory cells of the thoracic abdominal ganglion as being responsible for the production of bursicon, with the release occurring at a peripheral neurohaemal organ such as the corpus cardiacum or from the neurohaemal surfaces of abdominal nerves. The neurons that synthesise bursicon in the ventral nerve cord of *Manduca sexta* have been identified by a combination of surgical, physiological and anatomical techniques (Taghert and Truman 1979, 1980). Thus, individual neurosecretory cells in the abdominal ganglia have ben dissected out and shown to contain bursicon.

Four pairs of these cells have been identified in each of the ganglia and, by cobalt staining, it has been show that three of the pairs have axons projecting to the neurohaemal transverse nerve, previously identified as a bursicon release site (Truman 1973a). Intracellular recordings of the somata of the bursicon cells show that they have large (60–85 mV), overshooting action potentials of long duration (15–40 ms). Taghert (1980) suggested that during bursicon release in vivo, the cells are driven by specific excitatory inputs.

4.2 Eclosion Hormone

The physiology of the eclosion hormone (EH) has been studied in several different moths, including *Hyalophora cecropia, Antheraea pernyi* and *Manduca sexta* (e.g. Reynolds and Truman 1980). Recently, a partial sequence for the eclosion hormone of *Bombyx mori* was reported by Nagasawa et al. (1986) (see below).

This neurohormone, together with the other category B peptide discussed in this chapter, bursicon, controls two major events in the transformation from the pupa to the adult, viz the eclosion process itself and the sclerotization of the cuticle.

The timing of pupa-adult eclosion is determined by a decline in ecdysone levels and also by a circadian clock, located in the brain and entrained by a set of environmental variables. This clock provides the stimulus for the release of EH. Once the EH is in the blood, the performance of eclosion behaviour is either relatively invariant, as in saturniid moths (Truman 1971, 1973b), or, as in the sphingid moth *Manduca sexta*, the initiation of eclosion behaviour is subject to the influence of environmental variables (Reynolds et al. 1979).

The behaviour pattern, which appears to be preprogrammed in the CNS, has the function of extracting the moth from its pupal case. Experiments have shown that EH is able to elicit the pattern of behaviour from the CNS without any sensory feedback.

In addition to its effect on eclosion behaviour, EH has a number of other effects, e.g. the plasticisation of the cuticle of the wings (Reynolds 1977, 1980) and the initiation of the atrophy of the abdominal intersegmental muscles. Indeed, EH most probably influences a wide range of ecdysial physiology.

The eclosion hormone is produced in the pupal brain, probably in the median neurosecretory cells, transported to the corpus cardiacum and released into the haemolymph (Truman 1973). It is released rapidly and in very large amounts a short while before eclosion (2–3 h in *Manduca sexta* according to Reynolds et al. 1979). In *Manduca*, the hormone is rapidly removed from the blood, having a half-life of about 45 min. Target tissues are insensitive to the hormone except at or near to the normal time of release. The rapid release and subsequent destruction of EH shows that the hormone acts essentially as a trigger for ecdysis, with the timing of the release being more important than the precise amount present in the blood.

In larva-larva and larva-pupa ecdysis of Manduca it has now been shown that EH is active and, surprisingly, the release site at these times is not the brain, but the ventral ganglia (Truman et al. 1981). In these ecdyses, the release of EH depends only on the time when the titre of ecdysone falls below a certain level, not on a circadian clock.

The EH of *Bombyx mori* was purified from 180000 pupal heads according to a 16-step procedure resulting in a 2×10^6-fold purification (Nagasawa et al. 1985). The peptide was monitored by its ability to elicit precocious eclosion behaviour in pharate adult *Bombyx* and the peptide was shown to be active at a dose of 0.83 ng/animal. The yield was 1.2 nmol (10 μg) and the sequence of the first 13 N-terminal amino acid residues is given in Table 2. The molecular weight of the *Bombyx* EH has been estimated at ca. 8400 daltons, suggesting that only about a fifth of the molecular structure has so far been determined. As Nagasawa and his colleagues have pointed out, the chemical characterization of EH is the first step towards understanding its mode of action more precisely, discovering its cellular origins and understanding the mechanism of control of biosynthesis and release.

5 Category C Peptides

An interesting recent development in insect neuroendocrinology is the discovery that vertebrate-type peptides are present in the central and autonomic nervous systems. Thus, a range of antisera raised against the biologically active peptides of vertebrates has revealed the presence of immunoreactive neurons widespread in insect nervous tissues (Table 3). Although these findings only give evidence of common antigenic determinants, in several instances the results have been sup-

Table 3. Category C peptides

Trivial name	Species investigated	Immuno-cyto-chemical studies	Tissue/cell localisation	Purifi-cation studies	RIA of purified extracts and/or haemo-lymph	Bio-assay	Com-position and/or sequence	References
Insulin-immunoreactive peptide	*Calliphora*	+	MNC	+	+	+	+	Duve and Thorpe (1979), Duve et al. (1979), Thorpe and Duve (1984)
	Eristalis	+	MNC	–	–	–	–	El-Salhy et al. (1980)
	Bombyx	+	MNC, CC	–	–	–	–	Yui et al. (1980), Ishizaki et al. (1986)
	Manduca	+	MNC, LNC, frontal ganglion	+	+	+	+	El-Salhy et al. (1983, 1984), Tager et al. (1976), Kramer et al. (1982), Kramer (1985), Kramer et al. (1980)
	Ostrinia	+	MNC	+	+	+	–	Lavenseau et al. (1984)
	Periplaneta	+	MNC, CC	–	–	–	–	Orchard and Loughton (1980),
	Locusta	+		–	–	–	–	
	Carausius	+		–	–	–	–	Raabe (1986)
	Tenebrio	–	–	+	+	+	–	Teller et al. (1983), Teller and Pilc (1985)
	Apis	–	MNC, CC intestine	+	+	+	–	Ishay et al. (1976), O'Connor and Baxter (1985), Raoelison (1980), Maier et al. (1978), Moreau et al. (1981)
	Drosophila	–	–	+	+	+	–	Maier et al. (1978), Le Roith et al. (1981), Meneses and Ortiz (1975), Seecof and Dewhurst (1974), Veenstra et al. (1985b)
	Leptinotarsa	–	MNC	–	–	–	–	

Table 3 (continued)

Trivial name	Species investigated	Immuno-cyto-chemical studies	Tissue/cell localisation	Purifi-cation studies	RIA of purified extracts and/or haemo-lymph	Bio-assay	Com-position and/or sequence	References
Glucagon-immunoreactive peptide	*Calliphora*	–	–	+	+	–	–	Thorpe and Duve (1984), Duve and Thorpe (1984b)
	Manduca	+	Brain, CC, midgut					Kramer et al. (1980), Tager et al. (1976, 1975), Tager and Kramer (1980)
	Eristalis	+	Brain	–	–	–	–	El-Salhy et al. (1980, 1983)
	Periplaneta	+	Brain, CC, midgut	–	–	–	–	Iwanaga et al. (1981)
	Carausius	+	Brain, CC	–	–	–	–	Raabe (1986)
	Locusta	+	Brain, CC	–	–	–	–	Raabe (1986)
Pancreatic polypeptide-immunoreactive peptide	*Calliphora*	+	Brain (wide-spread), SOG, TG, hypocere-bral ganglion	+	+	–	+	Duve and Thorpe (1980, 1982), Duve et al. (1981, 1982), Duve and Thorpe (1984b)
	Eristalis	+	Brain, ventral ganglia	–	–	–	–	El-Salhy et al. (1980), El-Salhy et al. (1981)
	Bombyx	+	Brain	–	–	–	–	Yui et al. (1980)
	Periplaneta	+	Brain, SOG, ventral ganglia, midgut	–	–	–	–	Endo et al. (1982), Iwanaga et al. (1981)
	Manduca	+	Brain, CC	–	–	–	–	El-Salhy et al. (1983)
	Aeshna	+	Midgut					Andries and Tramu (1984)
	Schistocera	+	Ventral nerve cord	–	–	–	–	Myers and Evans (1985a, b)
	Leptinotarsa	+	Brain, SOG	–	–	–	–	Veenstra and Schooneveld (1984), Veenstra (1984)

Table 3 (continued)

Trivial name	Species investigated	Immuno-cyto-chemical studies	Tissue/cell localisation	Purifi-cation studies	RIA of purified extracts and/or haemo-lymph	Bio-assay	Com-position and/or sequence	References
Gastrin/CCK	*Calliphora*	+	Brain, CC, TG	+	+	–	–	Duve and Thorpe (1981, 1984a), Duve et al. (1983), Dockray et al. (1981), Duve et al. (1985)
	Bombyx	+	Brain, TG	–	–	–	–	Yui et al. (1980)
	Manduca	+	Brain, CC	+	+	–	–	Kramer et al. (1977), El-Salhy et al. (1983)
	Eristalis	+	Brain, ventral ganglia	–	–	–	–	El-Salhy et al. (1980)
	Leptinotarsus	+	Brain	–	–	–	–	Veenstra et al. (1985b)
Opioids (POMC-derived peptides)								
a) Enkephalins	*Calliphora*	+	Brain	+	+	–	–	Duve et al. (1986), Duve and Thorpe (1988)
	Eristalis	+	Brain, ventral ganglia	–	–	–	–	El-Salhy et al. (1980)
	Locusta	+	Brain	+	+	–	–	Rémy and Dubois (1981), Gros et al. (1978), Romeuf and Rémy (1984)
	Leucophaea	+	CC	–	–	–	–	Hansen et al. (1982)
	Manduca	+	Brain, CC, CA	–	–	–	–	El-Salhy et al. (1983)
	Drosophila	+	SOG, TG	–	–	–	–	Pages et al. (1983)
	Aeshna	+	Midgut	–	–	–	–	Andries and Tramu (1984)
	Periplaneta	+	Brain, CC, CA	–	–	–	–	Verhaert and De Loof (1985b)

Table 3 (continued)

Trivial name	Species investigated	Immuno-cyto-chemical studies	Tissue/cell localisation	Purifi-cation studies	RIA of purified extracts and/or haemo-lymph	Bio-assay	Com-position and/or sequence	References
b) α-Endorphins	*Calliphora*	+	Brain, CC	+	+	–	–	Duve and Thorpe (1983), Duve et al. (1986)
	Thaumetopoea	+	SOG	–	–	–	–	Rémy et al. (1978)
	Bombyx	+	SOG	–	–	–	–	Rémy et al. (1979)
β-Endorphins	*Eristalis*	+	Brain					El-Salhy et al. (1980)
	Manduca	+	Brain, CC	–	–	–	–	El-Salhy et al. (1983)
	Leptinotarsa	+	Brain, CC	–	–	–	–	Veenstra et al. (1985)
c) ACTH	*Leucophaea*	+	CC	–	–	–	–	Hansen et al. (1982, 1986)
	Periplaneta	+	Brain, SOG	–	–	–	–	Verhaert et al. (1984)
	Leptinotarsa	+	Brain	–	–	–	–	Veenstra et al. (1985b)
d) α-MSH	*Leptinotarsa*	+	SOG	–	–	–	–	Veenstra (1984)
	Locusta	+	SOG	–	–	–	–	Veenstra (1984)
Vasopressin/ oxytocin/ neurophysins	*Leucophaea*	+	CC	–	–	–	–	Hansen et al. (1982)
	Periplaneta	+	Brain, CC, CA	–	–	–	–	Verhaert et al. (1984)
	Locusta	+	SOG	–	–	–	–	
	Clitumnus	+	SOG	–	–	–	–	Rémy et al. (1977)
	Aceta	+	SOG	–	–	–	–	Strambi et al. (1979)
	Leptinotarsa	+	Brain, SOG	–	–	–	–	Veenstra et al. (1984)
Substance P	*Eristalis*	+	Brain	–	–	–	–	El-Salhy et al. (1980)
	Locusta	+	Brain	–	–	–	–	Benedeczky et al. (1982)
	Leucophaea	+	CC	–	–	–	–	Hansen et al. (1982)
	Manduca	+	Brain, CC, CA	–	–	–	–	El-Salhy et al. (1983)
	Aeshna	+	Midgut	–	–	–	–	Andries and Tramu (1984)
	Blaberus	+	Midgut	–	–	–	–	Andries and Tramu (1985)

Table 3 (continued)

Trivial name	Species investigated	Immuno-cyto-chemical studies	Tissue/cell localisation	Purifi-cation studies	RIA of purified extracts and/or haemo-lymph	Bio-assay	Com-position and/or sequence	References
Bombesin	*Leucophaea* seven different species)	+	CC, brain, SOG	–	–	–	–	Hansen et al. (1982), Veenstra and Yanaihara (1984)
Pituitary hormones and hypothalamic releasing hormones								
a) LH-RH	*Aeshna*	+	Midgut	–	–	–	–	Andries and Tramu (1984)
	Blaberus	+	Midgut	–	–	–	–	Andries and Tramu (1985)
b) SRIF	*Locusta*	+	Brain, CC	–	–	–	–	Doerr-Schott et al. (1978)
	Eristalis	+	Brain, ventral ganglion	–	–	–	–	El-Salhy et al. (1980)
	Periplaneta	+	Midgut	–	–	–	–	Iwanaga et al. (1981)
	Leucophaea	+	CC	–	–	–	–	Hansen et al. (1982)
	Apis	+	Midgut	–	–	–	–	Bounias and Dubois (1982)
	Manduca	+	Brain, CC	–	–	–	–	El-Salhy et al. (1983)
c) CRF	*Periplaneta*	+	Brain, SOG, CC	–	–	–	–	Verhaert and De Loof (1984a)
d) GRF	*Aeshna*	+	Brain, SOG, midgut	–	–	–	–	Andries et al. (1984), Andries and Tramu (1984)
	Blaberus	+	Midgut	–	–	–	–	Andries and Tramu (1985)
FMRF amide	*Leptinotarsa*	+	Brain, CC, SOG	–	–	–	–	Boer et al. (1980)
	Locusta	+	Brain, CC, SOG	–	–	–	–	Veenstra (1984)
	Periplaneta	+	Brain, CC, SOG	–	–	–	–	Verhaert et al. (1985)
	Pieris	+		–	–	–	–	Boer et al. (1980)
	Schistocerca	+	SOG, TG	–	–	–	–	Myers and Evans (1985a, b)

ported and verified by biochemical studies in which the vertebrate-type peptides have been isolated by means of RIA, purified and partially characterised. To those working in this field of research, it comes as no surprise that classical insect neuropeptides known for a long period of time only by virtue of their physiological roles have now been shown to have a degree of sequence homology with biologically active vertebrate peptides, e.g. PTTH-insulin (Nagasawa et al. 1986), hyperglycaemic hormone-glucagon (Scarborough et al. 1984).

Some of the general practical details and problems in applying immunological techniques to the study of insect neuropeptides of vertebrate type will be illustrated here by reference to the CCK- and endorphin-related peptides of the blowfly, *Calliphora vomitoria*.

5.1 The CCK-Related Peptides

The neuroendocrine system of *Calliphora* contains neurons immunoreactive to antisera directed against the common C-terminal pentapeptide sequence of gastrin and CCK.

Immunoreactive cells are present in several areas of the brain, including the median neurosecretory cells (Duve and Thorpe 1981). Certain of these cells have been shown by combined ICC and cobalt-backfilling techniques to send material to the *corpus cardiacum*, whilst others innervate specific targets in the brain, including the central body (Duve et al. 1983). The CCK-like material entering the neurohaemal organ, the corpus cardiacum, is presumably liberated into the haemolymph for general circulation as a neurohormone, whilst that confined to the brain is most likely acting as a neurotransmitter or neuromodulator. This duality of occurrence of the insect CCK-related peptide(s) is closely analagous to the dual occurrence of the CCK peptides of mammals where they are separately produced, in neurons of the brain and also in endocrine cells of the gut. It could well be that the insect CCK-related peptides exemplify the more primitive condition in which all biologically active peptides were initially produced solely within the nervous system as neurosecretory products, which were liberated from neurohaemal organs in order that they could have a more widespread effect on aspects of physiology and metabolism within the rest of the body. As body organisation became more gross and more complex during evolution, specialised cells would have been developed outside the confines of the brain, in closer proximity to the areas over which they had control, e.g. the gut. In the context of stimulus-secretion coupling the organisation of the insect neuropeptides is also homologous to certain situations in mammals. Thus, in insects, the external and internal stimuli to the brain elicit peptidergic responses through a simple neuroendocrine reflex, i.e. a neuronal input to the brain followed by a neurosecretory (neurohormonal) output from the neurohaemal organ. In mammals, this same relatively simple reflex occurs, e.g. neuronal input to the hypothalamus followed by neurohormonal output (oxytocin – vasopressin – various releasing factors to the pituitary). In both groups of animals the response can be considerably more complex, with second- and even third-order secretory mechanisms being involved. In mammals the thyroid gland is modulated by output from the TSH-secreting cells of the pituitary, and as an example in insects, the activity of the *corpus allatum* in producing juvenile hormone is regulated to some extent by neurosecretion from the brain.

In addition to the brain as a source of CCK-related peptides in *Calliphora*, the fused thoracic ganglionic mass has been shown to be a primary area of production (Duve and Thorpe 1984a). As with the brain, CCK-immunoreactive neurons have been shown to be linked with a neurohaemal organ situated in the dorsal neural sheath in the thoracic and abdominal ganglia, providing a means of access of the CCK-like material to the haemolymph.

As stated earlier, ICC evidence is not, in itself, proof of the existence of the full sequence of the peptide against which the antiserum was raised. The antigenic determinant that is being recognised is generally believed to be a short sequence of from three to eight residues (Larsson 1980). Since there is a possibility that this same sequence could be present in an otherwise dissimilar peptide, it is necessary to purify and characterise the peptide by biochemical means.

For the CCK peptides of *Calliphora*, several attempts at purification have been made (Dockray et al. 1981; Duve et al. 1985). Although the peptides are still not fully characterised, we have been able to confirm the ICC findings and provide some additional information as to their identity and chemical properties. Firstly, we have shown by different extraction methods followed by Sephadex gel filtration that the CCK material is heterogeneous and exists in a variety of different forms. These forms all appear to possess the C-terminus immunoreactive region of mammalian CCK in that they cross-react with a range of C-terminus-specific antibodies. Additional evidence from sequence-specific RIAs is that at least one form of the material (that extracted in 0.2 *M* HCl) has a greater degree of similarity to CCK than to gastrin. (Most ICC studies of insect CCK-like peptides, including our own, make use of antibodies raised against the common C-terminus of both gastrin and CCK, with the result that the immunoreactive material identified is best described as gastrin/CCK-like.) Thus, in a recent purification study (Duve et al. 1985) with a series of antibodies directed progressively towards the N-terminus, we were able to show that C-terminal directed antibodies were strongly recognised by the partially purified material in the RIA, those directed towards mid-core regions of CCK were less well recognised and N-terminal antisera were not recognised at all.

It is of interest in this regard that the CCK hormonal activity in mammals is known to reside in the C-terminus of the molecule including the sulphated tyrosine at C-terminal position 7. It would appear from these results that selection pressures have operated in evolution to conserve the functionally important amino acid sequence of this C-terminus.

Our purification studies of the CCK-like peptides of *Calliphora* are continuing, but meanwhile it is of great interest that the myotropic peptides of the cockroach *Leucophaea*, the so-called leucosulfakinins (LSKs), have been identified as having a degree of CCK sequence homology (Nachman et al. 1986a, b). It could well be that the *Calliphora* peptides that we are studying are, in turn, homologous to the *Leucophaea* peptides (as well as to CCK). One significant point, however, is that the C-terminal tetrapeptide sequence of the LSKs reads His-Met-Arg-Phe-NH_2, whereas that of CCK is Trp-Met-Asp-Phe-NH_2. Since the C-terminal antibodies of CCK that we have been using require (as does the biological activity of CCK) both the tryptophan and aspartic acid residues, it is very doubtful whether we are dealing with precisely the same molecules in *Calliphora* as in *Leucophaea*.

One final point of interest in the CCK-related peptides of insects relates to their possible function. We have previously suggested (Duve and Thorpe 1984a) that they could well have a role in feeding, analagous to that of CCK in mammals where they are known to cause gall bladder contraction and pancreatic enzyme secretion and to have a general effect on gut motility. Their presence in a neurohaemal area on the dorsal neural sheath of the thoracic ganglion puts them in close proximity to the salivary glands, the crop duct and the foregut of *Calliphora*, all of which are important structure in the feeding and digestion process. Knowledge that the newly identified CCK-like LSKs in *Leucophaea* are myotropic reinforces the view that as well as chemical homology, the CCK-related peptides of insects could have a degree of functional homology with those of their vertebrate counterparts.

5.2 The Enkephalin/Endorphin-Related Peptides

Since the initial discovery of Met- and Leu-enkephalin by Hughes et al. (1975), considerable scientific interest has been generated in the opioid peptides of mammals. The precursor of the endorphins is proopio-Melanocortin (POMC), which also gives rise to a series of other biologically active peptides, including ACTH and the MSHs.

Although the Met-enkephalin sequence also appears in POMC (61-65 of β-lipotrophin), it is generally considered now that the precursor of Met-enkephalin is preproenkephalin A (four sequences of Met-enkephalin, one of Leu-enkephalin and one each of the extended enkephalins Met-enk-Arg-Gly-Leu and Met-enk-Arg-Phe), whilst that of Leu-enkephalin (three sequences) is preproenkephalin B (Noda et al. 1982; Kakidani et al. 1982).

The enkephalins and endorphins were considered initially not to be produced in invertebrates (Simantov et al. 1979), but since then a steady stream of reports, particularly from studies of insects and molluscs, has indicated evidence to the contrary.

In *Calliphora* we have studied, by means of ICC, the presence of an α-endorphin-like peptide (Duve and Thorpe 1983) and, more recently, both Met- and Leu-enkephalin (Duve and Thorpe 1988). The α-endorphin-like peptide does not have such a wide distribution in the nervous system of *Calliphora* as, say, the CCK-like peptides, being restricted to approximately six pairs of median neurosecretory cells. These cells are different from those that produce either insulin (Duve and Thorpe 1979) or CCK (Duve and Thorpe 1981). The axons bearing α-endorphin-immunoreactive material join the median nerve bundle which passes ultimately via the cardiac recurrent nerve to enter the *corpus cardiacum*. Some fibres end in contact with the aorta, and hence have provision for releasing material into the haemolymph, while other fibres continue on dorsally into posterior regions, supplying possibly the heart and gut.

Both Met- and Leu-enkephalin-immunoreactive material have recently been identified in *Calliphora* (Duve et al. 1986, 1988) with a complex distribution pattern in both the brain and thoracic ganglion, and it has been possible to trace certain enkephalinergic neuronal pathways. It is suggested that at least one Met-enkephalin pathway is linked with the visual system. One interesting aspect of the enkephalin ICC study is the finding of a complex pattern of coexistence involving Met- and Leu-enkephalins, CCK and pancreatic polypeptide. By means of carefully controlled experiments with antigen-inactivated antisera, it has been possible to identify certain neurons with a single peptidergic substance and others with a combination of two, three or even all four of the aforementioned peptides.

Similar coexistence of these particular biologically active peptides has been noted both in molluscs (Gesser and Larsson 1983, 1985) and in mammals (Larsson and Stengaard-Pedersen 1981, 1982). The coexistence of gastrin/CCK and enkephalin/endorphin peptides seems particularly well documented, and it will be of great interest and importance for future studies to discover the functional significance of such a relationship, depending as it does upon the processing of two different precursors.

The identification of the precise chemical nature of the enkephalin/endorphin-like peptides has not kept pace with the ICC studies. (This is true for virtually any vertebrate-type peptide in any invertebrate and is due to the very great difficulties in attempting to isolate the very small amounts of active peptide from the correspondingly large amounts of non-active contaminating proteins and peptides.) We have carried out a preliminary purification study on the α-endorphin peptide of *Calliphora* (Duve et al. 1986) and are currently engaged on a reinvestigation of the problem with much larger quantities of starting material than we have used hitherto. In addition to the general problem of having to effect something like a 2×10^6 purification, there are more specific problems, including low yield due to losses at each chromatographic step.

6 Conclusion

The identification of more of the insect neuropeptides represents an important challenge for future scientific research. These peptides control fundamental physiological and metabolic processes, and apart from the intrinsic scientific value in identifying the substances, there are obvious potential rewards in the field of insect control. In the Third World and also in the USA, crop damage by insect pests is a major threat to the economy. Knowledge of the neurochemistry of insects is an essential first step in the development of much-needed new insect control measures.

Acknowledgement. The original work cited in this article was supported by a grant from the Science and Engineering Research Council of Great Britain to A.T. (GR/D/03383)

References

Agricola H, Eckert M, Ude J, Birkenbeil H, Penzlin H (1985) The distribution of a proctolin-like immunoreactive material in the terminal ganglion of the cockroach, *Periplaneta americana*. Cell Tissue Res 239:203–209

Agui N, Granger NA, Gilbert LI, Bollenbacher WE (1979) Cellular localisation of the insect prothoracicotropic hormone: in vitro assay of a single neurosecretory cell. Proc Natl Acad Sci USA 76:5694–5698

Amer MS (1969) Studies with cholecystokinin. II. Cholecystokinetic potency of porcine gastrins I and II and related peptides in three systems. Endocrinology 84:1277–1281

Andries J, Tramu G (1984) Détection immunohistochimique de substances apparentées des hormones peptidiques de Mammifères dans le mésentéron d'*Aeshna cyanea* (Insecte, Odonate). CR Acad Sci (Paris) 299(III):181–184

Andries J, Tramu G (1985) Ultrastructural and immunohistochemical study of endocrine cells in the midgut of the cockroach *Blaberus craniifer* (Insecta, Dictyoptera). Cell Tissue Res 240:323–332

Andries J, Belemtougri G, Tramu G (1984) Immunohistochemical identification of growth hormone-releasing factor-like material in the nervous system of an insect, *Aeshna cyanea* (Odonata). Neuropeptides 4:519–528

Aston RJ, Hughes L (1980) Diuretic hormone – extraction and chemical properties. In: Miller TA (ed) Neurohormonal techniques in insects. Springer, Berlin Heidelberg New York, pp 91–115

Bargmann W (1967) Neurosecretion. Int Rev Cytol 19:183–201

Baumann E, Gersch M (1981) Purification and identification of neurohormone D, a heart-accelerating peptide from the corpora cardiaca of the cockroach *Periplaneta americana*. J Insect Biochem 12:7–14

Beenakkers AMTh (1969) The influence of corpus allatum and cardiacum on lipid metabolism in *Locusta*. Gen Comp Endocrinol 13:492

Benedeczky I, Kiss J, Somogyi P (1982) Light and electron microscopic localization of substance P-like immunoreactivity in the cerebral ganglion of locust with a monoclonal antibody. Histochemistry 75:123–131

Bishop CA, O'Shea M (1982) Neuropeptide proctolin (H-Arg-Tyr-Leu-Pro-Thr-OH): immunocytochemical mapping of neurons in the central nervous system of the cockroach. J Comp Neurol 207:223–238

Bishop CA, O'Shea M, Miller RJ (1981) Neuropeptide proctolin (H-Arg-Tyr-Leu-Pro-Thr-OH): immunological detection and neuronal localisation in insect central nervous system. Proc Natl Acad Sci USA 78:5899–5902

Boer H, Schot L, Veenstra J, Reichelt D (1980) Immunocytochemical identification of neural elements in the central nervous systems of a snail, some insects, a fish, and a mammal with an antiserum to the molluscan cardio-excitatory tetrapeptide FMRF-amide. Cell Tissue Res 213:21–27

Bollenbacher WE, Agui N, Granger NA, Gilbert LI (1980) Insect prothoracic glands in vitro: a system for studying the prothoracicotropic hormone. In: Kurstak E, Maramorosch KK, Dubendorfer A (eds) Invertebrate systems in vitro. Elsevier, North Holland, Amsterdam, pp 253–271

Bounias M, Dubois M (1982) Inhibition par la somatostatine de l'action hypoglycémiante de l'insuline chez l'abeille in vivo et localisation cytochimique d'un antigène apparenté a la somatostatine dans l'épithélium digestif ainsi que les tubes de Malpighi de l'abeille. CR Acad Sci (Paris) Ser III 294:1029–1034

Brown BE (1967) Neuromuscular transmitter substance in insect visceral muscle. Science 15:595–597

Brown BE (1975) Proctolin: a peptide transmitter candidate in insects. Life Sci 17:1241–1252

Brown BE, Starratt AN (1975) Isolation of proctolin, a myotropic peptide, from *Periplaneta americana*. J Insect Physiol 21:1879–1881

Camier M, Girardie J, Rémy C, Girardie A, Cohen P (1980) Identification of immunoreactive neurophysin-like proteins in the central nervous system of an insect, *Locusta migratoria*. Biochem Biophys Res Commun 93:792–796
Carlsen J, Herman WS, Christensen M, Josefsson L (1979) Characterization of a second peptide with adipokinetic and red pigment-concentrating activity from the locust corpora cardiaca. Insect Biochem 9:497–501
Cheeseman P, Goldsworthy GJ, Mordue W (1977) Studies on the purification of locust adipokinetic hormone. Life Sci 21:231–236
Chippendale GM (1983) Larval and pupal diapause. In: Downer RGH, Laufer H (eds) Endocrinology of insects. Liss, New York, pp 343–356
Cottrell CB (1962) The imaginal ecdysis of blowflies. The control of cuticular tanning and darkening. J Exp Biol 39:395–411
Davey KG, Kuster JE (1981) The source of an antigonadotropin in the female of *Rhodnius prolixus*. Stal. Can J Zool 59:761–764
Denlinger DL, Chaudhury MFB, Dhadialla TS (1978) Cyclic AMP is a likely mediator of ovulation in the tsetse fly. Experientia 34:1296–1297
de Wilde J (1983) Endocrine aspects of diapause in the adult stage. In: Downer RGH, Laufer H (eds) Endocrinology of insect. Liss, New York, pp 357–367
Dockray GJ, Duve H, Thorpe A (1981) Immunochemical characterisation of gastrin/cholecystokinin-like peptides in the brain of the blowfly *Calliphora vomitoria*. Gen Comp Endocrinol 45:491–496
Dodd J, Kelly JS (1981) The actions of cholecystokinin and related peptides on pyramidal neurones of the mammalian hippocampus. Brain Res 205:337–350
Doerr-Schott J, Joly L, Dubois M (1978) Sur l'existence dans la pars intercerebralis d'un insecte (*Locusta migratoria* R. et F.) de cellules neurosécrétrices fixant un antisérum antisomatostatine. CR Acad Sci (Paris) 286:93–95
Downer RGH, Laufer H (1983) Invertebrates endocrinology vol 1. Endocrinology of insects. Liss, New York
Duve H (1978) The presence of a hypoglucemic and hypotrehalocemic hormone in the neurosecretory system of the blowfly *Calliphora erythrocephala*. Gen Comp Endocrinol 36:102–110
Duve H, Thorpe A (1979) Immunofluorescent localisation of insulin-like material in the median neurosecretory cells of blowfly, *Calliphora vomitoria* (Diptera). Cell Tissue Res 200:187–191
Duve H, Thorpe A (1980) Localisation of pancreatic polypeptide (PP)-like immunoreactive material in neurones of the brain of the blowfly, *Calliphora erythrocephala* (Diptera). Cell Tissue Res 210:101–109
Duve H, Thorpe A (1981) Gastrin/cholecystokinin (CCK)-like immunoreactive neurones in the brain of the blowfly, *Calliphora erythrocephala* (Diptera). Gen Comp Endocrinol 43:381–391
Duve H, Thorpe A (1982) The distribution of pancreatic polypeptide in the nervous system and gut of the blowfly, *Calliphora vomitoria* (Diptera). Cell Tissue Res 227:67–77
Duve H, Thorpe A (1983) Immunocytochemical identification of α-endorphin-like material in neurones of the brain and corpus cadiacum of the blowfly, *Calliphora vomitoria* (Diptera). Cell Tissue Res 233:415–426
Duve H, Thorpe A (1984 a) Immunocytochemical mapping of gastrin/CCK-like peptides in the neuroendocrine system of the blowfly *Calliphora vomitoria* (Diptera). Cell Tissue Res 237:309–320
Duve H, Thorpe A (1984 b) Comparative aspects of insect-vertebrate neurohormones. In: Borkovec AB, Kelly TJ (eds) Insect neurochemistry and neurophysiology. Plenum, New York, pp 171–196
Duve H, Thorpe A (1988) Mapping of enkephalin-related peptides in the nervous system of the blowfly *Calliphora vomitoria* and their co-localization with cholecystokonin (CCK)- and pancreatic polypeptide (PP)-like peptides. Cell Tissue Res 251:399–415
Duve H, Thorpe A, Lazarus NR (1979) Isolation of material displaying insulin-like immunological and biological activity from the brain of the blowfly *Calliphora vomitoria*. Biochem J 184:221–227

Duve H, Thorpe A, Neville R, Lazarus N (1981) Isolation and partial characterization of pancreatic polypeptide-like material in the brain of the blowfly *Calliphora vomitoria*. Biochem J 197:767–770

Duve H, Thorpe A, Lazarus N, Lowry P (1982) A neuropeptide of the blowfly *Calliphora vomitoria* with an amino acid composition homologous with vertebrate pancreatic polypeptide. Biochem J 201:429–432

Duve H, Thorpe A, Strausfeld N (1983) Cobalt-immunocytochemical identification of peptidergic neurons in *Calliphora* innervating central and peripheral targets. J Neurocytol 12:847–861

Duve H, Thorpe A, Rehfeld JF (1985) Localisation and characterisation of cholecystokinin (CCK)-like peptides in the brain of the blowfly, *Calliphora vomitoria*. In: Kobayashi H, Bern, HA, Urano A (eds) Neurosecretion and the biology of neuropeptides. Japan Scientific Societies Press, Tokyo/Springer, Berlin Heidelberg New York, pp 401–409

Duve H, Thorpe A, Scott A (1986) Localization and characterization of opioid-like peptides in the nervous system of the blowfly *Calliphora vomitoria*. In: Stefano GB (ed) Handbook of comparative opioid and related neuropeptide mechanisms, vol 1. CRC Press, Boca Raton, pp 197–211

Duve H, Thorpe A, Nässel DR (1988) Light and electron microscopic immunocytochemistry of peptidergic neurons innervating thoracico-abdominal neurohaemal organs in the blowfly, *Calliphora vomitoria*. Cell Tissue Res (In Press)

Eckert M, Agricola H, Penzlin H (1981) Immunocytochemical identification of proctolin-like immunoreactivity in the terminal ganglion and hindgut of the cockroach *Periplaneta americana*. Cell Tissue Res 217:633–645

El-Salhy M (1981) Immunohistochemical localization of pancreatic polypeptide (PP) in the brain of the larval instar of the hoverfly, *Eristalis aeneus* (Diptera). Experienta 37:1009

El-Salhy M, Abou-El-Ela R, Falkmer S, Grimelius L, Wilander E (1980) Immunohistochemical evidence of gastro-entero-pancreatic neurohormonal peptides of vertebrate type in the nervous system of the larva of a dipteran insect, the hoverfly, *Eristalis aeneus*. Regul Pept 1:187–204

El-Salhy M, Falkmer S, Kramer K, Speirs R (1983) Immunohistochemical investigations of neuropeptides in the brain, corpora cardiaca, and corpora allata of an adult lepidopteran insect, *Manduca sexta* (L.). Cell Tissue Res 232:295–317

El-Salhy M, Falkmer S, Kramer K, Speirs R (1984) Immunocytochemical evidence for the occurrence of insulin in the frontal ganglion of a lepidopteran insect, the tobacco hornworm moth, *Manduca sexta* L. Gen Comp Endocrinol 54:85–88

Endo Y, Iwanaga T, Fujita T, Nishiitsutsuji-Uwo J (1982) Localization of pancreatic polypeptide (PP)-like immunoreactivity in the central and visceral nervous systems of the cockroach *Periplaneta*. Cell Tissue Res 227:1–9

Engelmann F (1970) The physiology of insect reproduction. Permagon, Oxford

Fraenkel G, Hsiao C (1962) Hormonal and nervous control of tanning in the fly. Science 138:27–29

Fraenkel G, Hsiao C (1963) Tanning in the adult fly: a new function of neurosecretion in the brain. Science 141:1057–1058

Fraenkel G, Hsiao C (1965) Bursicon a hormone which mediates tanning of the cuticle in the adult fly and other insects. J Insect Physiol 11:513–1516

Friedel T, Loughton BG (1983) Insect neurophysins. In: Downer RGH, Laufer H (eds) Endocrinology of insects. Liss, New York, pp 131–140

Friedel T, Loughton BG, Andrew RD (1980) A neurosecretory protein from *Locusta migratoria*. Gen Comp Endocrinol 41:487–498

Fuchs MS, Sundland BR, Kang SH (1980) In vivo induction of ovarian development in *Aedes atropalpus* by head extract from *Aedes aegypti*. Int J Invertebr Reprod 2:121–129

Fujita T (1985) Neurosecretion and new aspects of neuroendocrinology. In: Kobayashi H, Bern HA, Urano A (eds) Neurosecretion and the biology of neuropeptides. Japan Scientific Societies Press, Tokyo/Springer, Berlin Heidelberg New York, pp 521–528

Gäde G (1981) Studies on a possible hyperglycaemic factor from the corpus cardiacum of stick insects: characterization and preliminary purification. Zool J Physiol 85:266–277

Gersch M (1983) Chemistry of other neurohormonal factors. In: Downer RGH, Laufer H (eds) Endocrinology of insects. Liss, New York, pp 121–129

Gesser BP, Larsson L-I (1983) Localization of α-MSH-, endorphin- and gastrin/CCK-like immunoreactivities in the nervous system of invertebrates. In: Angelucci L, de Wied D, Endröczi E, Scapagnini U (eds) Integrative neurohormonal mechanisms. Elsevier Biomedical, Amsterdam

Gesser BP, Larsson L-I (1985) Changes from enkephalin-like to gastrin/cholecystokinin-like immunoreactivity in snail neurones. J Neurosci 5:6:1412–1417

Girardie A (1966) Contrôle de l'activité génitale chez *Locusta migratoria*. Mise én evidence d'un facteur gonadotrope et d'un facteur allatrope dans la pars intercerebralis. Bull Soc Zool Fr 91:423–439

Girardie A (1983) Neurosecretion and reproduction. In: Downer RGH, Laufer H (eds) Endocrinology of insects. Liss, New York, pp 305–317

Girardie J, Tobe SS, Girardie A (1981) Biosynthése de l'hormone juvenile C16 (JH-III) et maturation ovarienne chez le criquet migrateur. CR Acad Sci (Paris) 293:443–446

Goldsworthy GJ, Gäde G (1983) The chemistry of hypertrehalosemic factors. In: Downer RGH, Laufer H (eds) Endocrinology of insects. Liss, New York, pp 109–120

Goldsworthy GJ, Mordue W, Guthketch J (1972) Studies on insect adipokinetic hormones. Gen Comp Endocrinol 18:545–551

Gregory H, Hardy PM, Jones DS, Kenner GW, Sheppard RC (1964) The antral hormone gastrin. Nature 204:931–933

Gros C, Lafon-Cazal M, Dray F (1978) Présence de substances immunoréactivement apparentées aux enképhalines chez un insecte, *Locusta migratoria*. CR Acad Sci (Paris) 287(D):647–650

Hanaoka K, Hagedorn HH (1980) Brain hormone control of ecdysone secretion by the ovary in a mosquito. In: Hoffmann JA (ed) Progress in ecdysone research. Elsevier North Holland, Biomedical, Amsterdam, pp 467–480

Hansen B, Hansen G, Scharrer B (1982) Immunoreactive material resembling vertebrate neuropeptides in the corpus cardiacum and corpus allatum of the insect *Leucophaea maderae*. Cell Tissue Res 225:319–329

Hansen BL, Hansen GN, Scharrer B (1986) Immunocytochemical demonstration of a material resembling vertebrate ACTH and MSH in the corpus cardiacum – corpus allatum complex of the insect *Leucophaea maderae*. In: Stefano GB (ed) Handbook of comparative opioid and related neuropeptide mechanisms, vol 1. CRC, Boca Raton, pp 213–222

Hashiguchi T, Yoshitake N, Takahashi N (1965) Hormone determining the black pupal colour in the silkworm, *Bombyx mori*. Nature 206:215

Highnam KC (1962) Neurosecretory control of ovarian development in *Schistocerca gregaria*. Q JL Microsc Sci 103:57–72

Highnam KC, Hill L (1977) The comparative endocrinology of the invertebrates. Arnold, London

Holman GM, Cook BJ (1972) Isolation, partial purification and characterization of a peptide which stimulates the hindgut of the cockroach *Leucophaeae maderae* (Fabr.). Biol Bull 142:446–460

Holman GM, Cook BJ, Wagner RM (1984) Isolation and partial characterization of five myotropic peptides present in head extracts of the cockroach *Leucophaea maderae*. Comp Biochem Physiol 77[C]:1–5

Holwerda DA, Van Doorn J, Beenakkers AMT (1977) Characterization of the adipokinetic and hyperglycaemic substances from the locust corpus cardiacum. Insect Biochem 7:151–157

Houben NMD, Beenakkers AMT (1973) Regulation of diglyceride release from the fat body of the locust during flight. J Endocrinol 57:III–IV

Huber R, Hoppe W (1965) Zur Chemie des Ecdysons. VII. Die Kristall- und Molekülstrukturanalyse des Insektenverpuppungshormones Ecdyson mit der automatisierten Faltmolekülmethode. Chem Ber 98:2403

Hughes J, Smith LW, Kosterlitz HW, Fothergill LA, Morgan BA, Morris HR (1975) Identification of two related pentapeptides from the brain with potent opiate agonist activity. Nature 258:577–579
Ishay J, Gitter S, Galun R, Doron M, Laron Z (1976) The presence of insulin and some effects of insulin on Hymenoptera tissues and body fluids. Comp Biochem Physiol 54[A]:203–206
Ishizaki H, Suzuki A (1980) Prothoracicotropic hormone. In: Miller T (ed) Neurohormonal techniques in insects. Springer, Berlin Heidelberg New York, pp 244–276
Ishizaki H, Mizoguchi A, Hatta M, Suzuki A, Nagawawa H, Kataoka H, Isogai A, Tamura S, Fujino M, Kitada C (1986) Prothoracicotrophic hormone (PTTH) of the silkmoth, *Bombyx mori*: 4K-PTTH. In: Proceedings of the UCLA symposia, molecular and cellular biology, molecular entomology. (in press)
Isobe M, Goto T (1980) Diapause hormones. In: Miller TA (ed) Neurohormonal techniques in insects. Springer, Berlin Heidelberg New York, pp 216–243
Iwanaga T, Fujita T, Nishiitsutsuji-Uwo J, Endo Y (1981) Immunohistochemical demonstration of PP-, somatostatin-, enteroglucagon- and VIP-like immunoreactivities in the cockroach midgut. Biomed Res 2:202–207
Jaffe H, Raina AK, Riley CT, Fraser BA, Holman GM, Wagner RM, Ridgway RL, Hayes DK (1986) Isolation and primary structure of a peptide from the corpora cardiaca of *Heliothis zea* with adipokinetic activity. Biochem Biophys Res Commun 135:622–628
Kakidani H, Furutani Y, Takahashi H, Noda M, Morimoto Y, Hirose T, Asai M, Inayama S, Nakanishi S, Numa S (1982) Cloning and sequence of cDNA for porcine α-neo-endorphin/dynorphin. Nature 298:245–249
Karlson P, Hoffmeister H, Hummel H, Hocks P, Spiteller G (1965) Zur Chemie des Ecdysons. VI. Reaktionen des Ecdysonmoleküls. Chem Ber 98:2394
Kerkut GA, Gilbert LI (1985) Comprehensive insect physiology, biochemistry and pharmacology. Pergamon, Oxford
Kopec S (1922) Studies on the necessity of the brain for the inception of insect metamorphosis. Biol Bull 42:322–342
Kramer KJ (1985) Vertebrate hormones in insects. In: Kerkut GA, Gilbert LI (eds) Comprehensive insect physiology, biochemistry and pharmacology, vol 7: endocrinology I. Pergamon, Oxford, pp 511–536
Kramer KJ, Spiers RD, Childs CN (1977) Immunochemical evidence for a gastrin-like peptide in insect neuroendocrine systems. Gen Comp Endocrinol 32:423–426
Kramer KJ, Tager HS, Childs CN (1980) Insulin-like and glucagon-like peptides in insect haemolymph. Insect Biochem 10:179–182
Kramer KJ, Childs CN, Spiers RD, Jacobs RM (1982) Purification of insulin-like peptides from insect haemolymph and royal jelly. Insect Biochem 12:91–98
Krolak JN, Zimmerman ML, Mills RR (1977) Cardioaccelerating factors from the terminal abdominal ganglion of the American cockroach. J Insect Physiol 23:1343–1347
Kubota I, Isobe M, Goto T, Hasegawa K (1976) Molecular size of the diapause hormone of the silkworm, *Bombyx mori*. Z Naturforsch [C] 31:132–134
Larsson L-I (1980) Problems and pitfalls in immunocytochemistry of gut peptides. In: Glass GBJ (ed) Comprehensive endocrinology. Gastrointestinal hormones. Raven, New York
Larsson L-I, Stengaard-Pedersen K (1981) Enkephalin/endorphin-related peptides in antropyloric gastrin cells. J Histochem Cytochem 29:1088–1098
Larsson L-I, Stengaard-Pedersen K (1982) Immunocytochemical and ultrastructural differentiation between Met-enkephalin, Leu-enkephalin, and Met/Leu-enkephalin immunoreactive neurons of feline gut. J Neurosci 2:861–878
Lavenseau L, Gadenne C, Trabelsi M (1984) Immunofluorescent localization of a substance immunologically related to insulin in the protocerebral neurosecretory cells of the European corn borer. Cell Tissue Res 238:207–208
Lea AO (1967) The medial neurosecretory cells and egg maturation in mosquitoes. J Insect Physiol 13:419–429
LeRoith D, Lesniak MA, Roth J (1981) Insulin in insects and annelids. Diabetes 30:70–76

Liu TP, Davey KG (1974) Partial characterisation of a proposed antigonadotropin from the ovaries of the insect *Rhodnius prolixus*. Stal. Gen Comp Endocrinol 24:405–408
Maier V, Witznick G, Keller R, Pfeiffer EF (1978) Insulin-like and glucagon-like immunoreactivities in the honeybee (*Apis mellifera*). Acta Endocrinol (Copenh) 215:69–70
Mayer RJ, Candy RJ (1969) Control of haemolymph lipid concentration during locust flight: an adipokinetic hormone from the corpora cardiaca. J Insect Physiol 15:611–620
McCaffery AR (1976) Effects of electrocoagulation of cerebral neurosecretory cells and implantation of corpora allata on oöcyte development in *Locusta migratoria*. J Insect Physiol 22:1081–1092
Meneses P, Ortiz M (1975) A protein extract from *Drosophila melanogaster* with insulin-like activity. Comp Biochem Physiol [A] 51:483–485
Miller T (1979) Nervous versus neurohormonal regulation of insect heartbeat. Am Zool 19:77–86
Mizoguchi A, Ishizaki H, Nagawawa H, Kataoka H, Isogai A, Tamura S, Suzuki A, Fujino M, Kitada C (1987) A monoclonal antibody against a synthetic fragment of bombyxin (4K-prothoracicotropic hormone) from the silkmoth, *Bombyx mori*: characterisation and immunohistochemistry. Mol Cell Endocrinol (in press)
Mordue W (1965) Neuro-endocrine factors in the control of oöcyte production in *Tenebrio mollitor* L. J Insect Physiol 11:617–629
Mordue W (1970) Evidence for the existence of diuretic and antidiuretic hormones in locusts. J Endocrinol 46:119–120
Mordue W, Morgan PJ (1985) Chemistry of peptide hormones. In: Kerkut GA, Gilbert LI (eds) Comprehensive insect physiology, biochemistry and pharmacology, vol 7: endocrinology. Pergamon, Oxford, pp 153–183
Moreau R, Raoelison C, Sutter BCJ (1981) An intestinal insulin-like molecule in *Apis mellifera* L. (Hymenoptera). Comp Biochem Physiol [A] 69:79–83
Motta M (1980) Comprehensive endocrinology. The endocrine functions of the brain. Raven, New York
Myers C, Evans P (1985a) An FMRFamide antiserum differentiates between populations of antigens in the ventral nervous system of the locust, *Schistocerca gregaria*. Cell Tissue Res 242:109–114
Myers C, Evans P (1985b) The distribution of bovine pancreatic polypeptide/FMRFamide-like immunoactivity in the ventral nervous system of the locust. J Comp Neurol 234:1–16
Nachman RJ, Holman GM, Haddon WF, Ling N (1986a) Leucosulfakinin, a sulfated insect neuropeptide with homology to gastrin and cholecystokinin. Science 234:71–73
Nachman RJ, Holman GM, Cook BJ, Haddon WF, Ling N (1986b) Leucosulfakinin-II, a blocked sulfated insect neuropeptide with homology to cholecystokinin and gastrin. Biochem Biophys Res Commun 140:357–364
Nagasawa H, Kataoka H, Isogai A, Tamura S, Suzuki A, Ishizaki H, Mizoguchi A, Fujiwara Y, Suzuki A (1984) Amino-terminal amino acid sequence of the silkworm prothoracicotropic hormone: homology with insulin. Science 26:1344–1345
Nagasawa H, Kamito T, Takahashi S, Isogai A, Fugo H, Suzuki A (1985) Eclosion hormone of the silkworm *Bombyx mori*. Purification and determination of the N-terminal amino acid sequence. Insect Biochem 15:573–578
Nagasawa H, Kataoka H, Isogai A, Tamura S, Suzuki A, Mizoguchi A, Fujiwara Y, Suzuki A, Takahashi SY, Ishizaki H (1986) Amino acid sequence of a prothoracicotropic hormone of the silkworm *Bombyx mori*. Proc Natl Acad Sci USA 83:5840–5843
Nijhout HF, Williams CM (1974) Control of moulting and metamorphosis in the tobacco hornworm, *Manduca sexta* (L): growth of the last-instar larva and the decision to putate. J Exp Biol 61:481–491
Noda M, Furutani Y, Takahashi H, Toyosato M, Hirose T, Inayama S, Nakanishi S, Numa S (1982) Cloning and sequence analysis of cDNA for bovine adrenal preproenkephalin. Nature 295:202–206
Normann TC (1975) Neurosecretory cells in insect brain and production of hypoglycemic hormone. Nature 254:259–261

Normann TC, Duve H (1969) Experimentally induced release of a neuro-hormone influencing haemolymph trehalose level in *Calliphora erythrocephala* (Diptera). Gen Comp Endocrinol 12:449–459

Normann TC, Duve H (1978) Insulin-like and glucagon-like neurohormones in the blowfly. In: Galliard PJ, Boer HH (eds) Comparative endocrinology. Elsevier, Amsterdam, pp 441–444

O'Connor KJ, Baxter D (1985) The demonstration of insulin-like material in the honey bee, *Apis mellifera*. Comp Biochem Physiol [B] 3:755–760

Orchard I, Loughton BG (1980) A hypolipaemic factor from the corpus cardiacum of locusts. Nature 286:494–496

Orchard I, Loughton BG (1981 a) The neural control of release of hyperlipemic hormone from the corpus cardiacum of *Locusta migratoria*. Comp Biochem Physiol [A] 68:25–30

Orchard I, Loughton BG (1981 b) Is octopamine a transmitter mediating hormone release in insects? J Neurobiol 12:143–153

Pages M, Jimenez F, Ferrus A, Peralta E, Ramirez G, Gelpi E (1983) Enkephalin-like immunoreactivity in *Drosophila melanogaster*. Neuropeptides 4:87–98

Phillips JE (1983) Endocrine control of salt and water balance: excretion. In: Downer RGH, Laufer H (eds) Endocrinology of insects. Liss, New York, pp 411–425

Phillips JE, Mordue W, Meredith J, Spring J (1980) Purification and characteristics of the chloride transport stimulating factor from locust corpora cardiaca: a new peptide. Can J Zool 58:1851–1856

Piek T, Mantel P (1977) Myogenic contractions in locust muscle induced by proctolin and by wasp, *Philanthus triangulum* venom. J Insect Physiol 23:321–325

Proux J, Rougon-Rapuzzi G, Cupo A (1982) Enhancement of excretion across locust Malpighian tubules by a diuretic vasopressin-like hormone. Gen Comp Endocrinol 47:449–457

Raabe M (1982) Insect neurohormones. Plenum, New York

Raabe M (1986) Comparative immunocytochemical study of release sites in *Locusta migratoria, Periplaneta americana* and *Carausius morosus*. Cell Tissue Res 245:267–271

Rademakers LHPM (1977) Identification of a secretomotor centre in the brain of *Locusta migratoria*, controlling the secretory activity of the adipokinetic hormone producing cells of the corpus cardiacum. Cell Tissue Res 184:381–395

Raoelison R (1980) Isolation, charactérisation et propriétés biologiques d'une molécule insulino-semblable chez l'abeille. Thesis, University of Bordeaux

Rehfeld JF (1982) The influence of antiserum properties on radioimmunoassay characteristics. In: Thorell JI (ed) Radioimmunoassay design and quality control. Pergamon, U.K., 19–27

Rémy C, Dubois M (1981) Immunohistological evidence of methionine enkephalin-like material in the brain of the migratory locust. Cell Tissue Res 218:271–278

Rémy C, Girardie J, Dubois M (1977) Exploration immunocytologique des ganglions cérébroïdes et sous-oesophagien due phasme *Clitumnus extradentatus*: existence d'une neurosécrétion apparentée à la vasopressine-neurophysine. CR Acad Sci (Paris) 285(D):1495–1497

Rémy C, Girardie J, Dubois M (1978) Présence dans le ganglion sousoesophagien de la chenille processionnaire du pin (*Thaumetopoea pityocampa* Schiff) de cellules révélées en immunofluorescence par un anticorps anti-α-endorphine. CR Acad Sci Paris Série D 286:651–653

Rémy C, Girardie J, Dubois M (1979) Vertebrate neuropeptide-like substances in the suboesophageal ganglion of two insects: *Locusta migratoria* R. and F. (Orthoptera) and *Bombyx mori* L. (Lepidoptera). Immunocytological investigation. Gen Comp Endocrinol 37:93–100

Reynolds SE (1976) Hormonal regulation of cuticle extensibility in newly emerged adult blowflies. J Insect Physiol 22:529–534

Reynolds SE (1977) Control of cuticle extensibility in the wings of adult *Manduca* at the time of eclosion: effects of eclosion hormone and bursicon. J Exp Biol 70:27–39

Reynolds SE (1980) Cuticle plasticizing factors. In: Miller TA (ed) Neurohormonal techniques in insects. Springer, Berlin Heidelberg New York, pp 179–195 (Springer series in experimental entomology)

Reynolds SE (1983) Bursicon. In: Downer RGH, Laufer H (eds) Endocrinology of insects. Liss, New York, pp 235–248

Reynolds SE, Truman JW (1980) Eclosion hormones. In: Miller TA (ed) Neurohormonal techniques in insects. Springer, Berlin Heidelberg New York, pp 196–215

Reynolds SE, Truman JW (1983) Eclosion hormone. In: Downer RGH, Laufer H (eds) Endocrinology of insects. Liss, New York, pp 217–233

Reynolds SE, Taghert PH, Truman JW (1979) Eclosion hormone and bursicon titres and the onset of hormonal reponsiveness during the last day of adult development in *Manduca sexta* (L). J Exp Biol 78:77–86

Riddiford LM, Williams CM (1971) Role of the corpora cardiaca in the behaviour of Saturniid moths I. Release of sex pheromone. Biol Bull Woods Hole 140:1–7

Röller H, Bierke JS, Holthaus LM, Norgard DW, McShan WH (1969) Isolation and biological properties of the juvenile hormone. J Insect Physiol 15:379–389

Romeuf M, Rémy C (1984) Early immunohistochemical detection of somatostatin-like and methionine-enkephalin-like neuropeptides in the brain of the migratory locust embryo. Cell Tissue Res 236:289–292

Scarborough RM, Jamieson GC, Kalish F, Kramer SJ, McEnroe GA, Miller CA, Schooley DA (1984) Isolation and primary structure of two peptides with cardioacceleratory and hyperglycemic activity from the corpora cardiaca of *Periplaneta americana*. Proc Natl Acad Sci USA 81:5575–5579

Schooneveld H, Tesser GI, Veenstra JA, Romberg-Privee HM (1983) Adipokinetic hormone and AKH-like peptide demonstrated in the corpora cardiaca and nervous system of *Locusta migratoria* by immunocytochemistry. Cell Tissue Res 230:67–76

Seecof RL, Dewhurst S (1974) Insulin is a *Drosophila* hormone and acts to enhance the differentiation of embryonic *Drosophila* cells. Cell Differentiation 3:63–70

Seligman IM (1980) Bursicon. In: Miller TA (ed) Neurohormonal techniques in insects. Springer, Berlin Heidelberg New York, pp 137–153

Siegert K, Morgan P, Mordue W (1985) Primary structure of locust adipokinetic hormones II. Biol Chem 366:723–726

Simantov R, Goodman R, Aposhian D, Snyder SH (1979) Phylogenetic distribution of a morphine-like peptide enkephalin. Brain Res 111:204–211

Starrat AN, Brown BE (1975) Structure of the pentapeptide proctolin, a proposed neurotransmitter in insects. Life Sci 17:1253–1256

Steel CGH, Harmsen R (1971) Dynamics of the neurosecretory system in the brain of an insect, *Rhodnius prolixus* during growth and moulting. Gen Comp Endocrinol 17:125–141

Steele JE (1961) Occurrence of a hyperglycaemic factor in the corpus cardiacum of an insect. Nature 192:680–681

Steele JE (1963) The site of action of insect hyperglycaemic hormone. Gen Comp Endocrinol 3:46–52

Steele JE (1980) Hormonal modulation of carbohydrate and lipid metabolism in the fat body. In: Locke M, Smith DS (eds) Insect biology in the future. Academic, New York, pp 253–271

Steele JE (1983) Endocrine control of carbohydrate metabolism in insects. In: Downer RGH, Laufer H (eds) Endocrinology of insects. Liss, New York, pp 427–439

Stone JV, Mordue W, Batley KE, Morris HR (1976) Structure of locust adipokinetic hormone, a neurohormone that regulates lipid utilisation during flight. Nature 263:207–211

Strambi C, Rougon-Rapuzzi G, Cupo A, Martin N, Strambi A (1979) Mise en évidence immunocytologique d'un composé apparenté à la vasopressine dans le système nerveux du grillon *Acheta domesticus*. CR Acad Sci (Paris) 288(D):131–133

Suzuki A, Matsumoto S, Ogura N, Isogai A, Tamura S (1976) Extraction and partial purification of the hormone inducing cuticular melanization in armyworm larvae. Agric Blood Chem (Jpn) 40:2037

Tager HS, Kramer KJ (1980) Insect glucagon-like peptides: evidence for high molecular weight form in midgut from *Manduca sexta* (L.). Insect Biochem 10:617–619

Tager HS, Markese J, Spiers RD, Kramer KJ (1975) Glucagon-like immunoreactivity in insect corpus cardicum. Nature 254:707–708

Tager HS, Markese J, Kramer KJ, Spiers RD, Childs CN (1976) Glucagon-like and insulin-like hormones of the insect neurosecretory system. Biochem J 156:515–520

Taghert PH (1980) The identification and analyses of specific peptide-containing neurons in the moth *Manduca sexta*. Dissertation, University of Washington

Taghert PH, Truman JW (1979) Identification and morphological variability of a peptidergic neuron in the tobacco hawkmoth *Manduca sexta*. Soc Neurosci Abstr 5:263

Taghert PH, Truman JW (1980) Physiological properties of identified peptidergic neurons in an insect. Am Zool 20:867

Taghert PH, Truman JW, Reynolds SE (1980) Physiology of pupal ecdysis in the tobacco hornworm *Maduca sexta*. II. Chemistry, distribution and release of eclosion hormone at pupal ecdysis. J Exp Biol 88:339–349

Teller JK, Pilc L (1985) Insulin in insects: analysis of immunoreactivity in tissue extracts. Comp Biochem Physiol [B] 81:493–497

Teller JK, Rosinski G, Pilc L, Kasprzyl A, Lesicki A (1983) The presence of insulin-like hormone in heads and midguts of *Tenebrio mollitor* L . (Coleoptera) larvae. Comp Biochem Physiol [A] 74:463–465

Thomsen E (1952) Functional significance of the neurosecretory brain cells and corpus cardiacum in the female blowfly, *Calliphora erythrocephala* (Meig.). J Exp Biol 29:137–172

Thomsen E, Møller (1963) Influence of neurosecretory cells and corpus allatum on intestinal protease activity in the adult *Calliphora erythrocephala* Meig. J Exp Biol 40:301–321

Thorpe A, Duve H (1984) Insulin- and glucagon-like peptides in insects and molluscs. Mol Physiol 5:235–260

Truman JW (1971) Physiology of insect ecdysis. I. The eclosion behaviour of saturniid moths and its hormonal release. J Exp Biol 54:805–814

Truman JW (1972) Physiology of insect rhythms. 1. Circadian organization of the endocrine events underlying the moulting cycle in larval tobacco hornworms. J Exp Biol 57:805–820

Truman JW (1973a) Physiology of insect ecdysis. II. The assay and occurrence of the eclosion hormone in the Chinese oak silkmoth, *Antheraea pernyi*. Biol Bull 144:200–211

Truman JW (1973b) Physiology of insect ecdysis. III. Relationship between the hormonal control of eclosion and of tanning in the tobacco hornworm (*Manduca sexta*). J Exp Biol 58:821–829

Truman JW, Riddiford LM (1974) Physiology of insect rhythms. III. The temporal organisation of the endocrine events underlying pupation of the tobacco hornworm. J Exp Biol 60:371–382

Truman JW, Taghert PH, Copenhaver PF, Tublitz NJ, Schwartz LM (1981) Eclosion hormone may control all ecdyses in insects. Nature 291:70–71

Veenstra J (1984) Immunocytochemical demonstration of a homology in peptidergic neurosecretory cells in the suboesophageal ganglion of a beetle and a locust with antisera to bovine pancreatic polypeptide, FMRFamide, vasopressin and α-MSH. Neurosci Lett 48:185–190

Veenstra J, Schooneveld H (1984) Immunocytochemical localization of neurons in the nervous system of the Colorado potato beetle with antisera against FMRFamide and bovine pancreatic polypeptide. Cell Tissue Res 235:303–308

Veenstra J, Yanaihara N (1984) Immunocytochemical localization of gastrin-releasing peptide/bombesin-like immunoreactive neurons in insects. Histochemistry 81:133–138

Veenstra J, Romberg-Privee H, Schooneveld H (1984) Immunocytochemical localization of peptidergic cells in the neuro-endocrine system of the Colorado potato beetle *Leptinotarsa decemlineata*, with antisera against vasopressin, vasotocin and oxytocin. Histochemistry 81:29–34

Veenstra JA, Romberg-Privee HM, Schooneveld H (1985a) A proctolin-like peptide and its immunocytochemical localisation in the Colorado potato beetle, *Leptinotarsa decemlineata*. Cell Tissue Res 240:535–540

Veenstra JA, Romberg-Privee HM, Schooneveld H, Polak JM (1985b) Immunocytochemical localization of peptidergic neurons and neurosecretory cells in the neuro-endocrine system of the Colorado potato beetle with antisera to vertebrate regulatory peptides. Histochemistry 82:9–18

Verhaert P, De Loof A (1985a) Substance P-like immunoreactivity in the central nervous system of the blattarian insect *Periplaneta americana* L revealed by a monoclonal antibody. Histochemistry 83:501–507

Verhaert P, De Loof A (1985b) Immunocytochemical localization of a Methionine-Enkephalin-resembling neuropeptide in the central nervous system of the American cockroach, *Periplaneta americana* L. J Comp Neurol 239:54–61

Verhaert P, Geysen J, De Loof A, Vandesande F (1984) Immunoreactive material resembling vertebrate neuropeptides and neurophysins in the brain, suboesophageal ganglion, corpus cardiacum and corpus allatum of the dictyopteran *Periplaneta americana* L. Cell Tissue Res 238:55–59

Verhaert P, Grimmelikhuijzen C, De Loof A (1985) Distinct localization of FMRF amide and bovine pancreatic polypeptide-like material in the brain, retrocerebral complex and suboesophageal ganglion on the cockroach *Periplaneta americana* L. Brain Res 348:331–338

Wigglesworth VB (1964) The hormonal regulation of growth and reproduction in insects. Adv Insect Physiol 2:268–335

Williams CM (1956) The juvenile hormone of insects. Nature 178:212–213

Williams CM, Adkisson PL (1964) Physiology of insect diapause. XIV. An endocrine mechanism for the photoperiodic control of pupal diapause in the oak silkworm, *Antherea pernyi*. Biol Bull 127:511–525

Yamashita O (1983) Egg diapause. In: Downer RGH, Laufer H (eds) Endocrinology of insects. Liss, New York, pp 337–342

Yui R, Fujita T, Ito S (1980) Insulin-, gastrin-, pancreatic polypeptide-like immunoreactive neurones in the brain of the silkworm *Bombyx mori*. Biomed Res 1:42–46

Žďárek I (1980) Neurohormonal factors involved in the control of pupariation. In: Miller TA (ed) Neurohormonal techniques in insects. Springer, Berlin Heidelberg New York, pp 154–178

Ziegler R, Eckart K, Schwarz H, Keller R (1985) Amino acid sequence of *Manduca sexta* adipokinetic hormone elucidated by combined fast atom bombardment (FAB)/tandem mass spectrometry. Biochem Biophys Res Commun 133:337–342

Stimulus-Secretion Coupling in the Pancreatic B Cell

W. J. MALAISSE

Contents

1 Introduction

The maintenance of fuel homeostasis is critically dependent on a constant and constantly adjusted supply of insulin from the endocrine pancreas. An output of insulin adequate to meet extrapancreatic insulin requirements is ensured by a

Laboratory of Experimental Medicine, Brussels Free University, 115, Boulevard de Waterloo, B-1000 Brussels, Belgium

Current Topics in Neuroendocrinology, Vol. 9

series of nutritional, hormonal, neural, and ontogenic factors, which all participate in the control of insulin secretion (Malaisse 1972). Most of these factors have, in either an immediate or delayed fashion, direct effects upon pancreatic B cells located in the islets of Langerhans. B cells must both be equipped with a series of suitable sensor systems in order to identify each regulatory factor, and be suitably organized to integrate the information provided by each sensor system, in order eventually to respond with an adequate rate of hormonal release. This situation can be visualized as a multifactorial control of a single release process (Malaisse 1973). Among the factors conceivably involved in the immediate regulation of insulin release under physiological conditions, four major types can be identified. They are circulating nutrients, cholinergic neurotransmitters, adrenergic agents, and peptidergic hormones. The present contribution deals mainly with the mechanisms for the insulinotropic action of these four types of factors. A brief description of the overall functional organization of the B cell will, however, be presented first.

2 Functional Organization of the B Cell

2.1 The Islet Syncytium

The pancreatic B cell is located in the islets of Langerhans, where it is surrounded by other B cells and non-B islet cells including glucagon-, somatostatin-, and pancreatic polypeptide-producing cells. It is conceivable that the local release of the latter hormones affects, in a paracrine process, the secretory activity of adjacent B cells (Pipeleers 1984). Moreover, B cells and non-B islet cells are interconnected by gap junctions, which represent a pathway for metabolic, ionic and bioelectrical intercellular coupling (Orci et al. 1975). Hence, it may be unwise to consider the B cell as an isolated secretory unit. Instead, all cells within the same islet could be viewed as a functional syncytium displaying coordinated and synchronized secretory activity (Leclercq-Meyer et al. 1987). This concept may have several implications. To cite only one example, one could question whether the difference in the kinetics of D-glucose transport into B and non-B islet cells, as documented in purified populations of isolated cells, is operative in intact islets, when it is possible for D-glucose to move from the cytosol of one cell to another (Giroix et al. 1984; Gorus et al. 1984).

2.2 Proinsulin Biosynthesis and Insulin Release

For the organism as a whole, the release of insulin into the bloodstream represents the sole relevant variable of B cell physiology, at least if it is assumed that C peptide, which is released in equimolar amounts to insulin, and proinsulin, which is normally released in a molar amount much lower than insulin, do not act as first endocrine messengers upon extrapancreatic target tissues. From this perspective, the biosynthesis of proinsulin and its conversion to insulin and C peptide can be considered independently of the release of insulin, even more so since the immediate regulation of insulin secretion does not depend on a change in biosynthetic activity. It is nevertheless obvious that, over a prolonged period of time, a sufficient synthesis of proinsulin is required to allow for a sufficient release of insulin. Moreover, the respective rates at which proinsulin and insulin – as well as preformed and newly synthesized insulin – are secreted can be altered during sustained exposure of the B cell to several secretagogues (Gold and Grodsky 1984). Furthermore, a comparison between the respective effects of a given secretagogue on proinsulin biosynthesis and insulin release may help to elucidate the mechanism of action involved (Malaisse et al. 1973). Finally, in certain models of B cell dysfunction, anomalies can be found in the chemical structure of (pro)insulin, in the conversion of the prohormone, or in the capacity of the cell to store these secretory products (Chan et al. 1986; Pipeleers et al. 1975). Although these aspects of B cell physiology will not be discussed further in this review, it would be unwise to overlook them.

2.3 Long-Term Regulation of Insulin Release

Along a comparable line of thinking, it should be emphasized that the degree of the secretory response of the endocrine pancreas to a given secretagogue may be affected by the amount of insulin stored in the islet cells and by the total mass of pancreatic B cells; hypo- or hypertrophy of islets is usually related to cell hypo- or hyperplasia. These differences are especially relevant when considering the long-term regulation of insulin release, e.g., through ontogenic factors (Malaisse and Malaisse-Lagae 1969). Yet a change in insulin content or islet size is obviously not the sole factor involved in such a long-term regulation. Thus, the modulation of insulin release, as observed during fetal and neonatal periods, growth, aging, pregnancy, and lactation, and the slow changes in islet function encountered in fasting, obesity, and several endocrinopathies are also attributable, at least in part, to site-specific alterations in the secretory sequence. To cite only one example, fasting appears to be associated with a rather selective repression of key glycolytic enzymes in pancreatic islet cells, such as glucokinase and phosphofructokinase (Malaisse et al. 1976a).

2.4 The Effector System of Insulin Release

Whatever the physiological factor participating in the immediate regulation of insulin release and, hence, whatever the sensor system involved, the resulting change in insulin output is thought to be mediated by a common effector system for the intracellular translocation of secretory granules and their access to the site of exocytosis. The definition and properties of this effector system will be considered, therefore, at this point, rather than as part of a specific class of secretagogues. This is not meant to deny, however, that suitable experimental agents used in the study of insulin release may act primarily upon a selective component of this effector system. Moreover, agents such as D-glucose may in their role as secretagogue alter the intrinsic properties of the effector system, e.g., by favoring the assembly of microtubules (Pipeleers et al. 1976).

The current view ascribes a dual role to the effector system for insulin release: it gives the secretory granules access to the exocytotic site and is responsible for the fusion and fission of membranes at the latter site. The first of these two roles seems to be under the control of a microtubular-microfilamentous system, which is thought to be responsible for the functional segregation of secretory granules within the B cell and to provide the motive force for both the back-and-forth saltatory movements of secretory granules along oriented microtubular pathways and their channelling to the plasma membrane through the microfilamentous cell web (Malaisse et al. 1975; Malaisse and Orci 1979). Since the contractile activity of the latter network of microfilaments may be triggered by an increase in cytosolic Ca^{2+} concentration (Somers et al. 1979), the cell web could be looked upon as a target system for changes in cytosolic Ca^{2+} activity. The second mechanical event and final step of the secretory sequence consists in the fusion of the granule limiting-membrane and the plasma membrane, followed by the fission of these membranes and the subsequent dissolution in the extracellular medium of the insulin microcrystal stored in each granule. An anion osmotic process has been proposed to account for this step and, hence, for the chain release of several secretory granules at the same exocytotic site (Somers et al. 1980; Orci and Malaisse 1980). Under normal conditions, the exocytosis of β granules appears to be coupled with an increased endocytosis of microvesicles, allowing inter alia for the recirculation of membranes in the stimulated B cell (Orci et al. 1973).

3 The Nutrient Pathway of Insulin Release

Circulating nutrients, especially D-glucose, play a critical role in the control of insulin release. The stimulation of insulin secretion by these secretagogues is currently being considered within the framework of a fuel concept for insulin release. According to this concept, the response of a B cell to nutrient secretagogues reflects the capacity of the latter to augment oxidative fluxes and hence to increase ATP generation in the same cell (Malaisse et al. 1979; Malaisse 1983).

3.1 Identification of Nutrient Secretagogues

The fuel concept described above differs from a prior hypothesis according to which the stimulation of insulin release by D-glucose and other nutrient secretagogues was attributed to the activation of stereospecific receptors, possibly located at the B cell plasma membrane (Matschinsky et al. 1975). In order to choose between these two theories, it was necessary to elucidate such items as the anomeric specificity of the secretory response to D-glucose and D-mannose, and the insulinotropic action of a nonmetabolized analog of L-leucine, 2-aminobicyclo-[2,2,1]heptane-2-carboxylic acid (BCH), as reviewed elsewhere (Malaisse et al. 1981, 1983a). It was eventually determined that the degree of insulin release could be accounted for by the metabolic response of the islet cells. For instance, the greater efficiency of the α-anomers of both D-glucose and D-mannose in stimulating insulin release coincides with a higher rate of glycolysis in the islet cells (Malaisse et al. 1976b; Sener et al. 1982). Likewise, the insulinotropic action of BCH was found to be due to the activation of glutamate dehydrogenase, resulting in the accelerated catabolism of endogenous amino acids (Sener and Malaisse 1980; Sener et al. 1981).

The fuel concept of insulin release stresses the importance of such phenomena as the regulation of nutrient catabolism in the islet cells, and the implicit alignment between the rate of ATP generation and hydrolysis in both resting and stimulated islet cells. Yet, since the present review deals mainly with the mechanism of stimulus-secretion coupling, the discussion here will be restricted to the generation of those second messengers conceivably coupling the metabolism of nutrients to more distal cellular events in the secretory sequence.

3.2 Coupling of Metabolic to Distal Events

The second messengers coupling metabolic to more distal events in the secretory sequence remain to be identified. One of the difficulties encountered is the selection, from among a great number of distal events, of those events which may be directly regulated by metabolic mechanisms. In this respect, emphasis is currently being placed on a decrease in K^+ conductance resulting from the closure of a class of K^+ channels located at the B cell plasma membrane. Several coupling factors could be considered. Indeed, an increase in nutrient oxidation usually coincides with an increase in the generation rate of reduced nicotinamide adenine dinucleotide (NADH) and reduced nicotinamide adenine dinucleotide phosphate (NADPH), high-energy phosphate intermediates (ATP) and protons (H^+). Alternatively, metabolites generated in suitable catabolic pathways could act as coupling factors. It is also conceivable that the coupling between metabolic and more distal events in the secretory sequence represents a multifactorial process, with distinct coupling factors acting separately or in concert to affect distinct distal targets.

3.2.1 Metabolic Intermediates

A few years ago, when it was still a matter of debate whether glucose must be metabolized in islet cells in order to stimulate insulin release, one view which was being considered was that an early metabolite of glucose, e.g., glucose-6-phosphate, acted as a signal for insulin release. Now it seems evident that distinct nutrient secretagogues, which are metabolized by quite different pathways, owe their insulinotropic capacity to their ability to act as a fuel in islet cells, and the idea that a critical metabolite acts as the major coupling factor is viewed with greater skepticism. Nevertheless, such an idea should not be ruled out. For instance, phosphoenol pyruvate may affect the mitochondrial handling of Ca^{2+} or the activity of enzymes such as adenylate cyclase and protein kinase (Capito and Hedeskov 1977; Sugden and Ashcroft 1978).

3.2.2 Reducing Equivalents and Protons

The possible role played by either an increased generation of reducing agents, such as NADH, NADPH and reduced glutathione, or by the changes in intracellular pH evoked by nutrient secretagogues in the coupling of metabolic to distal events was examined in detail in two recent reviews (Malaisse et al. 1984a; Malaisse and Sener 1987b). Recent findings have cast some doubt on the view that either of these two processes represents the key second messenger in nutrient-induced insulin release. As far as the redox state is concerned, no parallelism could be found between the changes in cytosolic $NADH/NAD^+$ and $NADPH/NADP^+$ ratios evoked by distinct nutrient secretagogues and their insulinotropic action (Sener and Malaisse 1987). Concerning the role of intracellular pH, a recent report (Lindström and Sehlin 1986) emphasizes that intracellular alkalinization may provoke insulin release at very low glucose concentrations (1.0 m*M*). Since D-glucose indeed increases intracellular pH, this would be compatible with a stimulus-secretion coupling role for such a pH. However, the increase of cellular pH evoked by D-glucose apparently does not represent a primary consequence of the acceleration in glucose catabolism but may instead result from the secondary activation of processes such as Na^+/H^+ and HCO_3^-/Cl^- exchange (Deleers et al. 1985a). Hence, it might be unwise to consider the rise in cell pH as a coupling factor immediately generated through the catabolism of nutrients in islet cells.

3.2.3 ATP

Over the last few years, considerable attention has been paid to the possible role of a rise in cytosolic ATP concentration as the major factor coupling the catabolism of nutrients to ionic events in the secretory sequence. This concept is based mainly on the following three series of findings.

First, electrophysiological studies by the patch clamp technique have identified in islet cell membranes a class of K^+ channels that can be inhibited by intracellular ATP (Cook and Hales 1984; Ashcroft et al. 1984; Rorsman and Trube 1985). In islet cells stimulated by D-glucose or D-glyceraldehyde, the closure of these channels is thought to cause membrane depolarization, which is required for opening the voltage-gated Ca^{2+} channels and, hence, facilitates influx of Ca^{2+}. In excised inside-out membrane patches, a concentration of 1.0 m*M* ATP suffices to abolish all K^+ channel activity. Since the resting cytosolic ATP concentration is not lower than 1.0 m*M*, it may appear unlikely that a nutrient-induced increase in the latter concentration would indeed affect the open-state probability of the ATP-sensitive K^+ channels. However, a recent study suggests that, in saponin-permeabilized insulin-secreting cells of the RINm5F line, ADP (0.1–0.5 m*M*) markedly activates K^+ channels, as judged from single-channel current recording (Dunne and Petersen 1986). The effect of ADP (0.5 m*M*) in activating K^+ channels was also operative in the presence of ATP (0.5 m*M*). Hence, the open-state probability of these K^+ channels may be dependent on changes in the ATP/ADP ratio, rather than solely on the ATP concentration.

Second, I have recently indicated (Malaisse and Sener 1987a) that D-glucose indeed increases markedly the cytosolic ATP/ADP ratio in normal pancreatic islets, whereas previous studies were restricted to measuring the total cellular concentrations of adenine nucleotides.

Lastly, exposure of tumoral islet cells of the RINm5F line to the nonmetabolized analogue of L-leucine, BCH provided a unique opportunity to distinguish between changes in cytosolic redox state and ATP availability (or ATP/ADP ratio), as a determinant of nutrient-stimulated insulin release (Sener et al. 1987). In these cells, BCH unexpectedly inhibited insulin release despite the induction of a more reduced cytosolic redox state. The inhibition of insulin release by BCH coincided with a decrease in O_2 uptake and a lowering of ATP concentration and ATP/ADP ratio, and was accompanied by an increase in ^{86}Rb outflow from prelabeled cells. Thus, in this system, the change in ATP generation rate, which is attributable to a sparing action on the catabolism of endogenous fatty acids (Blachier et al. 1987b) was apparently responsible for the functional response of these tumoral cells.

Another additional mechanism by which ATP might affect insulin release consists in the exocytotic release of the adenine nucleotide present in the secretory granules, which leads to a further amplification of the secretory response (Hellman 1986) due to the intervention of purinergic receptors. It should again be stressed that although only the role of ATP is under consideration in the present review, the participation of other factors generated through the catabolism of nutrients, e.g. reducing equivalents and protons, in the coupling of metabolic to distal events should not be entirely neglected.

3.3 Amplification Devices

In Sects. 4.1 and 6.1 two modalities for the modulation of nutrient-stimulated insulin release by nonnutrient environmental agents will be dealt with, namely the activation of either phospholipase C or adenylate cyclase. It should be realized, however, that in intact pancreatic islets exposed solely to D-glucose, the generation of cyclic AMP and hydrolysis of phosphoinositides are apparently also involved in the secretory response to this hexose. As a working hypothesis, it can be proposed that the effect of D-glucose upon such processes represents a suitable device for the amplification of the functional response to nutrient secretagogues.

Apparently, D-glucose and other nutrient secretagogues augment the rate of cyclic AMP generation in islet cells (Malaisse and Malaisse-Lagae 1984). This is best demonstrated in the presence of phosphodiesterase inhibitors. The modelling of cyclic AMP turnover suggests, however, that the activation of adenylate cyclase by nutrients is not dependent on the presence of such inhibitors (Valverde et al. 1983). The nutrient-induced increase in cyclic AMP formation is considerably impaired when the islets are incubated in the absence of extracellular Ca^{2+} (Valverde et al. 1983). This raises the possibility that the effect of nutrients upon adenylate cyclase is secondary to the increase in cytosolic Ca^{2+} activity observed in glucose-stimulated islet cells exposed to a normal concentration of extracellular Ca^{2+} (Deleers et al. 1985b). The discovery that, in a subcellular particulate fraction prepared from isolated islets, calmodulin causes calcium-dependent activation of adenylate cyclase also makes clear a pathway for the acceleration of cyclic AMP generation in nutrient-stimulated islet cells (Valverde et al. 1979).

A somewhat comparable proposal was recently advanced to account for the stimulation by nutrient secretagogues of the hydrolysis of inositol-containing phospholipids. This effect was documented in islets exposed to such nutrient secretagogues as D-glucose, 2-ketoisocaproate, 3-phenylpyruvate and 2-*endo*-amino-norbornane-2-carboxylic acid (Best and Malaisse 1983 a). The response of D-glucose is suppressed in the presence of mannoheptulose. These findings indicate that the activation of phospholipase C in islets exposed to nutrient secretagogues is dependent on the integrity of their metabolic effects. The effect of these nutrients upon the hydrolysis of inositol-containing lipids is suppressed at extracellular Ca^{2+} concentrations equal or below 10^{-5} *M*, and can be duplicated by a rise in extracellular K^+ concentration (from 5 to 30 m*M* or more), which is known to cause cell-membrane depolarization and, hence, facilitates Ca^{2+} inflow into islet cells (Best 1986). Moreover, in digitonin-permeabilized islets, a marked stimulation of phosphoinositide hydrolysis is observed when the Ca^{2+} concentration of the medium is raised from 10^{-7} to 10^{-5} *M* (Best 1986). All these data are consistent with the view that the effect of nutrient secretagogues upon phospholipase C in islet cells is secondary to an increase in cytosolic Ca^{2+} activity.

The two examples just mentioned do not exhaust the list of cellular mechanisms possibly involved in the stimulus-secretion coupling in nutrient-induced insulin release. For instance, the activation of phospholipase A_2 and the resulting generation of eicosanoids in the arachidonate cascade (Mathias et al. 1985 b), the influence of a change in both redox state and cytosolic Ca^{2+} concentration upon the activity of transglutaminase (Gomis et al. 1986), or a decrease in plasma membrane fluidity (Deleers et al. 1981) could be cited as further cytophysiological processes participating in the stimulation of islet cells by D-glucose. In this respect, it remains a challenge to assess the relative importance, in both qualitative and quantitative terms, of each of these coupling processes when considering the overall magnitude – and time course – of the secretory response to D-glucose and other nutrient secretagogues.

4 The Cholinergic Pathway of Insulin Release

It has been known for more than two decades that cholinergic agents exert an immediate and direct stimulatory effect upon insulin release by the pancreatic B cell (Malaisse et al. 1967 b). Moreover, it has long been postulated that vagal stimulation of insulin secretion participates in the response of the endocrine pancreas to food intake, including a cephalic phase of insulin release (Malaisse 1972). However, it was only recently that the cytophysiological events mediating the response to cholinergic neurotransmitters were elucidated.

4.1 Muscarinic Receptors and Activation of Phospholipase C

Islet cells are equipped with muscarinic receptors (Grill and Östenson 1983; Östenson and Grill 1985; Malaisse et al. 1985 b). In membranes isolated from dispersed islet cells, carbamylcholine causes a concentration-related decrease in the amount of [^{32}P]phosphatidylinositol 4-phosphate and [^{32}P]phosphatidylinositol 4,5-bisphosphate. In these experiments, the polyphosphoinositides were prelabeled by exposing the isolated membranes to [γ–^{32}P]ATP, and carbamylcholine was then added 10 s prior to lipid extraction (Dunlop and Malaisse 1986). The formation of diacylglycerol was documented by preincubating the islet cells with [U–^{14}C]arachidonate. These experiments support the view that activation of a plasma membrane associated phospholipase C directed against polyphosphoinositides represents an early event in the cholinergic stimulation of insulin release. Moreover, the modulation of the response to carbamylcholine by atropine, calcium chelators and calcium antagonists in the isolated membranes points to a key role for membrane-bound Ca^{2+} in the coupling between muscarinic receptor occupancy and polyphosphoinositide hydrolysis. It was recently proposed that a GTP-binding regulatory protein participates in the activation of phospholipase C by cholinergic agents in islet cells (Blachier and Malaisse 1987 a, b). This regulatory protein is apparently distinct from either Ns or Ni. Thus, none of the agents acting upon the latter two regulatory proteins (glucagon, clonidine, cholera toxin) affect the hydrolysis of inositol-containing phospholipids, whether in resting or carbamylcholine-stimulated normal or tumoral islet cells (Blachier et al. 1987 a; Blachier and Malaisse 1987 b). It should be noted, however, that clonidine suppresses the insulin-secretory response of the islets to cholinergic agents (Malaisse and Sener 1986).

4.2 Hydrolysis of Polyphosphoinositides in Intact Islet Cells

In intact islets, carbamylcholine also stimulates the hydrolysis of polyphosphoinositides (Best and Malaisse 1984 a). This coincides with a rise in the production of inositol 1,4,5-triphosphate, myo-inositol 1,4-bisphosphate and myo-inositol 1-phosphate (Best and Malaisse 1983 b, 1984 a). The carbamylcholine-induced hydrolysis of phosphoinositides appears to be closely coupled with their resynthesis from phosphatidic acid (Best and Malaisse 1983 c). Moreover, cholinergic stimuli apparently also favor the de novo synthesis of phosphatidic acid and phosphatidylinositol (Best and Malaisse 1984 b). The enhanced turnover of inositol-containing phospholipids caused by cholinergic agents in islet cells represents a calcium-dependent process, though apparently it is not triggered by an increase in Ca^{2+} fluxes into the islet cells (Best and Malaisse 1983 b, c, 1984 b; Mathias et al. 1985 a).

The effect of cholinergic agents on phospholipid metabolism in islet cells is not restricted to the turnover of phosphoinositides. Carbamylcholine also apparently causes activation of phospholipase A_2 (Mathias et al. 1985 b). By analogy with findings obtained in other tissues (Lapetina 1982), the suggestion was made that such an activation may be mediated, in part at least, through the hydrolysis of polyphosphoinositides. Since the activation of phospholipase A_2 is more marked in response to cholinergic agents than D-glucose, the liberation of arachidonate and the generation of messengers in the arachidonate cascade could play a greater role in the cholinergic stimulation of the B cell than in nutrient-induced insulin release.

4.3 Activation of Protein Kinase C

As reviewed in greater detail elsewhere (Best and Malaisse 1983d), there are a number of mechanisms by which the above-mentioned changes in phospholipid metabolism could participate in the secretory response of the B cell to cholinergic neurotransmitters. A current hypothesis postulates that diacylglycerol and inositol 1,4,5-triphosphate, which are liberated from phosphatidylinositol 4,5-bisphosphate, may lead, respectively, to the activation of protein kinase C and mobilization of Ca^{2+} from nonmitochondrial organelles.

The presence of a phospholipid-dependent, Ca^{2+}-responsive, and diacylglycerol-activated protein kinase activity in islet homogenates has been documented by several investigators. The sensitivity of this enzyme to increasing concentrations of Ca^{2+} is modulated by the extent of activation by either diacylglycerol or its substitute 12-O-tetradecanoylphorbol 13-acetate (Malaisse et al. 1985c; Hubinont and Malaisse 1985). It is conceivable, therefore, that activation of the enzyme leads to stimulation of insulin release even at a resting level of cytosolic Ca^{2+} activity (Hubinont et al. 1984). This is supported by comparison between the cationic and secretory responses, respectively, to such agents as tumor-promoting phorbol esters and the membrane-accessible diglyceride 1-oleyl-2-acetylglycerol (Malaisse et al. 1980, 1983b, 1985c). A selective inhibitor of protein kinase C (H-7) was used to further document the participation of this enzyme in the secretory response to cholinergic agents (Malaisse and Sener 1985).

4.4 Mobilization of Intracellular Ca^{2+}

The ionic response of islet cells to cholinergic agents differs in several respects from that evoked by nutrient secretagogues (Gagerman et al. 1980; Wollheim et al. 1980). For instance, whereas the latter usually decrease ^{86}Rb outflow from prelabeled islets, carbamylcholine increases ^{86}Rb outflow (Nenquin et al. 1984; Mathias et al. 1985c). This effect persists in the absence of extracellular Ca^{2+} and at low glucose concentrations, under which conditions the neurotransmitter does not change the B cell membrane potential (Gagerman et al. 1978).

Cholinergic agents also provoke a rapid increase in ^{45}Ca outflow from prelabeled islets. This effect, which is blocked by atropine, is seen both in the absence and in the presence of either D-glucose or extracellular Ca^{2+} (Nenquin et al. 1984; Mathias et al. 1985c). It is thought, therefore, to reflect mobilization of ^{45}Ca from cellular sites by inositol 1,4,5-triphosphate, in a manner comparable to that described in rat insulinoma microsomes (Prentki et al. 1984).

4.5 Modulation of Secretory Response to Cholinergic Agents

In the light of the information so far reviewed, the stimulation of insulin release by cholinergic agents could be viewed as resulting from a dual mechanism, namely the activation of protein kinase C and the mobilization of intracellular Ca^{2+}. According to some authors (Rasmussen et al. 1984; Zawalich et al. 1983), such a dual mechanism may account for the biphasic pattern of insulin release. It should be stressed, however, that cholinergic agents fail to stimulate insulin release in the absence of an exogenous nutrient or at low concentrations of D-glucose (Malaisse et al. 1967b; Nenquin et al. 1984; Loubatières-Mariani et al. 1973). The permissive role of D-glucose was tentatively ascribed to the capacity of the sugar to cause membrane depolarization and, hence, to allow for stimulation of Ca^{2+} inflow by the cholinergic agent (Nenquin et al. 1984). Incidentally, cholinergic agents fail to exert any obvious effect upon glucose oxidation (Gagerman et al. 1980), although they may increase the NADH content of islet cells (Trus et al. 1978). The secretory response to acetylcholine is amplified by eserine, simulated by muscarine, and suppressed by atropine or methylscopolamine (Malaisse et al. 1967b; Grill and Östenson 1983; Loubatières-Mariani et al. 1973).

In conclusion, the cholinergic pathway for the stimulation of insulin release apparently involves a sophisticated sequence of cellular events, starting with the occupation of muscarinic receptors, followed by the activation of phospholipase C and the liberation of diacylglycerol and inositol phosphate from membrane phosphoinositides. These biochemical processes eventually lead to a remodeling of ionic fluxes, induction of bioelectrical activity, and the activation of enzymes such as protein kinase C and phospholipase A_2.

Although the functional response of the pancreatic B cell to cholinergic agents differs in some respects from that evoked by insulinotropic nutrients, these two types of secretagogues may act synergistically upon insulin release. This may be essential for the anabolic disposal of nutrients in extrapancreatic tissues at the time of food intake.

5 The Adrenergic Pathway of Insulin Release

Adrenergic agents either increase or inhibit glucose-stimulated insulin release. The enhancing action provoked by isoproterenol appears to be mediated by the intervention of β-adrenoceptors and may hence be linked to an increased production of cyclic AMP (Malaisse et al. 1967a). This process will not be further considered here. The inhibitory and prevailing action of catecholamines is thought to play a role in the control of insulin release during stress and exercise (Brisson et al. 1971). It is mediated by the intervention of α_2-adrenoceptors. There is no convincing evidence for the presence of α_1-adrenoceptors in the pancreatic B cell (Malaisse and Moratinos 1986).

5.1 Activation of Adrenergic Receptors

The presence of adrenergic receptors in islet cells has already been documented (Cherksey et al. 1982, 1983). Studies based on the use of selected adrenergic agonists and antagonists indicate that α_2-adrenergic receptors mediate the inhibitory action of catecholamines on insulin release. Such an inhibitory action is suppressed when the islets are exposed in vivo or in vitro to the islet-activating protein isolated from the culture medium of *Bordetella pertussis*. This treatment results in typical changes in the activity of adenylate cyclase in islet homogenates or subcellular fractions. In addition to a decrease in basal enzyme activity, these changes include an increased responsiveness to GTP relative to stable GTP analogs, such as GTPγS, and resistance to the inhibitory action of α_2-adrenergic agonists. These findings suggest the presence in islet cells of the regulatory protein Ni. This was confirmed by the demonstration that the islet-activating protein catalyzes in the islet cell membrane the ADP-ribosylation of a single protein with a M_r close to 41 000, which corresponds to the α subunit of Ni (Malaisse et al. 1984b).

5.2 Changes in Cyclic AMP Generation

Several studies have shown that adrenergic agents inhibit islet adenylate cyclase in acellular systems. This effect is best seen in crude homogenates and in the presence of NaCl (Garcia-Morales et al. 1984). It coincides with a decreased production of cyclic AMP in intact islets. In purified B cells exposed to both D-glucose (20 mM) and glucagon (10 nM), the lowering action of epinephrine upon the cell content of cyclic AMP is dose-related in the 0.1 nM-0.1 μM range (Schuit 1987). The effect of epinephrine is reproduced by norepinephrine and clonidine but not by isoproterenol or methoxamine, and is prevented by yohimbine and phentolamine, but not by prazosin or propranolol.

Apart from their effects upon cyclic AMP content and insulin release, adrenergic agents do not cause any obvious change in other functional variables, such as the oxidation of glucose and the net uptake of ^{45}Ca by intact islets (Leclercq-Meyer et al. 1980). Likewise, clonidine fails to prevent the rapid changes in ^{45}Ca efflux evoked by D-glucose in prelabeled islets and, although severely decreasing insulin output, does not alter the biphasic time course of the secretory response to the hexose. These negative findings suggest that the primary site of action of adrenergic agents is located distally to those metabolic and ionic events involved in the secretory response to nutrient secretagogues.

5.3 Interference with Distal Events in the Secretory Sequence

In the light of the experimental data so far reviewed, the most naive hypothesis concerning the interference of adrenergic agents in the secretory sequence would be that they lower the cyclic AMP content of islet cells. Since adrenergic agents inhibit the release of insulin evoked by virtually all secretagogues, this hypothesis would imply that a sufficient cyclic AMP content plays a permissive role in insulin release. This proposal is compatible with a recent mathematical model for the interaction between Ca^{2+} and cyclic AMP in the control of insulin release (Owen and Malaisse 1987). Indeed, in this model, it was postulated that the cyclic AMP concentration must exceed a critical threshold value in order to allow stimulation of insulin release. The threshold value was determined as that found in glucose-stimulated islets incubated for 90 min in the absence of $CaCl_2$ and ethylene glycol tetra-acetic acid (EGTA). Moreover, it has recently been proposed that the ample secretory response to D-glucose as observed in intact islets can only be duplicated in purified B cell when the latter are concomitantly exposed to exogenous glucagon which markedly augments the cyclic AMP content of glucose-stimulated cells (Schuit 1987).

A number of findings, however, strongly suggest that the inhibitory effect of adrenergic agents upon insulin release cannot be accounted for solely by a change in the cyclic AMP content of the B cell. This is best illustrated by the following two observations. First, in 1970 it was reported that exogenous dibutyryl cyclic AMP, when used at a concentration (0.2 m*M*) sufficient to double insulin release evoked by D-glucose (16.7 m*M*) in rat pancreatic islets, failed to prevent the inhibitory action of epinephrine (10 μ*M*) upon insulin release (Malaisse et al. 1970). Second, quite recently, it was reported that epinephrine (0.1 μ*M*) suppresses insulin release evoked in purified B-cells by the tumor-promoting phorbol ester tetradecanoyl-phorbol-acetate (TPA, 10 n*M*), whether at low (1.0 m*M*) or high (20 m*M*) concentrations of D-glucose, although the cyclic AMP content of the cells was identical in the presence of TPA alone and of both TPA and epinephrine (Schuit 1987). Thus, in the first instance epinephrine blocked insulin release despite the provision of exogenous dibutyryl cyclic AMP, while in the second instance epinephrine again inhibited secretion despite unaltered cyclic AMP cell content.

The possibility must thus be considered that catecholamines affect insulin release through a mechanism distal to the generation of cyclic AMP. This proposal is not incompatible with the postulated role of Ni in the response to adrenergic agents, since the regulatory protein could conceivably affect the activity of enzyme(s) other than adenylate cyclase. This proposal is also consistent with the view that the α subunits released from GTP-regulatory proteins can act as programmable messengers (Rodbell 1985). Distal events possibly affected by catecholamines may include the subcellular distribution of Ca^{2+} (Brisson and Malaisse 1973) or the responsiveness to the latter cation of target systems involved in the effector system of insulin release.

6 The Peptidergic Pathway of Insulin Release

Several peptide hormones affect insulin release in an immediate and direct fashion (Ahren et al. 1986). The effect of these hormones may be either stimulation or inhibition of insulin release.

Regarding the physiological regulation of insulin release in vivo, emphasis has for several decades been placed on the effect of gastrointestinal hormones which may be released as a consequence of food intake and would increase insulin release (e.g., in response to prandial hyperglycemia) to a greater extent than observed when a comparable hyperglycemic profile is achieved by the intravenous administration of the hexose. It is currently believed that these positive insulinotropic hormonal agents, which would participate in the function of a so-called enteroinsular axis, may act upon the B cell in a manner comparable to that observed for pancreatic glucagon, which also enhances insulin release from isolated islets or purified B cells (Moody et al. 1970). In my opinion, a crucial feature of the insulinotropic action of glucagon consists in the failure, except under unusual experimental conditions, of the hormone to affect insulin output at low extracellular concentrations of D-glucose, while it efficiently augments insulin release evoked by higher concentrations of the hexose or other secretagogues (Malaisse et al. 1967a). Such a situation, which I have defined as glucose potentiation (Malaisse 1973), is common to all secretagogues, including forskolin or phosphodiesterase inhibitors (Malaisse et al. 1984c), which are supposed to act on the B cell by specifically augmenting its cyclic AMP content.

The most classical example of a peptide with inhibitory action on insulin release is somatostatin. Both somatostatin 14 and somatostatin 28, as well as several other somatostatin analogues, efficiently inhibit insulin release in various experimental models. Dose-action relationships for the inhibition of insulin release from purified B cells by the two somatostatins and their analogues suggest somatostatin receptor heterogeneity (Schuit 1987). The physiological relevance of the inhibitory action of somatostatin upon insulin release remains to be documented, with current speculations dealing with a possible paracrine effect of the hormone released by the islet D cells upon adjacent B cells.

Both the enhancing action of glucagon and the inhibitory action of somatostatin upon insulin release coincide with parallel changes in the cyclic AMP content of purified B cells (Schuit 1987). Hence, the discussion on the peptidergic pathway is here limited to the modality of cyclic AMP generation and action in these cells. It should be noted, however, that, as is the case for adrenergic agents, somatostatin was proposed as inhibiting insulin release by both cyclic AMP-dependent and -independent mechanisms (Schuit 1987).

6.1 Generation of Cyclic AMP

We have already mentioned that nutrient secretagogues exert a modest effect upon cyclic AMP generation in islet cells, this effect possibly being secondary to a cytosolic Ca^{2+} accumulation and mediated by Ca-calmodulin (Valverde and Malaisse 1984). The effect of nutrients in increasing the islet cell cyclic AMP content is much less marked than the effect observed in response to suitable activators of adenylate cyclase, such as forskolin or glucagon (Garcia-Morales et al. 1984).

In the case of the latter hormone, the occupancy of the glucagon receptor (Goldfine et al. 1972; Patel et al. 1982) is thought to be coupled to the activation of adenylate cyclase upon the intervention of the GTP-regulatory protein Ns. In rat pancreatic islet membrane exposed to [α-^{32}P]NAD, cholera toxin stimulates the labeling of both the light and heavy forms of the α subunit of Ns, with predominance of the heavy form (Svoboda et al. 1985). When intact islets are preincubated with cholera toxin, the adenylate cyclase activity of a subcellular particulate fraction is increased. The responsiveness of adenylate cyclase to GTP – but not to GTPγS – is also augmented, but that to NaF is decreased. In intact islets, the production of cyclic AMP and the glucose-stimulated release of insulin are both enhanced after pretreatment with cholera toxin (Svoboda et al. 1985). These findings thus indicate the presence in pancreatic islets of the guanyl nucleotide regulatory protein Ns, which mediates the hormonal activation of adenylate cyclase. We have already indicated in Sect. 5.1 that islet cells are also equipped with the regulatory protein Ni.

6.2 Mode of Action of Cyclic AMP

The mode of action of cyclic AMP in the pancreatic B cell was reviewed in detail in a recent publication (Malaisse and Malaisse-Lagae 1984). The essential information can be summarized as follows. It is currently assumed, but remains to be proved, that the functional effects of cyclic AMP are linked to the activation of a cyclic AMP-responsive protein kinase, which was indeed identified in islet homogenates (Harrison et al. 1984).

The bulk of the evidence suggests that, especially at high glucose concentrations, the enhancing action of cyclic AMP upon insulin release is not attributable to any marked facilitation of nutrient catabolism in islet cells. An exceptional situation should be mentioned, however, in this respect. When pancreatic tissue is removed from rats maintained hyperglycemic by infusion of exogenous glucose (Malaisse et al. 1967a) or when pancreatic islets are first cultured at a very high concentration of the hexose (Malaisse et al. 1977), the normally glycogen-free B cells accumulate significant amounts of glycogen as judged by both ultrastructural and chemical criteria (Malaisse et al. 1977). In these preparations, agents augmenting the islet cell content in cyclic AMP, e.g., phosphodiesterase inhibitors, stimulate insulin release even in the absence of an exogenous nutrient. The secretory response coincides with and seems attributable, in part at least, to stimulation of glycogenolysis and acceleration of glycolysis (Malaisse et al. 1977).

An increase in cyclic AMP content may affect either the intracellular distribution or net uptake of Ca^{2+} in islet cells. The intracellular redistribution of Ca^{2+} was first postulated after findings indicated that agents raising the cyclic AMP content in islet cells tended to restore, at least to a limited extent, the secretory response to glucose of islets incubated in the nominal absence of Ca^{2+} (Brisson et al. 1972). When forskolin was used as an activator of adenylate cyclase, such a partial restoration was even observed in islets incubated in the absence of Ca^{2+} and presence of EGTA (Malaisse et al. 1984c). The view that cyclic AMP may exert a modest effect upon Ca^{2+} net uptake by islet cells is based mainly on the bioelectrical effects of forskolin or dibutyryl cyclic AMP in mouse pancreatic B cells (Henquin and Meissner 1983).

A last but possibly most important modality for the insulinotropic action of endogenous cyclic AMP could be increased responsiveness of the effector system to Ca^{2+}. This view is supported by recent findings suggesting that a rise in cyclic AMP content may coincide with an unaltered cytosolic Ca^{2+} activity in these cells (Wollheim et al. 1984). It is also consistent with a model for the mathematical simulation of stimulus-secretion coupling in the B cell. Indeed, in this model the major mode of action of cyclic AMP is precisely to augment the output of insulin at any given concentration of cytosolic Ca^{2+}, provided that the latter concentration exceeds the threshold value required for stimulation of insulin output (Malaisse et al. 1985 a). Lastly, forskolin augments Ca^{2+}-induced insulin release in rat islets permeabilized with digitonin, again suggesting a mode of action of cyclic AMP distal to the provision of Ca^{2+} (Tamagawa et al. 1985).

7 Concluding Remarks

The present review documents that the major physiological factors involved in the immediate regulation of insulin release, i.e., nutrients, gastrointestinal hormones, cholinergic and adrenergic agents, affect the pancreatic B cell through distinct sensor systems. Nevertheless, the second messengers generated by each of these sensor systems are apt to interfere with cytophysiological events in such a manner that their messages are eventually integrated to ensure a single control of the most distal events in the secretory sequence.

It should be stressed that this information does not concern either the mode of action of other agents acting immediately upon insulin release (e.g., hypoglycemic sulfonylureas) or the delayed regulation of secretion by ontogenic and nutritional factors, and is restricted to the release process to the exclusion of biosynthetic events whenever these are associated with the secretory response. Moreover, no information is provided on the alteration in stimulus-secretion coupling found in various models of B cell dysfunction. Finally, even on those issues under consideration here, several aspects have not been dealt with exhaustively. This applies, for instance, to the regulation of nutrient metabolism in islet cells or to the biophysics of insulin release, including electrical, mechanical, and motile events. Hence, it should be realized that the present review does not reflect the full extent of actual knowledge on the physiology and pathophysiology of the pancreatic B cell.

References

Ahren B, Taborsky GJ Jr, Porte D Jr (1986) Neuropeptidergic versus cholinergic and adrenergic regulation of islet hormone secretion. Diabetologia 29:827–836

Ashcroft FM, Harrison DE, Ashcroft SJH (1984) Glucose induces closure of single potassium channels in isolated rat pancreatic B-cells. Nature 312:446–448

Best L (1986) A role for calcium in the breakdown of inositol phospholipids in intact and digitonin-permeabilized pancreatic islets. Biochem J 238:773–779

Best L, Malaisse WJ (1983a) Effects of nutrient secretagogues upon phospholipid metabolism in rat pancreatic islets. Mol Cell Endocrinol 32:205–214

Best L, Malaisse WJ (1983b) Stimulation of phosphoinositide breakdown in rat pancreatic islets by glucose and carbamylcholine. Biochem Biophys Res Commun 116:9–16

Best L, Malaisse WJ (1983c) Phosphatidylinositol and phosphatidic acid metabolism in rat pancreatic islets in response to neurotransmitter and hormonal stimuli. Biochem Biophys Acta 750:157–163

Best L, Malaisse WJ (1983d) Phospholipids and islet function. Diabetologia 25:299–305

Best L, Malaisse WJ (1984a) Nutrient and hormone-neurotransmitter stimuli induce hydrolysis of polyphosphoinositides in rat pancreatic islets. Endocrinology 115:1814–1820

Best L, Malaisse WJ (1984b) Enhanced de novo synthesis of phosphatidic acid and phosphatidyl inositol in rat pancreatic islets exposed to nutrient and neurotransmitter stimuli. Arch Biochem Biophys 234:253–257

Blachier F, Malaisse WJ (1987a) Phospholipase C activation via a GTP binding protein in tumoral islet cells stimulated by carbamylcholine. Experienta 43:601–602

Blachier F, Malaisse WJ (1987b) Possible role of a GTP-binding protein in the activation of phospholipase C by carbamylcholine in tumoral insulin-producing cells. Res Commun Chem Pathol Pharmacol 58:237–255

Blachier F, Segura MC, Malaisse WJ (1987a) Unresponsiveness of phospholipase C to the regulatory proteins Ns and Ni in pancreatic islets. Res Commun Chem Pathol Pharmacol 55:335–355

Blachier F, Sener A, Malaisse WJ (1987b) Interference of a nonmetabolized analog of L-leucine with lipid metabolism in tumoral pancreatic islet cells. Biochim Biophys Acta 921:494–501

Brisson GR, Malaisse WJ (1973) The stimulus-secretion coupling of glucose-induced insulin release. XI. Effects of theophylline and epinephrine on ^{45}Ca efflux from perifused islets. Metabolism 22:455–465

Brisson GR, Malaisse-Lagae F, Malaisse WJ (1971) Effect of phentolamine upon insulin secretion during exercise. Diabetologia 7:223–226

Brisson GR, Malaisse-Lagae F, Malaisse WJ (1972) The stimulus-secretion coupling of glucose-induced insulin release. VII. A proposed site of action of adenosine-3′,5′-cyclic monophosphate. J Clin Invest 51:232–241

Capito K, Hedeskov CJ (1977) Effects of glucose, glucose metabolites and calcium ions on adenylate cyclase activity in homogenates of mouse pancreatic islets. Biochem J 162:569–573

Chan SJ, Nanjo K, Miyano M, Lu Y-S, Welsh M, Nielsen D, Haneda M, Kwok SCM, Tager HS, Rubenstein AH, Steiner DF (1986) Abnormalities of insulin gene structure and expression. A minireview. In: Serrano-Rios M, Lefèbvre PJ (eds) Diabetes 1985. Excerpta Medica, Amsterdam, pp 486–494

Cherksey B, Mendelsohn S, Zadunaisky J, Altzuler N (1982) Demonstration of α_2-adrenergic receptors in rat pancreatic islets using radioligand binding. Proc Soc Exp Biol Med 171:196–200

Cherksey B, Mendelsohn S, Zadunaisky J, Altzuler N (1983) Displacement of alpha- and beta-radioligands by specific adrenergic agonists in rat pancreatic islets. Pharmacology 27:95–102

Cook DL, Hales CN (1984) Intracellular ATP directly blocks K^+ channels in pancreatic B-cells. Nature 311:271–273

Deleers M, Ruysschaert JM, Malaisse WJ (1981) Glucose induces membrane changes detected by fluorescence polarization in endocrine pancreatic cells. Biochem Biophys Commun 98:255–260

Deleers M, Lebrun P, Malaisse WJ (1985a) Nutrient-induced changes in the pH of pancreatic islet cells. Horm Metab Res 17:391–395

Deleers M, Mahy M, Malaisse WJ (1985b) Glucose increases cytosolic Ca^{2+} activity in pancreatic islet cells. Biochem Int 10:97–103

Dunlop ME, Malaisse WJ (1986) Phosphoinositide phosphorylation and hydrolysis in pancreatic islet cell membrane. Arch Biochem Biophys 244:421–429

Dunne MJ, Petersen OH (1986) Intracellular ADP activates K^+ channels that are inhibited by ATP in an insulin-secreting cell line. FEBS Lett 208:59–62

Gagerman E, Idahl L-A, Meissner HP, Täljedal I-B (1978) Insulin release, cGMP, cAMP and membrane potential in acetylcholine-stimulated islets. Am J Physiol 235:E493–E500

Gagerman E, Sehlin J, Täljedal I-B (1980) Effects of acetylcholine on ion fluxes and chlorotetracycline fluorescence in pancreatic islets. J Physiol (Lond) 300:505–513

Garcia-Morales P, Dufrane SP, Sener A, Valverde I, Malaisse WJ (1984) Inhibitory effect of clonidine upon adenylate cyclase activity, cyclic AMP production and insulin release in rat pancreatic islets. Biosci Rep 4:511–521

Giroix M-H, Sener A, Pipeleers DG, Malaisse WJ (1984) Hexose metabolism in pancreatic islets. Inhibition of hexokinase. Biochem J 223:447–453

Gold G, Grodsky GM (1984) Kinetic aspects of compartmental storage and secretion of insulin and zinc. Experientia 40:1105–1114

Goldfine ID, Roth J, Birnbaumer L (1972) Glucagon receptors in β-cells. Binding of ^{125}I-glucagon and activation of adenylate cyclase. J Biol Chem 247:1211–1218

Gomis R, Arbos MA, Sener A, Malaisse WJ (1986) Glucose-induced activation of transglutaminase in pancreatic islets. Diabetes Res 3:115–117

Gorus FK, Malaisse WJ, Pipeleers DG (1984) Differences in glucose handling by pancreatic A- and B-cells. J Biol Chem 259:1196–1200

Grill V, Östenson CG (1983) Muscarinic receptors in pancreatic islets of the rat: demonstration and dependence on long term glucose environment. Biochim Biophys Acta 756:159–162

Harrison DE, Ashcroft SJH, Christie MR, Lord JM (1984) Protein phosphorylation in the pancreatic B-cell. Experientia 40:1075–1084

Hellman B (1986) External ATP initiates receptor-mediated mobilisation of calcium from pancreatic islets. Diabetologia 29:548A

Henquin JC, Meissner HP (1983) Dibutyryl cyclic AMP triggers Ca^{2+} infux and Ca^{2+}-dependent electrical activity in pancreatic B-cells. Biochem Biophys Res Commun 112:614–620

Hubinont CJ, Malaisse WJ (1985) Protein kinase C in pancreatic islets: effects of Ca^{2+}, calmodulin and retinoic acid. Biochem Int 10:557–584

Hubinont C, Best L, Sener A, Malaisse WJ (1984) Activation of protein kinase C by a tumor-promoting phorbol ester in pancreatic islets. FEBS Lett 170:247–253

Lapetina EG (1982) Regulation of arachidonic acid production: role of phospholipases C and A_2. Trends Pharmacol Sci 3:115–118

Leclercq-Meyer V, Herchuelz A, Valverde I, Couturier E, Marchand J, Malaisse WJ (1980) Mode of action of clonidine upon islet function. Diabetes 29:193–200

Leclercq-Meyer V, Woussen-Colle MC, Lalieu C, Marchand J, Malaisse WJ (1987) Anomeric specificity of glucose-induced somatostatin secretion. Experientia 43:1216–1218

Lindström P, Sehlin J (1986) Effect of intracellular alkalinization on pancreatic islet calcium uptake and insulin secretion. Biochem J 239:199–204

Loubatières-Mariani MM, Chapal J, Alrich R, Loubatières A (1973) Studies of the cholinergic receptors involved in the secretion of insulin using isolated perfused rat pancreas. Diabetologia 9:439–446

Malaisse WJ (1972) Hormonal and environmental modification of islet activity. In: Steiner DF, Freinkel N (eds) Endocrine pancreas. American Physiological Society, Washington, pp 237–260 (Handbook of physiology, sect. 7, vol 1)

Malaisse WJ (1973) Insulin secretion: multifactorial regulation for a single process of release. Diabetologia 9:163–167

Malaisse WJ (1983) Insulin release: the fuel concept. Diabete Metab 9:313–320

Malaisse WJ, Malaisse-Lagae F (1969) Influences nutritionnelles et hormonales chroniques sur la fonction insulaire. In: Journées de diabétologie de l'Hôtel-Dieu 1969. Flammarion, Paris, pp 131–138

Malaisse WJ, Malaisse-Lagae F (1984) The role of cyclic AMP in insulin release. Experientia 40:1068–1075

Malaisse WJ, Moratinos J (1986) Are pancreatic B-cells equipped with α_1-adrenoceptors? IRCS Med Sci 14:1194–1195

Malaisse WJ, Orci L (1979) The role of the cytoskeleton in pancreatic B-cell function. In: Gabbiani G (ed) Methods of achievements in experimental pathology, vol 9. Karger, Basel, pp 112–136

Malaisse WJ, Sener A (1985) Inhibition by 1-(5-isoquinolinesulfonyl)-2-methylpiperazine (H-7) of protein kinase C activity and insulin release in pancreatic islets. IRCS Med Sci 13:1239–1240

Malaisse WJ, Sener A (1986) Opposite effects of adrenergic and cholinergic agents in pancreatic islets. Exp Clin Endocrinol (Life Sci Adv) 5:43–49

Malaisse WJ, Sener A (1987a) Glucose-induced changes in cytosolic ATP content in pancreatic islets. Biochem Biophys Acta 927:190–195

Malaisse WJ, Sener A (1987b) (to be published) The redox potential. In: Akkerman JWN (ed) The energetics of secretion responses. CRC Press, Boca Raton

Malaisse WJ, Malaisse-Lagae F, Mayhew DA (1967a) A possible role for the adenyl cyclase system in insulin secretion. J Clin Invest 46:1724–1734

Malaisse WJ, Malaisse-Lagae F, Wright PH, Ashmore J (1967b) Effects of adrenergic and cholinergic agents upon insulin secretion in vitro. Endocrinology 80:975–978

Malaisse WJ, Brisson G, Malaisse-Lagae F (1970) The stimulus-secretion coupling of glucose-induced insulin release. I. Interaction of epinephrine and alkaline earth cations. J Lab Clin Med 76:895–902

Malaisse WJ, Pipeleers DG, Van Obberghen E, Somers G, Devis G, Marichal M, Malaisse-Lagae F (1973) The glucoreceptor mechanism in the pancreatic beta-cell. Am Zool 13:605–612

Malaisse WJ, Malaisse-Lagae F, Van Obberghen E, Somers G, Devis G, Ravazzola M, Orci L (1975) Role of microtubules in the phasic pattern of insulin release. Ann NY Acad Sci 253:630–652

Malaisse WJ, Sener A, Levy J (1976a) The stimulus-secretion coupling of glucose-induced insulin release. XXI. Fasting-induced adaptation of key glycolytic enzymes in isolated islets. J Biol Chem 251:1731–1737

Malaisse WJ, Sener A, Koser M, Herchuelz A (1976b) The stimulus-secretion coupling of glucose-induced insulin release. XXIV. The metabolism of α- and β-D-glucose in isolated islets. J Biol Chem 251:5936–5943

Malaisse WJ, Sener A, Koser M, Ravazzola M, Malaisse-Lagae F (1977) The stimulus-secretion coupling of glucose-induced insulin release. XXV. Insulin release due to glycogenolysis in glucose-deprived islets. Biochem J 164:447–454

Malaisse WJ, Sener A, Herchuelz A, Hutton JC (1979) Insulin release: the fuel hypothesis. Metabolism 28:373–386

Malaisse WJ, Sener A, Herchuelz A, Carpinelli AR, Poloczek P, Winand J, Castagna M (1980) Insulinotropic effect of the tumor promotor 12-O-tetradecanoylphorbol-12-acetate in rat pancreatic islets. Cancer Res 40:3827–3831

Malaisse WJ, Sener A, Malaisse-Lagae F (1981) Insulin release: reconciliation of the receptor and metabolic hypotheses. Nutrient receptors in islet cells. Mol Cell Biochem 37:157–165

Malaisse WJ, Malaisse-Lagae F, Sener A (1983a) Anomeric specificity of hexose metabolism in pancreatic islets. Physiol Rev 63:773–786

Malaisse WJ, Lebrun P, Herchuelz A, Sener A, Malaisse-Lagae F (1983b) Synergistic effect of a tumor-promoting phorbol ester and a hypoglycemic sulfonylurea upon insulin release. Endocrinology 113:1870–1873

Malaisse WJ, Malaisse-Lagae F, Sener A (1984a) Coupling factors in nutrient-induced insulin release. Experientia 40:1035–1043

Malaisse WJ, Svoboda M, Dufrane SP, Malaisse-Lagae F, Christophe J (1984b) Effect of Bordetella pertussis toxin on ADP-ribosylation of membrane proteins, adenylate cyclase activity and insulin release in rat pancreatic islets. Biochem Biophys Res Commun 124:190–196

Malaisse WJ, Garcia-Morales P, Dufrane SP, Sener A, Valverde I (1984c) Forskolin-induced activation of adenylate cyclase, cyclic adenosine monophosphate production and insulin release in rat pancreatic islets. Endocrinology 115:2015–2020

Malaisse WJ, Scholler Y, De Maertelaer V (1985a) Mathematical modelling of stimulus-secretion coupling in the pancreatic B-cell. IV. Dissociated time course for the glucose-induced changes in distinct Ca^{2+} movements. Diabetes Res 2:195–199

Malaisse WJ, Mahy M, Mathias PCF (1985b) Binding of [^{3}H]methylscopolamine to rat pancreatic islets. IRCS Med Sci 13:503–504

Malaisse WJ, Dunlop ME, Mathias PCF, Malaisse-Lagae F, Sener A (1985c) Stimulation of protein kinase C and insulin release by 1-oleyl-2-acetyl-glycerol. Eur J Biochem 149:23–27

Mathias PCF, Best L, Malaisse WJ (1985a) Stimulation by glucose and carbamylcholine of phospholipase C in pancreatic islets. Cell Biochem Funct 3:173–177

Mathias PCF, Best L, Malaisse WJ (1985b) Stimulation by glucose and carbamylcholine of phospholipase A_2 in pancreatic islets. Diabetes Res 2:267–270

Mathias PCF, Carpinelli AR, Billaudel B, Garcia-Morales P, Valverde I, Malaisse WJ (1985c) Cholinergic stimulation of ion fluxes in pancreatic islets. Biochem Pharmacol 34:3451–3457

Matschinsky FM, Ellerman J, Stillings S, Raybaud F, Pace C, Zawalich W (1975) Hexoses and insulin secretion. In: Hasselblatt A, Bruchhausen Fv (eds) Insulin, part 2. Springer, Berlin Heidelberg New York, pp 79–114

Moody AJ, Markussen J, Schaich Fries A, Steenstrup C, Sundby F, Malaisse WJ, Malaisse-Lagae F (1970) The insulin releasing activities of extracts of pork intestine. Diabetologia 6:135–140

Nenquin M, Awouters P, Mathot F, Henquin JC (1984) Distinct effects of acetylcholine and glucose on ^{45}calcium and ^{86}rubidium efflux from mouse pancreatic islets. FEBS Lett 176:457–461

Orci L, Malaisse WJ (1980) Hypothesis: single and chain release of insulin secretory granules is related to anionic transport at exocytotic sites. Diabetes 29:943–944

Orci L, Malaisse-Lagae F, Ravazzola M, Amherdt M, Renold AE (1973) Exocytosis-endocytosis coupling in the pancreatic beta cell. Science 181:561–562

Orci L, Malaisse-Lagae F, Ravazzola M, Rouiller D, Renold AE, Perrelet A, Unger RH (1975) A morphological basis for intercellular communication between α- and β-cells in the endocrine pancreas. J Clin Invest 56:1066–1070

Östenson CG, Grill V (1985) Glucose exerts opposite effects on muscarinic receptor binding to A and B cells of the endocrine pancreas. Endocrinology 116:1741–1744

Owen A, Malaisse WJ (1987) Mathematical modelling of stimulus-secretion coupling in the pancreatic B-cell. V. Threshold phenomenon for the response to cyclic AMP. Diabete Metab 13:514–519

Patel YC, Amherdt M, Orci L (1982) Quantitative electron microscopic autoradiography of insulin, glucagon and somatostatin binding sites on islets. Science 217:1155–1156

Pipeleers DG (1984) Islet cell interactions with pancreatic B-cells. Experientia 40:1114–1126

Pipeleers DG, Levy J, Malaisse-Lagae F, Malaisse WJ (1975) In vitro biosynthesis and release of three immunoreactive insulin-like components by a human insulinoma. Diabete Metab 1:7–11

Pipeleers DG, Pipeleers-Marichal MA, Kipnis DM (1976) Microtubule assembly and the intracellular transport of secretory granules in pancreatic islets. Science 191:88–90

Prentki M, Biden TJ, Janjic D, Irvin RF, Berridge MJ, Wollheim CB (1984) Rapid mobilization of Ca^{2+} from rat insulinoma microsomes by inositol-1,4,5-trisphosphate. Nature 309:562–564

Rasmussen H, Kojima I, Zawalich W (1984) The calcium messenger system in endocrine systems. Abstracts 7th international congress of endocrinology. Excerpta Medica, Amsterdam, p 157

Rodbell M (1985) Programmable messengers: a new theory of hormone action. Trends Biochem Sci 10:461–464

Rorsman P, Trube G (1985) Glucose dependent K^+-channels in pancreatic B-cells are regulated by intracellular ATP. Pflugers Arch 405:305–309

Schuit FC (1987) Functional characterization of purified pancreatic B-cells. Regulatory role of cyclic AMP. Thesis, Vrije Universiteit Brussel, Brussels

Sener A, Malaisse WJ (1980) L-leucine and a non-metabolized analogue activate pancreatic islet glutamate dehydrogenase. Nature 288:187–189

Sener A, Malaisse WJ (1987) The coupling of metabolic to secretory events in pancreatic islets: comparison between insulin release and cytosolic redox state. Biochem Int 14:897–902

Sener A, Malaisse-Lagae F, Malaisse WJ (1981) Stimulation of islet metabolism and insulin release by a non-metabolizable amino acid. Proc Natl Acad Sci USA 78:5460–5464

Sener A, Malaisse-Lagae F, Lebrun P, Herchuelz A, Leclercq-Meyer V, Malaisse WJ (1982) Anomeric specificity of D-mannose metabolism in pancreatic islets. Biochem Biophys Res Commun 108:1567–1573

Sener A, Leclercq-Meyer V, Giroix M-H, Malaisse WJ, Hellerström C (1987) Opposite effects of D-glucose and a nonmetabolized analogue of L-leucine on respiration and secretion in insulin-producing tumoral cells (RINm5F) Diabetes 36:187–192

Somers G, Blondel B, Orci L, Malaisse WJ (1979) Motile events in pancreatic endocrine cells. Endocrinology 104:255–264

Somers G, Sener A, Devis G, Malaisse WJ (1980) The stimulus-secretion coupling of glucose-induced insulin release. XLV. The anion-osmotic hypothesis for exocytosis. Pflugers Arch 388:249–253

Sugden MC, Ashcroft SJH (1978) Effects of phosphoenol-pyruvate, other glycolytic intermediates and methylxanthines on calcium uptake by a mitochondrial fraction from rat pancreatic islets. Diabetologia 15:173–180

Svoboda M, Garcia-Morales P, Dufrane SP, Sener A, Valverde I, Christophe J, Malaisse WJ (1985) Stimulation by cholera toxin of ADP-ribosylation of membrane proteins, adenylate cyclase and insulin release in pancreatic islets. Cell Biochem Funct 3:25–32

Tamagawa T, Niki H, Niki A (1985) Insulin release independent of a rise in cytosolic free Ca^{2+} by forskolin and phorbol ester. FEBS Lett 183:430–432

Trus MD, Hintz CS, Weinstein JB, Williams AD, Pagliara AS, Matschinsky FM (1978) Effects of glucose and acetyl choline on islet tissue NADH and insulin release. Life Sci 22:809–816

Valverde I, Malaisse WJ (1984) Calmodulin and pancreatic B-cell function. Experientia 40:1061–1068

Valverde I, Vandemeers A, Anjaneyulu R, Malaisse WJ (1979) Calmodulin activation of adenylate cyclase in pancreatic islets. Science 206:225–227

Valverde I, Garcia-Morales P, Ghiglione M, Malaisse WJ (1983) The stimulus-secretion coupling of glucose-induced insulin release. LII. Calcium dependency of the cyclic AMP response to nutrient secretagogue. Horm Metab Res 15:62–68

Wollheim CB, Siegel EG, Sharp GWG (1980) Dependency of acetylcholine-induced insulin release on Ca^{2+} uptake by rat pancreatic islets. Endocrinology 107:924–929

Wollheim CB, Ullrich S, Pozzan T (1984) Glyceraldehyde, but not cyclic AMP-stimulated insulin release is preceded by a rise in cytosolic free Ca^{2+}. FEBS Lett 177:17–22

Zawalich W, Brown C, Rasmussen H (1983) Insulin secretion: combined effects of phorbol ester and A23187. Biochem Biophys Res Commun 117:448–455

Subject Index